New Perspectives in Equine Colic

Guest Editor

FRANK M. ANDREWS, DVM, MS

VETERINARY CLINICS OF NORTH AMERICA: EQUINE PRACTICE

www.vetequine.theclinics.com

Consulting Editor
A. SIMON TURNER, BVSc, MS

August 2009 • Volume 25 • Number 2

SAUNDERS an imprint of ELSEVIER, Inc.

W.B. SAUNDERS COMPANY

A Division of Elsevier Inc.

1600 John F. Kennedy Boulevard • Suite 1800 • Philadelphia, Pennsylvania 19103

http://www.vetequine.theclinics.com

VETERINARY CLINICS OF NORTH AMERICA: EQUINE PRACTICE Volume 25, Number 2
August 2009 ISSN 0749-0739, ISBN-13: 978-1-4377-1280-3

Editor: John Vassallo; j.vassallo@elsevier.com
Developmental Editor: Donald Mumford

Veterinary Clinics of North America: Equine Practice (ISSN 0749-0739) is published in April, August, and December by Elsevier Inc., 360 Park Avenue South, New York, NY 10010-1710. Business and Editorial Offices: 1600 John F. Kennedy Blvd., Suite 1800, Philadelphia, PA 19103-2899. Customer Service office: 11830 Westline Industrial Drive, St. Louis, MO 63146. Subscription prices are $200.00 per year (domestic individuals), $332.00 per year (domestic institutions), $100.00 per year (domestic students/residents), $233.00 per year (Canadian individuals), $415.00 per year (Canadian institutions), $269.00 per year (international individuals), $415.00 per year (international institutions), and $136.00 per year (international and Canadian students/residents). To receive student/resident rate, orders must be accompanied by name of affiliated institution, date of term, and the signature of program/residency coordinator on institution letterhead. Orders will be billed at individual rate until proof of status is received. Foreign air speed delivery is included in all *Clinics* subscription prices. All prices are subject to change without notice. **POSTMASTER:** Send address changes to *Veterinary Clinics of North America: Equine Practice,* 11830 Westline Industrial Drive, St. Louis, MO 63146. Customer Service (orders, claims, online, change of address): Elsevier Periodicals Customer Service, 11830 Westline Industrial Drive, St. Louis, MO 63146. Tel: 1-800-654-2452 (U.S. and Canada); 314-453-7041 (outside U.S. and Canada). Fax: 314-523-5170. E-mail: journalscustomerservice-usa@elsevier.com (for print support); E-mail: journalsonlinesupport-usa@elsevier (for online support).

Reprints. For copies of 100 or more of articles in this publication, please contact the Commercial Reprints Department, Elsevier Inc., 360 Park Avenue South, New York, NY 10010-1710. Tel.: 212-633-3812; Fax: 212-462-1935; E-mail: reprints@elsevier.com.

Veterinary Clinics of North America: Equine Practice is covered in *MEDLINE/PubMed (Index Medicus), Excerpta Medica, Current Contents/Agriculture, Biology and Environmental Sciences,* and *ISI.*

Printed and bound in the United Kingdom
Transferred to Digital Print 2011

Contributors

CONSULTING EDITOR

A. SIMON TURNER, BVSc, MS
Diplomate, American College of Veterinary Surgeons; Professor, Department of Clinical Sciences, College of Veterinary Medicine and Biomedical Sciences, Colorado State University, Fort Collins, Colorado

GUEST EDITOR

FRANK M. ANDREWS, DVM, MS
Diplomate, American College of Veterinary Internal Medicine; Director, Equine Health Studies Program; and LVMA Equine Committee Professor, Department of Veterinary Clinical Sciences, School of Veterinary Medicine, Louisiana State University, Baton Rouge, Louisiana

AUTHORS

RAFAT A.M. AL JASSIM, BSc, MSc, PhD
School of Animal Studies, The Faculty of Natural Resources, Agricultural and Veterinary Science, The University of Queensland, Queensland, Australia

FRANK M. ANDREWS, DVM, MS
Diplomate, American College of Veterinary Internal Medicine; Director of the Equine Health Studles Program; and LVMA Equine Committee Professor, Department of Veterinary Clinical Sciences, School of Veterinary Medicine, Louisiana State University, Baton Rouge, Louisiana

CARLA CESARINI, DVM
Diplomate, American College of Veterinary Internal Medicine (Large Animals); Diplomate, European College of Equine Internal Medicine; Assistant Professor of Equine Medicine, Servei de Medicina Interna Equina, Departament de Medicina i Cirurgia Animals, Facultat de Veterinària, Universitat Autònoma de Barcelona, Barcelona, Spain

ANN M. CHAPMAN, DVM, MS
Diplomate, American College of Veterinary Internal Medicine; Assistant Professor of Veterinary Medicine, Department of Veterinary Clinical Sciences, School of Veterinary Medicine, Louisiana State University, Baton Rouge, Louisiana

THOMAS J. DOHERTY, MVB, MSc
Diplomate, American College of Veterinary Anesthesiologists; Professor, Department of Large Animal Clinical Sciences, The University of Tennessee College of Veterinary Medicine, Knoxville, Tennessee

SARAH DUKTI, DVM
Diplomate, American College of Veterinary Surgeons; Clinical Assistant Professor in Emergency Medicine and Surgery, Marion duPont Scott Equine Medical Center, Virginia-Maryland Regional College of Veterinary Medicine, Virginia Tech, Leesburg, Virginia

KAREN A. KALCK, DVM
Diplomate, American College of Veterinary Medicine; Clinical Instructor of Equine Medicine, Department of Large Animal Clinical Sciences, The University of Tennessee College of Veterinary Medicine, Knoxville, Tennessee

GAL KELMER, DVM, MS
Diplomate, American College of Veterinary Surgeons; Instructor of Equine Surgery, Large Animal Department, Koret Veterinary Teaching Hospital, Koret School of Veterinary Medicine; Faculty of Agriculture, Hebrew University of Jerusalem, Rehovot, Israel; Formerly, Clinical Assistant Professor, Department of Large Animal Clinical Sciences, College of Veterinary Medicine, The University of Tennessee, Knoxville, Tennessee

ANDREAS KLOHNEN, DVM
Diplomate, American College of Veterinary Surgeons; Chino Valley Equine Hospital, Chino Hills, California

TIM MAIR, BVSc, PhD
Bell Equine Veterinary Clinic, Mereworth, Maidstone, Kent; Visiting Professor, Royal Veterinary College, London, United Kingdom

LUIS MONREAL, DVM, PhD
Diplomate, European College of Equine Internal Medicine; Professor of Equine Medicine, Servei de Medicina Interna Equina, Departament de Medicina i Cirurgia Animals, Facultat de Veterinària, Universitat Autònoma de Barcelona, Barcelona, Spain

MARTIN KRARUP NIELSEN, DVM, PhD
Department of Large Animal Sciences, Faculty of Life Sciences, University of Copenhagen, Taastrup, Denmark

REBECCA L. PIERCE, BVetMed, MRCVS
Clinical Assistant Professor, Department of Large Animal Clinical Sciences, The University of Tennessee College of Veterinary Medicine, Knoxville, Tennessee

AMY E. PLUMMER, DVM
Diplomate, American College of Veterinary Surgeons; Clinical Assistant Professor, Large Animal Clinical Sciences, The University of Tennessee, College of Veterinary Medicine, Knoxville, Tennessee

CHRIS J. PROUDMAN, MA, VetMB, PhD, FRCVS
Head, Department of Veterinary Clinical Science, Faculty of Veterinary Science, University of Liverpool, Leahurst, Neston, Wirral, England

CRAIG R. REINEMEYER, DVM, PhD
East Tennessee Clinical Research, Inc., Rockwood, Tennessee

RICARDO VIDELA, DVM
Medicine Resident, Department of Large Animal Clinical Sciences, The University of Tennessee College of Veterinary Medicine, Knoxville, Tennessee

NATHANIEL A. WHITE, DVM
Diplomate, American College of Veterinary Surgeons; Jean Ellen Shehan Professor and Director, Marion duPont Scott Equine Medical Center, Virginia-Maryland Regional College of Veterinary Medicine, Virginia Tech, Leesburg, Virginia

CLAIRE E. WYLIE, BVM&S, MSc, MRCVS
Epidemiology and Disease Surveillance, Animal Health Trust, Centre for Preventive Medicine, Kentford, Newmarket, Suffolk, England

Contents

> "Clinical governance" is the term used to describe a systematic approach
> to maintaining and improving the quality of patient care within a health
> system. This article introduces the concept of clinical governance as
> a tool for improving the quality of care. It also discusses the potential value
> of a large database of colic surgery in implementing some of the compo-
> nents of clinical governance in the field of equine colic surgery.

> The gastrointestinal tract of the horse has unique characteristics that make
> it well suited for the ingestion and utilization of roughage. The horse is con-
> sidered a simple-stomached herbivore and is classed as a hindgut fer-
> menter. The upper segments of the gastrointestinal tract resemble those
> of a typical simple-stomached animal. The lower have undergone modifi-
> cation to become voluminous and host to a large number of microbial pop-
> ulations similar to those of the compartmental stomach of ruminant
> animals. The main advantage of this arrangement is the ability of the horse
> to extract valuable nutrients from the diet before digesta reaches the hind-
> gut where the rigid structural components that resisted enzymatic diges-
> tion at the small intestinal level undergo extensive fermentation processes.

> Prognosticating survival in horses with colic is challenging because of the
> number of diseases and pathophysiologic processes that can cause the
> behavior. Although the treatment of horses with colic has improved dra-
> matically over the years, case fatality can still be high because of the delay
> in recognizing the problem, the time delay inherent in receiving veterinary
> care, and the lack of effective treatment for the more severe diseases. In-
> tensive case management and surgery for these horses may be expensive
> and emotionally draining for owners; therefore, providing an accurate
> prognosis is key to decisions needed for case management. This article
> is dedicated to recent advances in applying a prognosis for survival in
> horses at higher risk for a fatal outcome.

Equids are hosts to dozens of species of internal parasites that infect no other domestic animals. Virtually all horses, especially those exposed to pasture, experience some level of parasitism continuously. Despite pathologic evidence of parasitic damage in various organs and tissues, few parasitisms are manifested systemically in well-managed horses. Contrary to conventional wisdom, only three common parasitisms of horses are likely to be manifested as colic: *Strongylus vulgaris*, *Parascaris equorum*, and *Anoplocephala perfoliata*. This article discusses the life cycles, pathophysiology, manifestations and clinical findings, treatment, and management of these three common parasitisms. It also discusses related aspects of several other parasitisms that are unlikely to cause colic.

The most common coagulopathy in horses with colic is a hypercoagulable state associated with disseminated intravascular coagulation. The intensity of this coagulopathy depends on the severity and duration of the gastrointestinal lesion, with the ischemic and inflammatory problems and peritonitis being the most frequently affected by coagulopathies. Early initiation of prophylactic therapy significantly reduces the severe hypercoagulable state in horses with intestinal conditions which are recognized to be at high risk for disseminated intravascular coagulation. In addition to the systemic coagulopathy observed in horses with colic, a peritoneal coagulopathy independent from that occurring in blood has been observed, and its recognition and assessment may have clinical usefulness in the diagnosis of the gastrointestinal diseases and outcome.

Endotoxemia is a major cause of morbidity and mortality in horses affected by colic. This article briefly reviews the pathogenesis of endotoxemia in horses with colic, reviews current established treatments, and describes new advances in the treatment of endotoxemia.

In recent years important advancements in colic surgery have led to improved prediction of survival rates, better survival rates, and decreased complication rates. This article describes several modalities to combat and prevent incisional hernia and intestinal adhesion formation in horses undergoing colic surgery. These modalities have had a positive impact on reducing complications in horses after surgery.

Equine gastric ulcer syndrome (EGUS) is common in horses. A history of mild intermitted recurrent colic signs after eating is noted in many horses. Management of horses with abdominal pain caused by gastric ulcers is especially difficult, because non-steroidal anti-inflammatory agents, typically used to control abdominal pain, may exacerbate this condition. Effective pharmacologic agents are available to treat EGUS and eliminate abdominal pain, but more comprehensive measures of environmental and dietary management are needed to manage horses with EGUS and prevent recurrence. This article focuses on the history, clinical signs, diagnosis, and management of horses with abdominal pain associated with gastric ulcers. The primary goal is to provide an understanding of EGUS and to review effective pain management and specific antiulcer treatments and management strategies in horses with EGUS.

This article discusses types of inflammatory bowel disease in horses, including pathologic findings and proposed causes. The diagnosis of inflammatory bowel disease is presented in detail, including minimum database, rectal palpation, abdominal ultrasound, abdominocentesis, biopsy procedures, and absorption tests. Treatment recommendations and prognosis are also discussed.

Impactions of the small and large intestines are frequently diagnosed as the cause of colic in horses. An impaction is an accumulation of dehydrated ingesta in a portion of the digestive tract, typically at sites where the intestinal diameter decreases. The specific pathogenesis for impactions is not fully understood, although risk factors have been identified for several types of impactions. Treatment for impactions includes withholding feed until the impaction passes, rehydrating the ingesta, and, if necessary, administering analgesic agents. In severe cases, surgery may be necessary to relieve the impaction. This article discusses clinical signs, diagnosis, treatment (both drug and surgical options), and prognosis for impactions of the duodenum, jejunum, ileum, cecum, and small and large colons in horses.

This article focuses on obstructive diseases of the large intestine (large and small colons) caused by intraluminal bodies. Large intestinal obstructions from intraluminal bodies can be divided into the following categories:

Equine grass sickness (EGS) is recognized as a debilitating and predominantly fatal neurodegenerative disease affecting grazing equids. The gastrointestinal tract is the most severely affected body system, resulting in the main clinical signs of colic (acute grass sickness), weight loss, or dysphagia (chronic grass sickness). EGS predominantly occurs within Great Britain, although it is also recognized in regions of mainland Europe, and mainly affects young horses with access to pasture in the springtime. There is strong evidence of an association between EGS and the type C toxins produced by the bacterium *Clostridium botulinum*. This article covers the clinical aspects, epidemiology, and global distribution of EGS, along with comparisons with botulism and developments in disease prevention.

FORTHCOMING ISSUES

RECENT ISSUES

THE CLINICS ARE NOW AVAILABLE ONLINE!

Access your subscription at:
www.theclinics.com

Preface

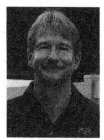

Frank M. Andrews, DVM, MS
Guest Editor

According to the National Animal Health Monitoring System studies in 1998 and 2005, colic is the second leading cause of death in horses, second only to old age. Almost every equine practitioner deals with colicky horses on a daily basis. Unfortunately, the actual cause of a colic episode is found only in approximately half of these cases. This finding makes recommending preventive measures difficult and leaves the client frustrated, especially if the horse experiences recurring episodes. Furthermore, once colic is recognized, prognosis of that individual case is difficult, and giving the owner an idea regarding outcome is difficult. If surgery is required, post-operative complications (such as ileus, incisional infections, and diarrhea) may occur and can frustrate the most seasoned equine clinician. That being said, recovery from colic episodes is quite high, and in recent years, the equine clinician's ability to diagnose and treat horses with colic has improved dramatically. Recent advancements in diagnosis and treatment has led to this dramatic improvement in outcome and improved the health of horses with colic.

This issue, "New Perspectives in Equine Colic," provides the most recent information on pathogenesis, diagnosis, treatment, and prognosis of colic in horses. There is also information on development of a colic auditing system in which hospitals can monitor and assess outcomes and adjust procedures and techniques to improve recovery and survival rates. The stimulus for this issue came from the 2008 Colic Research Symposium held in Liverpool, England. Every 3 years, the Colic Research Symposium brings together leading researchers and clinicians from around the world to present and discuss the latest research and clinical information on colic and laminitis in horses. In-depth oral and poster presentations provide state-of-the-art information on colic and laminitis in horses. The meeting lasts for 3 days and results in an enormous body of information that could not be duplicated in this issue. Therefore, this issue captures only a small portion of the symposium, but it provides clinicians with essential information to diagnose and treat colic in horses. The authors do a wonderful job putting together well-referenced material that will help equine clinicians become better clinician-scientists, with the ultimate goal of helping the horse.

I acknowledge and thank the gifted authors for their contributions to this issue. Without the authors and their expertise, this issue would not have been possible.

Vet Clin Equine 25 (2009) xiii–xiv
doi:10.1016/j.cveq.2009.05.002
0749-0739/09/$ – see front matter © 2009 Elsevier Inc. All rights reserved.

I am also grateful for the authors' willingness to share their insights with the equine community. A special acknowledgment goes out to the series editor, John Vassallo, and the Elsevier/Saunders crew for their help in putting this issue together and keeping me on time. Finally, thanks to Dr. Simon Turner, Consulting Editor, for the idea and his gentle "arm-twisting" to make this issue a reality.

Frank M. Andrews, DVM, MS
Equine Health Studies Program
Department of Veterinary Clinical Sciences
School of Veterinary Medicine
Louisiana State University
Skip Bertman Drive
Baton Rouge, LA 70803, USA

E-mail address:
fandrews@lsu.edu (F.M. Andrews)

Clinical Governance, Clinical Audit, and the Potential Value of a Database of Equine Colic Surgery

Tim Mair, BVSc, PhD[a,b,*]

KEYWORDS

• Clinical governance • Clinical audit • Colic surgery • Horse

What is the mortality rate of horses undergoing colic surgery at your hospital? How many of those deaths could be prevented? What is the rate of wound infections following colic surgery? What proportion of horses admitted to your hospital for treatment of small intestinal obstruction develop postoperative ileus, and how are they managed? What proportion of horses developing postoperative ileus recover? What is the average cost for treatment of a horse with right dorsal displacement at your hospital?

The answers to these and numerous other questions are vitally important to every clinician and equine hospital that undertakes colic surgery in horses. Such data provide baseline measurements of performance in relation to colic surgery that are required if any attempt is to be made to improve performance and maximize the quality of care that an individual veterinarian or hospital can provide. Sadly, most equine hospitals currently do not record such information,[1] thereby limiting the possibility of achieving improvement. Sustainable improvements can be achieved only by monitoring and critically appraising the results of clinical work.[2]

This article introduces the concept of clinical governance as a tool for improving quality of care and discusses the potential value of a large database of colic surgery in implementing some of the components of clinical governance in the field of equine colic surgery.[1]

CLINICAL GOVERNANCE

"Clinical governance" is the term used to describe a systematic approach to maintaining and improving the quality of patient care within a health system. The term is widely

[a] Bell Equine Veterinary Clinic, Mereworth, Maidstone, Kent, ME18 5GS, UK
[b] Royal Veterinary College, London, UK
* Corresponding author. Bell Equine Veterinary Clinic, Mereworth, Maidstone, Kent, ME18 5GS, UK.
E-mail address: tim.mair@btinternet.com

Vet Clin Equine 25 (2009) 193–198
doi:10.1016/j.cveq.2009.04.009
0749-0739/09/$ – see front matter © 2009 Elsevier Inc. All rights reserved.

vetequine.theclinics.com

used in the United Kingdom where, since April 1, 1999, all National Health Service (NHS) bodies have had the statutory duty of clinical governance placed upon them. The same standards also apply to the private sector. The most frequently cited formal definition of clinical governance is

A framework through which NHS organizations are accountable for continually improving the quality of their services and safeguarding high standards of care by creating an environment in which excellence in clinical care will flourish[3]

Clinical governance aims to integrate all the activities that affect patient care into one strategy. This integration involves improving the quality of information, promoting collaboration, teamwork, and partnerships, reducing variations in practice, and implementing evidence-based practice.

The system of clinical governance brings together all the elements that seek to promote quality of care. Clinical governance is composed of several different elements[4]:

- Education and training
- Clinical audit
- Clinical effectiveness
- Research and development
- Openness
- Risk management

Clinical effectiveness is a measure of the extent to which a particular intervention works. It means ensuring that interventions and treatments are based on the best available research evidence.[4] The measure on its own is useful, but it is enhanced by considering whether the intervention is appropriate and whether it represents value for money.

Poor performance and poor practice too often thrive behind closed doors. Processes that are open to public scrutiny, while respecting individual patient and practitioner confidentiality, and that can be justified openly are an essential part of quality assurance. Open proceedings and discussion about clinical governance issues should be a feature of the framework.

Medical clinicians are under increasing pressure to show that their services are safe, effective, and efficient.[5] Consideration and analysis of the quality of care are accepted as major responsibilities of all health care organizations.[6] In the United Kingdom, the high-profile discussions about the problems of pediatric cardiac deaths at the Bristol Royal Infirmary during the period from 1984 to 1995 raised public and political awareness of the issues. The experience of the pediatric cardiac surgical service in Bristol was a result not of flawed physicians[7] but rather of a lack of leadership and teamwork. The report of the Bristol Royal Infirmary Inquiry included 198 recommendations, 2 of which stated that patients must be able to obtain information about the relative performance of the hospital and of consultant units within the hospital.[8] These recommendations led to an increasing belief that the interests of the public and patients would be served by publication of individuals' surgical performance as reflected by postoperative mortality. A precedent for such reporting also exists in the United States: in 1990 the New York Department of Health published mortality statistics for coronary surgery for all hospitals in the state and has published comparable data each year since.[9,10]

At about the time of the Bristol Royal Infirmary inquiry, the Society of Cardiothoracic Surgeons of Great Britain and Ireland tried to redress perceived deficiencies in surgeons' approach to national data collection and audit, in addition to debate about how to measure their clinical performance, by producing unambiguous guidelines on data collection and clinical audit in cardiac surgical units.[7,11] After detailed discussion, the Society agreed to institute the collection of data on surgeon-specific activities and in-hospital mortality for several index procedures and to use a stringent set of limits to initiate an internal assessment. An annual mortality higher than a SD above the mean was set as the trigger for a review by local clinical governance. This review was intended to be a constructive process, not a trigger for criticism, blame, or ill-considered actions. The problem with this approach is that there always will be 2.5% of consultants under review, no matter how much improvement is gained.

Compelling arguments for performing systematic audits in human surgery have been documented more recently.[12,13] The Scottish Audit of Surgical Mortality is a voluntary, peer-reviewed, critical-event analysis that has become an established part of standard surgical practice in Scotland.[14] The scheme boasts a high level of support from Scottish surgeons, perhaps because it seems to be effective. After the analysis revealed errors in specific processes of care (eg, failure to use ICUs and failure to use prophylaxis for deep venous thrombosis) as contributing to surgical deaths, system-wide changes occurred, and the frequency of such errors declined greatly. The potential effectiveness of a program that focuses on death as the only critical event may be limited, however.[12] Although errors occur often in medicine, errors contributing to death occur in only 6% of cases identified by Scottish Audit of Surgical Mortality. Errors that do not occur often or that generally do not result in mortality are likely to be missed by such an analysis. In addition, the focus of the program on processes of care would indicate that feedback at the hospital level is at least as essential as feedback at the individual surgeon level.

CLINICAL AUDIT

Clinical audit is the process formally introduced in 1993 into the United Kingdom NHS and is defined as "a quality improvement process that seeks to improve patient care and outcomes through systematic review of care against explicit criteria and the implementation of change."[15] The key component of clinical audit is that clinical performance is reviewed (or audited) to ensure that what should be done is being done; if deficiencies are found, the clinical audit provides a framework to enable improvements to be made.

The essence of clinical audit is developing and improving clinical practice. Although clinical audit is a relatively new concept for the veterinary profession,[16] the belief that clinical staff constantly should seek to improve care is as old as the profession itself. Clinical audit takes this concept a step further and promotes the idea of continuous improvement, ensuring not just good care, but an on-going process of development; "a journey that never ends." Conducting a clinical audit means that you are comparing your actual performance in a defined area of clinical practice against targets/guidelines (which are, one hopes, evidence based) to see whether you are consistently achieving good practice (ie, you are meeting your targets and guidelines). If you are not meeting the targets, you then must investigate why not, create a plan of action to amend any shortcomings (often involving the modification or creation of clinical guidelines), implement the actions, and, once these steps have been successfully implemented, re-audit.

Clinical audit involves measuring your own practice and comparing it with what you consider to be best practice. Unless you can prove that you are indeed undertaking best practice in all areas that you study, you will use the results to identify areas in which your practice is deficient and then implement changes to improve; these changes will be followed by a re-audit. As a result, clinical audit usually develops as a cyclical process (**Fig. 1**).

The clinical audit process seeks to identify areas for service improvement, to develop and carry out action plans to rectify or improve service provision, and then to re-audit to ensure that these changes have an effect. Within the clinical audit cycle there are stages that follow the systematic process of establishing best practice, measuring against criteria (targets), taking action to improve care, and monitoring to sustain improvement. As the process continues, each cycle aspires to a higher level of quality.

Clinical audit is a technique that aims to measure and improve clinical performance, thereby improving the standards of patient care.[17] Clinical audit requires the comparison of data relating to a clinical issue from a specific clinician or institution with a standard set of data that describes the "normal" or "expected" results. The absence of readily available standards in many areas of veterinary clinical work (including colic surgery) makes it difficult to undertake an effective clinical audit. One of the major objectives of the proposed international audit/database of colic surgery[1,2] is to provide evidence-based data that can be used as the standards (or "targets") in clinical audit. Colic surgery is obviously only one area of equine practice that might benefit from assessment by clinical audit, but the high costs of colic surgery and the major implications for welfare make this area of equine surgery particularly suited to this process.

DATABASE OF EQUINE COLIC SURGERY

Equine colic surgery has been performed routinely by equine surgeons since the mid-1960s. Although the general success rates of colic surgery have improved significantly,[18] the surgery still carries significant rate of case fatality and risk of complications. It also is expensive surgery, especially in cases that require significant

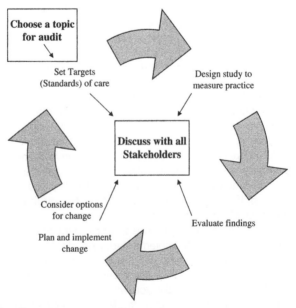

Fig. 1. The audit cycle.

postoperative intensive care. It is important that this type of surgery be undertaken efficiently and performed to the highest attainable standards. Owners (and insurers where appropriate) have a right to see evidence that surgeons are achieving these goals while treating patients (the horses) in the most humane and appropriate ways.

Many factors influence the death rates and complication rates of colic surgery. Most importantly, the delay between the onset of colic and the surgery, the nature of the underlying disease (ie, strangulating versus simple obstruction), and the severity and effects of shock and toxemia will have major influences on the success and complication rates.[18–23] Other factors, such as competence of the surgical team and the nature of postoperative intensive care, which are known to affect outcomes in human surgery,[24,25] are also likely to influence the outcomes of colic surgery.

With increasing awareness, both by the profession and by the general public, of the importance of clinical standards in human health care, it is appropriate that attempts be made to introduce protocols to measure and improve standards of care in veterinary surgery. The concept of an international audit and database of colic surgeries was proposed in an editorial leader published in the *Equine Veterinary Journal*.[2] The aims of this international audit and database would be (1) to improve the quality of care for colic patients by allowing appropriate comparison of clinical performance with local, national, and international standards, and (2) to provide useful data about changing trends within the specialty. These aims could be achieved by

1. Systematic collection at each contributing center of an agreed minimum dataset on a defined patient population
2. Aggregation and validation of data
3. Analysis and development of risk stratification models for outcome measures
4. Regular feedback to contributing centers

The creation of such a database of colic surgery obviously depends on the willingness and ability of equine hospitals and surgeons to provide the required data. A feasibility study was undertaken recently to assess the attitudes of equine colic surgeons toward potential participation in such a scheme.[1] The results indicated that there is a good level of interest among equine surgeons in developing a large-scale database for colic surgery, and most surgeons would be willing to contribute data from their own hospitals provided that the data collection is quick and easy and that confidentiality of the data is maintained.

If such a database became reality, it probably would not, at least initially, be placed in the public domain. Although many databases of human surgery are freely available on the Web, the major value of this database of equine colic surgery would be in allowing individual surgeons and hospitals to compare their own results with others undertaking similar procedures. The complexity of the numerous factors that affect outcome in individual cases means that the results would need to be interpreted with caution and with a detailed understanding of the disease processes and effects of treatments. To demonstrate improvements in quality, however, organizations need good information. Good data are essential to plan, commission, implement, manage, and evaluate services. It is hoped that a large-scale database of equine colic surgery would provide valuable data about complications, outcomes, and other variables that could be used to bring about real improvements in the standards of care for horses affected by colic.

REFERENCES

1. Mair TS, White NA. The creation of an international audit and database of equine colic surgery: survey of attitudes of surgeons. Equine Vet J 2008;40:400–4.

2. Mair TS, White NA. Improving the quality of care in colic surgery. Time for an international audit? Equine Vet J 2005;37:287–8.

3. Scally G, Donaldson LJ. Clinical governance and the drive for quality improvement in the new NHS in England. Br Med J 1998;317:61–5.

4. Swage T. Clinical governance in healthcare practice. 2nd edition. Edinburgh: Butterworth Heinemann; 2004.

5. Lord J, Littlejohns P. Evaluating healthcare policies: the case of clinical audit. Br Med J 1997;315:668–71.

6. Blumenthal D. Quality of care—what is it? Part one of six. N Engl J Med 1996;335: 891–4.

7. Keogh B, Dussek J, Watson D, et al. Public confidence and cardiac surgical outcome. Br Med J 1998;316:1759–60.

8. Bristol Royal Infirmary Enquiry. The enquiry into the management of care of children receiving complex heart surgery at the Bristol Royal Infirmary. Available at: www.bristol-inquiry.org.uk/. Accessed February 12, 2009.

9. New York State Department of Health. Available at: www.health.state.ny.us/. Accessed February 12, 2009.

10. Chassin MR, Hannan EL, DeBuono BA. Benefits and hazards of reporting medical outcomes publicly. N Engl J Med 1996;334:394–8.

11. Society for Cardiothoracic Surgery in Great Britain and Ireland. Available at: www.scts.org. Accessed February 12, 2009.

12. Baxter N. Monitoring surgical mortality. Br Med J 2005;330:1098–9.

13. Thompson AM, Stonebridge PA. Building a framework for trust: critical event analysis of deaths in surgical care. Br Med J 2005;330:1139–43.

14. Scottish Audit of Surgical Mortality. Available at: www.sasm.org.uk/. Accessed February 12, 2009.

15. Department of Health. Clinical audit—meeting and improving standards in health care. London: Department of Health; 1993.

16. Viner B. Clinical audit in veterinary practice—the story so far. In Pract 2005;27:215–8.

17. Teasdale S. The future of clinical audit: learning to work together. Br Med J 1996; 313:574.

18. Mair TS, Smith LJ. Survival and complication rates in 300 horses undergoing surgical treatment of colic. Part 1. Short-term survival following a single laparotomy. Equine Vet J 2005a;37:296–302.

19. Mair TS, Smith LJ. Survival and complication rates in 300 horses undergoing surgical treatment of colic. Part 2. Short-term complications. Equine Vet J 2005b;37:303–9.

20. Mair TS, Smith LJ. Survival and complication rates in 300 horses undergoing surgical treatment of colic. Part 3. Long-term complications and survival. Equine Vet J 2005c;37:310–4.

21. Mair TS, Smith LJ. Survival and complication rates in 300 horses undergoing surgical treatment of colic. Part 4. Early (acute) re-laparotomy. Equine Vet J 2005d;37:315–8.

22. Abutarbush SM, Carmalt JL, Shoemaker RW. Causes of gastrointestinal colic in horses in western Canada: 604 cases (1992 to 2002). Can Vet J 2005;46:800–5.

23. Proudman CJ, Dugdale AH, Senior JM, et al. Pre-operative and anaesthesia-related risk factors for mortality in equine colic cases. Vet J 2006;171:89–97.

24. Institute of Medicine. To err is human: building a safer health system. Washington, DC: National Academic Press; 1999.

25. Institute of Medicine. Crossing the quality chasm: a new health system for the 21st century. Washington, DC: National Academic Press; 2001.

The Bacterial Community of the Horse Gastrointestinal Tract and Its Relation to Fermentative Acidosis, Laminitis, Colic, and Stomach Ulcers

Rafat A.M. Al Jassim, BSc, MSc, PhD[a],*, Frank M. Andrews, DVM, MS[b]

KEYWORDS

- Bacterial community • Fermentative acidosis • Laminitis
- Colic • Stomach ulcer

Fermentation in the hindgut of the horse is similar to that in the rumen, resulting in the production of short-chain volatile fatty acids (VFAs), mainly acetic, propionic, and butyric acids. The proportion of these acids is influenced by the availability and type of substrate, the composition of the microbial community, and the hindgut physiologic conditions. The microbial community of the hindgut of the horse, particularly the fiber-degrading bacteria, is far less understood than that of the ruminant's compartmental stomach. VFAs are absorbed across the hindgut wall, transported by blood into different tissues, and used as an energy source. Horses are less efficient than ruminants in the digestion of fiber and therefore have a lower survival rate than ruminants under severe drought conditions. In addition to VFAs, a large volume of gases is produced and removed dorsally. Under normal feeding conditions, horses spend approximately 10 to 12 hours a day eating. Such feeding patterns allow them to maintain a full stomach and a continuous supply of nutrients both to the host animal and the microbial community residing the hindgut. This feeding behavior also helps the horse to overcome the problem of having a relatively small stomach compared with other herbivore species of a similar body size, such as the cow. This feeding behavior is

[a] School of Animal Studies, The Faculty of Natural Resources, Agricultural and Veterinary Science, The University of Queensland, Gatton Campus, Queensland 4343, Australia
[b] Equine Health Studies Program, Department of Veterinary Clinical Sciences, School of Veterinary Medicine, Louisiana State University, Skip Bertman Drive, Baton Rouge, LA 70803, USA
* Corresponding author.
E-mail address: r.aljassim@uq.edu.au (R.A.M. Al Jassim).

Vet Clin Equine 25 (2009) 199–215
doi:10.1016/j.cveq.2009.04.005
0749-0739/09/$ – see front matter © 2009 Elsevier Inc. All rights reserved.

vetequine.theclinics.com

important for health and for meeting horses' nutritional needs, especially energy. In contrast, racehorses are fed grain-rich diets twice daily and are withheld from feed for extended periods before exercise. The increase in gastric acid production during exercise, the reduction in saliva production caused by the low fiber content of the diet, and the periods of feed deprivation between meals lead to prolonged periods in which the unprotected non-glandular region of the stomach is exposed to acid. This exposure combined with typical indoor confinement and the stress of intense exercise is the probable cause of stomach ulcers in race and performance horses. The ingestion of a diet high in starch or rich in nonstructural carbohydrate also is associated with diseases such as fermentative acidosis, equine metabolic syndrome, equine Cushing's disease, laminitis, and colic. Maintaining health in horses under conditions of concentrate feeding is a real challenge facing nutritionists, veterinarians. and owners. Such challenge requires better understanding of the anatomic, physiologic, and functional features of the horse gastrointestinal (GI) tract. An understanding of the complexity of the microbial ecosystem, the interactions among the large and diverse microbial community and between microbes and the host animal, and the influences of diet on the microbes is equally important. This article focuses on the feeding conditions that maintain good health and on the dietary changes associated with diseases such as fermentative acidosis, laminitis, and colic that occur mainly in intensively managed horses.

The present horse belongs to the genus *Equus*, which evolved 1 million years ago from its ancestor *Eohippus*, an early type of mammal that began evolution 60 million years ago.[1] The evolution of the horse coincided with the development of grasslands that displaced forests. The environmental and geographic changes during that period led to anatomic and physiologic changes that enabled the horse's survival. It is not known exactly when the horse was domesticated, nor is it known whether its GI tract was modified to suit the available high-fiber grasses present at that time or whether the horse selected the type of feed most suited for its GI tract. Domestication that adapted horses to human use and captive life secured the survival of the species and assisted humankind in creating civilization.

Horses are best described as hindgut fermenters with an enlarged cecum and colon that harbors a complex microbial community. These microbes contribute to the digestion processes that enable the horse to extract energy from dietary components that otherwise would be wasted. In addition to hindgut fermentation, extensive fermentation occurs in the stomach when horses consume diets rich in nonstructural carbohydrates. The fermentation in the stomach, however, produces mainly lactic acid and small amounts of VFAs because of the acidic conditions of the stomach that support acid-tolerant bacteria (eg, lactic acid–producing bacteria). Horses are subject to nutritional disorders and diseases common to intensively managed animals such as acidosis, colic, gastric ulcers, and laminitis. The special anatomic and physiologic features of the horse's digestive system need to be considered when deciding what to feed horses. Improved pastures that have been developed to maximize microbial protein synthesis in the rumen of cattle and sheep[2] and to increase milk yield[3] may be deleterious to horses because of their high content of nonstructural carbohydrates and crude protein. Improved pastures may have an effect similar to that of grain or concentrate feeding for performance or racehorses.[4]

This article describes the GI tract of the horse, its bacterial community, the diets best suited for it, and the effects on health of feeding concentrate- or grain-based diets.

THE GASTROINTESTINAL TRACT OF THE HORSE

The GI tract of a typical herbivore consists of the oral cavity, the pharynx, the esophagus, the stomach, the small intestine, the large intestine, and rectum. It extends through the body and is located largely within the abdominal cavity. In addition to the main segments of the GI tract, several associated glands and organs that are situated outside the GI tract are involved in the digestion processes and empty their secretions into the tract. The next sections briefly describe the anatomic features and functions of the different segments of the GI tract of the horse.

THE UPPER SEGMENTS OF THE GASTROINTESTINAL TRACT
The Mouth and the Esophagus

The digestive system starts with the mouth, which is also called the "oral cavity." It contains structures that aid in the prehension and the mechanical breakdown of food.

These structures include the lips, tongue, teeth, and the associated salivary glands. The horse differs from cattle in that the horse has both upper and lower incisors that allow it to graze closer to the ground.[5] The upper jaw is wider than the lower jaw, and the horse chews with a side-to-side movement so that its teeth are brought together into a grinding apposition.[6] Three pairs of salivary glands secrete saliva, which aids in lubricating feeds and facilitates swallowing. The three pairs of salivary glands are the parotid glands, the mandibular or submaxillary glands, and the sublingual glands. The parotid glands, located just underneath the ear and below the jaw on each side, secrete saliva via a duct that is located near the third upper premolar. The mandibular glands, located deep to the parotid, discharge saliva into the mouth through a duct that opens in front of the tongue. The sublingual glands, located under the floor of the mouth on either side of the tongue, discharge saliva through a number of ducts that open alongside the tongue.

Saliva is secreted only in response to the chewing action and the presence of food in the mouth; it is not stimulated by the sight or smell of feed as happens in other animals. About 10 to 12 L of saliva is secreted daily; the amount depends on the texture and form of feed. The saliva seems to have no digestive enzyme activity but has a high mucus content that serves to saturate and lubricate food. Its bicarbonate (HCO_3^-) content provides it with a buffering capacity. The continuous secretion of saliva during feeding seems to buffer the digesta material in the proximal region of the stomach, to modify the decline in pH associated with VFA and lactic acid production to maintain mildly acidic conditions, and to permit acid-tolerant bacteria to ferment nonstructural carbohydrates with the production of lactate, which has important implications for the well-being of the horse.[7]

The Pharynx and the Esophagus

The pharynx is commonly called the "throat" and is the passageway for food and air. It is a funnel shaped musculo-membranous structure narrowing down to the trachea and esophagus. As food passes through the pharynx, the reflexive and mechanical factors associated with swallowing prevent the food from entering the larynx and nasal cavities.

The esophagus is a long muscular tube that passes from the pharynx down to the stomach, where it ends at the cardiac orifice a few centimeters beyond the diaphragm. The entry of food into the stomach is guarded by a sphincter muscle, which remains closed except during swallowing. Horses are incapable of vomiting or regurgitating gastric contents into the esophagus because the esophagus enters the stomach at a sharp angle, and a sphincter closes when the stomach expands. Fermentation of feed in the horse stomach and the accumulation of gases may increase the pressure dramatically and may cause the stomach to burst. The muscles of the esophagus consist of an inner circular layer and an outer longitudinal layer, similar in structure to the stomach and the intestine. In the horse, two thirds of the esophagus is striated muscle; smooth muscle is present in the lowest portion of the esophagus.[8]

The Stomach of the Horse

The stomach of the horse is relatively small compared with those of other large animal species, comprising only 8% to 10% of the GI tract with a net capacity of 7.5 to 15 L, depending on feed type. The stomach has two distinct regions: the upper half of the stomach consists of squamous epithelial cells that lack a mucous layer, whereas the lower part is glandular and consists of secretory tissue that produces acid and mucus, which helps protect this region from injury. Horses at pasture graze continuously and maintain a full stomach. The stomach is subdivided into continuous parts. The part located nearest the esophagus is called the "cardia" or the "esophageal part." Next is the fundus, which is the dome-shaped part of the stomach. The fundus is adjacent to the corpus, the rounded base, and together they constitute the middle portion, which is most subject to distension.[9] The part that joins the small intestine is the pylorus. The esophageal part is lined with a stratified squamous epithelium that is continuous with the lining of the esophagus. It is nonglandular and therefore produces no secretions. This portion represents approximately one third of the stomach. Food entering the stomach is poorly mixed, so there is a pH gradient between the entrance of the stomach, the cardiac region, and the pyloric glandular region. When roughage is consumed, chewing stimulates saliva secretion, and the continuous delivery of saliva to the stomach buffers the stomach contents and protects the nonglandular region from acid. The pH at the nonglandular region is about 5.4, whereas in the pyloric region it is about 1.8.

The Small Intestine

The small intestine is the major site for the chemical digestion of nutrients and absorption of digestion end products, including amino acids from proteins, simple sugars from carbohydrates, and fatty acids from fat. Apart from some nonstructural carbohydrates that are fermented in the nonglandular region of the stomach, the chemical nature of the chyme that leaves the stomach and enters the intestine is the same as that of the ingested feed. The small intestine comprises three sections, the duodenum, the jejunum, and the ileum (**Fig. 1**). The entry of chyme into the small intestine stimulates pancreatic secretions. The horse lacks a gall bladder, so bile is secreted directly into the duodenum. The secretion of bicarbonate from the pancreas and bile from the liver neutralizes the hydrochloric acid from the stomach and raises the pH of the digesta to 7.0. In grass-fed horses, the pH of the duodenum, jejunum, and ileum have been reported to be 6.32, 7.10, and 7.47, respectively.[10] Neutralization of the acidic chyme entering the duodenum provides an optimal pH for pancreatic enzymes. Pancreatic juice is secreted continuously in the horse, but in contrast to ruminant herbivores, secretion in the horse increases by three- to fourfold within 2 to 3 minutes after the horse has started eating. Also, in comparison with other herbivores such as the cow and sheep, horses produce larger amounts of pancreatic juice, 10 to 12 L/100 kg of body weight in a 24-hour period, compared with 5 L for cows and 1 L for sheep.[8] Because of the high amounts and continuous production of pancreatic juice, concentrations of pancreatic enzymes and HCO_3^- are always low. Nevertheless, the continuous production of pancreatic juice and bile ensures a steady flow of buffered intestinal contents to the large intestine. In addition to the buffering action

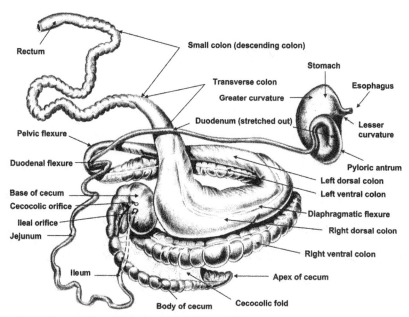

Fig. 1. Isolated stomach and intestines of the horse. (Sketched by Kate Andrews, University of Queensland Gatton Campus, Queensland, Australia. *Adapted from* McCracken TO, Kainer RA, Spurgeon TL. The horse. In: McCracken TO, Kainer RA, Spurgeon TL, editors. Spurgeon's color atlas of large animal anatomy: the essentials. Oxford: Wiley-Blackwell; 1999. p. 16; with permission.)

of the pancreatic juice, its high water content ensures that conditions favorable for the large and diverse microbial population in the cecum and colon are maintained. Bile also emulsifies fat and hence improves enzymatic digestion. Digestion and absorption of carbohydrates, proteins, and fat is more efficient in the duodenum than in the other two segments of the small intestine, the jejunum and ileum. Except for starch, most of the available nutrients are removed by the time digesta reaches the terminal ileum and enters the cecum. Digestion of starch in the small intestine of the horse is not very efficient, because the horse produces only 8% to 10% as much amylase as the pig.[11]

THE LOWER SEGMENTS OF THE GASTROINTESTINAL TRACT
The Large Intestine

The large intestine consists of the cecum, the colon, and the rectum (see **Fig. 1**), which harbor a complex microbial population. The conditions in the large intestine match the description of a continuous chemical reactor, in which the input of nutrients is continuous, mixing is adequate, products are removed, and reactants are in contact with enzymes produced either by the animal's body or by the GI tract microbes. Mixing of contents allows control over the temperature, pH, and the removal of gasses. The large intestine comprises approximately 64% of the volume of the equine GI tract but only 30% of its total length.[6] It is a voluminous but short organ, holding approximately 95 to 112 L of liquid, approximately the size of the compartmental stomach of an adult cow. It is similar to the rumen in that it is inhabited by a fermentative microbial community. The walls of the large intestine lack villi, and the epithelial cells lack microvilli, but they contain glands for secreting mucus. The walls of the large intestine also contain longitudinal and circular muscle fibers. Unlike other herbivores, the small intestine in the horse opens directly into the cecum, the first segment of the large intestine, through a muscular valve. Relatively close to this valve is a second valve where digesta passes from the cecum and into the right ventral colon.

The cecum is a large, blind, comma-shaped structure approximately 1 m in length with a capacity between 25 and 35 L. It extends from the pelvic inlet to the abdominal floor within the right flank area of the horse. The base of the cecum extends forward to lie under the cover of the last few ribs, with its tip just behind the diaphragm. The large intestine in the horse does not have a longitudinal muscle layer. Instead, it has bands of muscle (called the "tarnia") that follow the length of the cecum and gather the cecal wall into sacculations called "haustra." The haustra act like buckets, delaying the transport of chyme through the large intestine and contributing to the mixing of the colonic contents.

In the horse the ascending colon is called the "large colon" and consists of a ventral colon and a dorsal colon.[9] The first segment of the colon, the ventral colon, can hold a volume of approximately 150 L, has a diameter of 250 to 300 mm, and is about 2 to 4 m long. The transition between the ventral colon and dorsal colon is narrow. This narrow segment delays the transport of large particles from the ventral to the dorsal colon, increasing their retention time and fermentability. The diameter varies significantly between regions but is largest in the right dorsal colon, forming sacculations with a diameter of up to 500 mm. The large colon is folded so that it forms a double loop consisting of the right and left ventral colons and the left and right dorsal colons. The four parts of the large colon are connected by structures called the "sternal," "pelvic," and "diaphragmatic" flexures. Their importance probably lies in the differences in microbial populations and functions in the segments.[5] The small or descending colon joins the dorsal colon to the rectum and is approximately 3 m in length. The rectum is approximately 30 cm long and is the continuation of the small colon into the pelvic inlet, where it ends at the anus. Because of its size, location, and importance in digestion, the equine large intestine may be referred to as the "hindgut."

MICROBIOLOGY OF THE GASTROINTESTINAL TRACT OF THE HORSE

The microbial community of the equine GI tract has received very little attention despite its importance for the health of the animal and for the digestion of feed. Available information has dealt mainly with fermentation processes in the hindgut, especially those related to fiber digestion,[12–15] lactic acidosis,[16,17] and laminitis.[18,19] Early work by Mackie and Wilkins[10] reported a higher bacterial population in the distal parts of the GI tract between the duodenum and the colon. Horses that were fed a grass diet had a bacterial population of 2.9×10^6/g wet weight in the duodenum, 29.0×10^6 in the jejunum, 38.4×10^6 in the ileum, 2.05×10^9 in the cecum, and 1.26×10^9 in the colon. These investigators reported a relationship between mucosal and luminal counts. Bacteria associated with the mucosa were 73%, 22%, and 24% of the luminal counts in the duodenum, jejunum, and ileum, respectively. Using similar culturing techniques, the authors often obtain counts for total anaerobes around 4.3×10^8 in the stomach, 4.2×10^8 in the cecum, 1.0×10^8 in the proximal colon, 6.7×10^7 in the distal colon, and 1.7×10^8 in the rectum. Early work focused on bacterial groups and relied mainly on culture-dependent methods that had certain limitations. Molecular techniques have revealed the bacterial diversity within the equine large intestine[13,17] and the stomach.[7] The mildly acidic conditions in the nonglandular region of the stomach permit fermentation to occur and result in the production of lactic acid and VFAs (**Figs. 2** and **3**).

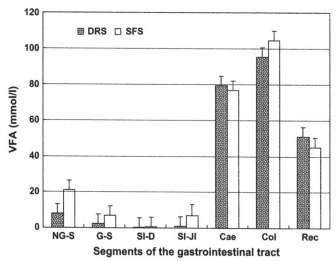

Fig. 2. Effect of supplementation of liverseed grass (*Urochloa panicoides*) hay with dry-rolled or steam-flaked sorghum grains on the concentration of VFA in the different segments of the GI tract. Cae, cecum; Col, colon; DRS, dry-rolled sorghum; G-S, glandular region of the stomach; NG-S, nonglandular region of the stomach; Rec, rectum; SFS, steam-flaked sorghum; SI-D, small intestine, duodenum; SI-JI, small intestine, jejunum and ileum. (*From* Al Jassim RAM. Supplementary feeding of horses with processed sorghum grains and oats. Anim Feed Sci Technol 2006;125:41; with permission.)

Fermentation may cease in the more acidic pyloric part of the stomach, but lactic acid–producing bacteria remain viable even when horses are deprived of food for 12 hours and seem to be able tolerate acid shock.[17] Bacteria observed in the stomach of horses fed diets rich in starch or nonstructural carbohydrates include *Streptococcus bovis* and *S. equinus*,[16,18,19] *Lactobacillus salivarius*, *L. mucosae*, *L. delbrueckii*, and *Mitsuokella jalaludinii*.[17] **Table 1** presents the origin and amount of L- and D-lactate produced in vitro by key isolates representative of the major groups and the recognized bacterial species to which they are most closely related. Of particular interest are the D-lactate producers that share between 97% and 98% sequence identity with *M. jalaludinii*. These isolates have not been identified previously in the GI tract of horses. *M. jalaludinii* was isolated first from the GI tract of cattle in Malaysia and was named after S. Jalaludin, an animal nutritionist at Putra University in Malaysia.[20] The organism was demonstrated to produce phytase and lactate. Unfortunately, the type of lactate produced was not determined. In a study by the first author and colleagues,[16] the isolates sharing 97% to 98% 16S rDNA sequence identity with *M. jalaludinii* were shown to ferment glucose and produce the D-isomer of lactate at quantities similar to the high amounts of L-lactate previously reported for *S. bovis*. Furthermore, these isolates were obtained from very high dilutions (10^{-7}–10^{-8}) of the GI tract contents of horses in which laminitis had been induced and in which there was evidence of an elevated blood D-lactate concentration.

Because the horse does not express the enzyme D-lactate dehydrogenase required for the conversion of pyruvate to D-lactate or lactate racemase that catalyzes the conversion of L-lactate to D-lactate, the D-lactate could come only from gut microbes that have such capacity. The relative population sizes of the isolated bacterial groups in vivo and their response to increased available carbohydrate, and hence the significance of lactic acidosis, are unknown at this time.

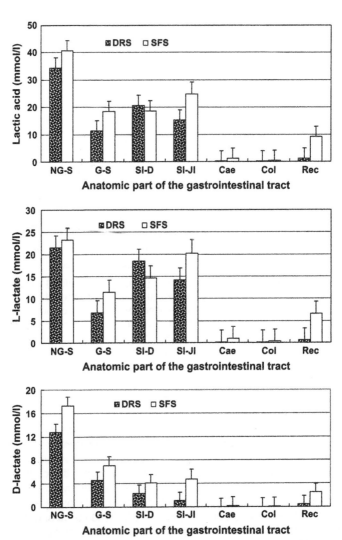

Fig. 3. Effect of supplementation of liverseed grass (*Urochloa panicoides*) hay with dry-rolled or steam-flaked sorghum grains on the concentration of total, L-, and D-lactate in the different anatomic parts of the GI tract. Cae, cacum; Col, colon; DRS, dry-rolled sorghum; G-S, glandular region of the stomach; NG-S, nonglandular region of the stomach; Rec, rectum; SFS, steam-flaked sorghum; SI-D, small intestine, duodenum; SI-JI, small intestine, jejunum and ileum. (*From* Al Jassim RAM. Supplementary feeding of horses with processed sorghum grains and oats. Anim Feed Sci Technol 2006;125:42; with permission.)

D-lactic acidosis is well documented in the literature, but little information is available about the identity of the bacteria producing D-lactic acid. Most of the work in the past focused on *S. bovis* and *S. equinus* because of their established role in acid build-up and their involvement in the sequence of events leading to the development of laminitis. In recent work, Milinovich and colleagues[19] monitored changes in the bacterial community of the cecum of horses using florescence in situ hybridization (FISH). Laminitis was induced in all horses following oral administration of oligofructose at

Table 1
16S rDNA identification of key lactic acid–producing bacteria that are distinct from *S bovis* and *S equinus* isolated from the different sites of the GI tract and their fermentation end products

Isolate	Origin	Closest Relatives[a]	Gram Reaction	L-Lactate (mM)	D-Lactate (mM)	Dietary Regimen
RA2053	Stomach	*Lactobacillus mucosae* 95%	+	1.0	2.2	Roughage fedad libitum
RA2062	Stomach	*Lactobacillus delbrueckii* 98%	+	Not detectable	3.5	Roughage fedad libitum
RA2113	Rectum	*Lactobacillus delbrueckii* 96%	+	2.0	3.7	Horse with induced laminitis
RA2070	Cecum	*Lactobacillus mucosae* > 99%	+	1.0	1.4	Horse with induced laminitis
RA2105	Colon and rectum	*Lactobacillus salivarius* > 99%	+	21.7	2.6	Horse with induced laminitis
T057	Stomach	*Lactobacillus salivarius* 94%	+	Not detectable	4.8	Roughage fed
RA2074	Cecum and rectum	*Mitsuokella jalaludinii* 98%	–	1.2	22.6	Horses with induced laminitis
RA2114	Rectum	*Veillonella atypica* 93%	–	3.0	5.3	Horse with induced laminitis

[a] The organisms named as closest relatives named are completely characterized bacterial species, but in some cases the true closest relative was an uncultured or incompletely described bacterium.
From Al Jassim R, McGowan T, Andrews F, et al. Gastric ulceration in horses, the role of bacteria and lactic acid. Rural Industries Research and Development Corporation 2008. Publication No. 08/033; with permission.

a relatively high rate of 10 g/kg body weight. All horses lost their appetite by 8 hours post oligofructose administration (POA) and developed profuse, watery diarrhea by 16 hours POA. Clinical signs of laminitis were observed in these horses (eg, lameness and shifting of weight from one foot to another) from 20 hours POA onwards. The population of the Gram-positive bacteria changed from less than 20% at time of administration to more than 70% between 4 and 8 hours POA and remained at high levels up to 32 hours POA. These findings were confirmed by FISH results that showed the relative abundance of *S bovis/S equinus* to be greater than 50% by 16 hours POA in all samples. These results confirm the association of *S bovis/S equinus* with acid build-up and sequential events leading to the development of laminitis in horses.

Recent work in our laboratory using culture-dependent and culture-independent techniques has revealed a diverse bacterial community in the stomach of the horse. The main bacterial groups were closely related to bacterial species belonging to the genera *Lactobacillus, Streptococcus, Clostridium, Prevotella, Pseudomonas,* and *Propionibacterium.* Other minor groups were closely related to *Escherichia, Legionella, Voraxella,* and *Pasteurella* (**Fig. 4**).[7] This study has shown that the acidic conditions

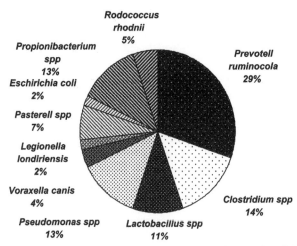

Fig. 4. Clones derived from denaturing gradient gel electrophoresis bands identified using the V3 region of 16S rDNA. Genomic DNA was extracted from stomach contents and stomach mucosa. (*From* Al Jassim R, McGowan T, Andrews F, et al. Gastric ulceration in horses, the role of bacteria and lactic acid. Rural Industries Research and Development Corporation 2008; Publication No. 08/033; with permission.)

of the stomach do not reduce the presence of a large number of bacteria in the stomach. The results also demonstrated the association of bacteria with mucous and squamous tissue in healthy and ulcerated stomachs.

ENERGY REQUIREMENTS OF THE HORSE

As mentioned earlier, horses spend long hours (10–12 hours a day) eating to satisfy their nutritional needs and to overcome the problem of having a relatively small stomach. This behavior is particularly important when considering the energy needs for a racehorse or a performance horse. Energy for the horse is derived from digestible nutrients, including carbohydrates, proteins, and fat. It therefore is logical to use digestible energy (DE) to express the energy needs of horses.[21] In addition, DE is easily measured from digestion trials. The DE values for feeds used by National Research Council[21,22] were derived from equations based on the acid detergent fiber and crude protein contents of feed and expressed as Mcal/kg of dry matter (DM). The use of acid detergent fiber and crude protein provides reliable estimates of DE, and the inclusion of other dietary chemical constituents resulted in little or no improvement in the prediction power of the constructed equations.[21,23] Although the two approaches produced similar results when dealing with common horse feedstuffs, Pagan (1998) suggested appropriate adjustments when dealing with nonconventional feedstuffs such as high-fiber or high-fat feeds. High-fat feed (>5%) raised particular concern, and additional 0.044 Mcal/kg body weight of DE was suggested for each additional 1% of fat above 5%. Problems caused by high fat contents also were acknowledged by Zeyner and Kienzle (2002).[24]

Energy requirements are categorized as those needed for maintenance and those required for growth, pregnancy, milk production, or performance. Energy requirement values are expressed on the basis of body weight to match the way requirements for other nutrients have been expressed and also to overcome problems associated with the use of a small number of horses to derive these values and validate them.[21] There seems, however, to be a need for feeding trials using large number of horses with ranges of body weight and size to validate the energy requirements values and to allow these requirements to be stated based on metabolic body weight ($BW^{0.75}$). The calculated DE requirements for maintenance (DE_m) ranged from 25.7 to 35.1 kcal/kg body weight.[21] These values are similar to the estimates reported for beef cattle by the Ministry of Agriculture, Fisheries and Food of the United Kingdom.[25] The United Kingdom estimates were based on calorimetric measurements of fasting metabolism (FM) and the use of fixed factors to convert FM to DE_m. The wide range for DE_m for horses reflects the numerous factors affecting DE_m, including heat production, the efficiency at which DE is utilized for metabolic activities, body composition, and other animal-related factors that often are referred to as "horse-to-horse variation." A horse eating medium-quality grass hay that has an average DE value of 1.79 Mcal/kg DM[21] needs to consume approximately 8.5 kg DM to meet its energy requirements for maintenance. More is needed to meet the additional physiologic requirements for gestation, lactation, or performance. Because the horse stomach has a limited capacity to hold feed, an alternative strategy of using digesta with a fast rate of passage through the GI tract was adopted to cope with such needs. This remarkable phenomenon, together with the enlargement of the cecum and the colon, gave the horse some advantages over other herbivores of similar feeding habits. There are some advantages, however, when the horse is fed less frequently on concentrate diets rich in starch. This approach is discussed further in the following sections.

ROUGHAGE FEEDING OF HORSES

Under normal feeding conditions, horses consume diets consisting mainly of cell wall polysaccharides including cellulose, hemicellulose, and pectin, the main structural constituents of the plant cell wall. Such diets often are bulky and low in energy content. For horses to meet their requirements for energy and other nutrients, they graze continually and spend approximately 10 to 12 hours eating during a 24-hour period, in sessions of 0.5 to 3 hours under free-range conditions.[8] Another report noted that a free-range horse spends 16 to 18 hours or more out of 24 hours searching for and selecting feed to meet its requirements.[6] Their continuous feeding ensures that horses maintain a full stomach, and continuous buffering from saliva protects the nonglandular stomach from acid injuries.

The digestive processes begin with acid hydrolysis in the stomach and enzymatic digestion by the host in the small intestine followed by extensive fermentation in the cecum and colon.

In horses fed grass or hay, fermentation of structural carbohydrates by the action of microbial enzymes in the cecum and the colon produces VFA, which are readily absorbed and used as an energy source. The contribution of VFA to the energy requirements of the horse can be as high as 70% to 80%. Under these conditions the environment of the large intestine remains buffered and supports the proliferation of the major groups of the microbial community. One disadvantage of the system is that considerable amounts of fermentation products, such as vitamins and amino acids, are retained by the microbes; hence these products are not utilized by the horse and appear in the feces. One way for the horse to benefit from products that are retained by bacteria is to consume its own feces. The incidence of coprophagy seems to be related to the quality of the horse's diet. In the other hand, feeding starch-rich diets, which is particularly a problem in intensively managed racehorses, disrupts the microbial ecosystem of the GI tract, particularly the large intestine.

Similar conditions may result from feeding grasses rich in the oligosaccharides fructans, which are polymers of fructose molecules. Temperate grasses contain three types of fructans: inulin, a linear fructan generally linked by β $(2 \rightarrow 1)$ glycosidic bonds; levan, a linear fructan generally linked by β $(2 \rightarrow 6)$ glycosidic bonds; and graminan, a branched fructan linked by both β $(2 \rightarrow 1)$ and β $(2 \rightarrow 6)$ glycosidic bonds.[26,27] Accumulation of fructans in grasses is influenced by grass type, environmental conditions, and stage of maturity.[26] Although, fructans are water soluble, the horse does not produce enzymes capable of digesting them, and thus they pass through the small intestine and enter the hindgut of the horse where they undergo fermentation by the hindgut microbes. Excessive intake of fructans can lead to acid build-up and metabolic disorders similar to those experienced under grain-overload conditions.[4] Little is known, however, about the interaction between the different bacterial species and the level of fructan intake.

SUPPLEMENTARY FEEDING OF HORSES, FERMENTATIVE ACIDOSIS, AND LAMINITIS

Dietary supplementation is essential to maintain good health and to satisfy the nutritional needs for growth and performance of various equine classes. Grain and mixed feeds contain large amounts of nonstructural carbohydrates, mainly as starch. The choice of cereal grain is based on its safety, palatability, energy value, and cost. Oat grain is palatable and relatively safe because it is lower in energy density and higher in fiber than other grains.

Starch is not well digested in the small intestine of the horse, and variable proportions of ingested starch that escape enzymatic digestion in the small intestine enter the large intestine and are rapidly fermented, increasing VFA and lactate production (see **Figs. 2** and **3**) and lowering the pH. An acidic environment favors the rapid proliferation of lactic acid–producing bacteria, resulting in increased lactic acid production and a further decline in the pH. Lactic acidosis often is accompanied by laminitis.

Accumulation of lactic acid in the hindgut of the horse results from the rapid fermentation by bacteria of starch that enters the cecum and colon. This fermentation occurs when the supply of starch in the diet exceeds the digestive capacity of the small intestine. The upper limit of 3.5 to 4.0 g starch/kg body weight per meal was suggested earlier by Potter and colleagues,[28] but studies on variations in the digestion of starch with increasing starch intake[28,29] suggest that the upper limit is less than 3.5 g/kg body weight per meal. Differences can be explained partly by the source of starch. An increase in the population of lactic acid–producing and lactic acid–using bacteria and a decrease in the concentration of cellulolytic bacteria in the cecal contents of horses were measured in horses fed a high-starch diet supplying 3.4 g starch/kg body weight per meal.[30] The lowest pH and highest lactic acid values were measured at 5 and 6 hours after feeding in the cecum (6.45; 532 mg/L) and the colon (6.38; 582 mg/L), respectively. A recent report by Hussein[31] showed a decrease in fecal pH level from 7.04 to an average of 6.74 and an increase in the concentration of lactate in horses fed alfalfa cubes supplemented with various grains (eg, barley, corn, naked oats, and oats). Lactate concentration was notably high for the barley-supplemented diet (2.82 μmol/g versus 0.96 μmol/g of DM). This report supports earlier results reported by Meyer and colleagues,[32] which showed a very low pre-ileal digestibility for rolled barley starch in horses (eg, 0.21). The source of starch and the processing method of the cereal grain also were emphasized by McLean and colleagues[33] and by McCracken and colleagues,[34] who observed unfavorable changes in intracecal fermentation in ponies fed a diet of hay and rolled barley (50:50) that was formulated to supply 2.1 g/kg body weight per meal. These unfavorable changes were not observed with micronized or extruded barley. Processing of grain to improve the extent of enzymatic hydrolysis in the small intestine should reduce the amount of starch reaching the large intestine.[32] Work by de Fombelle and colleagues,[35] however, indicated that the presence of significant numbers of lactic acid–producing and lactic acid–using bacteria in the horse stomach suggests that such grain processing might have the undesirable effect of increasing starch fermentation and hence lactic acid production in the stomach. Such a situation could contribute to lactic acidemia, a condition associated with laminitis.[36-38] Fermentation in the stomach also was shown to be extensive under concentrate-feeding conditions, particularly in the nonglandular region of the stomach. In horses fed 4 kg grass hay and 4 kg dry-rolled or steam-flaked sorghum per day, the lactic acid concentration in the nonglandular region of the stomach was greater than 40 mmol/L.[7] Another important feature of the fermentation process in the stomach is the high proportion of the D-lactate isomer, because in other anaerobic fermentations the L-isomer is the more prominent. In addition to the two isomers of lactate, which are the main products, small amounts of VFA are produced. The study also showed that lactic acid is absorbed from the GI tract before the digesta reaches the cecum.

COLIC

It is widely acknowledged by veterinarians, horse owners, and keepers that colic is a serious medical problem that affects horses worldwide and can be life threatening. Among the several potential causes of the problem internal parasites, change of diet, dietary management, housing conditions, lack of access to pasture and water, increasing exercise, and transport are the most common.[39,40] Factors that cause rapid fermentation and excessive build-up of gasses could lead to distention of the digestive tract and consequently cause colic. Inadequate supply of dietary fiber and high concentrate with less frequent feeding are man-made problems of modern horse husbandry systems. Bad teeth also can contribute to colic: ineffective chewing and the resultant ingestion of long feed particles can disrupt the passage of the digesta.

The effect of seasons also has been documented, with the equine grass sickness, which is considered acute colic, being a good example. An increase in the incidence of colic during spring and autumn months was reported in the United Kingdom.[41] Spring pastures are known to be rich in soluble carbohydrates and nonprotein nitrogenous compounds and sometimes have unbalanced mineral contents. If recovered in the hindgut, soluble carbohydrates undergo rapid fermentation, which leads to a build-up of gases and acids. Little is known about the link between green spring pastures and the incidence of colic, and there is a real need to investigate this association experimentally. Most of the available information is derived from epidemiologic studies based on statistical analysis of veterinary records that often reference nutrition. Although most reports emphasize the dietary factor and its implication in the development of colic, these reports lack solid experimental evidence derived from well-defined nutritional trials with controls. As a result, these associations remain as speculations that need to be verified.

The advances in veterinary care that led to the development of more effective methods of parasitic control[42] have not been matched by achievements in nutrition to reduce the risks of modern feeding of the captive and domesticated horse.

A review of the relevant literature on the incidence of colic by Archer and Proudman[39] showed that colic episodes could be as high as 10.7% per year and vary considerably within any horse population. They also indicated that the majority of cases (69%–72%) were spasmodic/gas colic or colic of unknown nature, and only a small portion of these cases (7%–9%) required surgery. Apart from the well-documented parasitic causes, all other factors in the available literature are based on observation and are not experimentally confirmed. Interesting evidence from studies on horses diagnosed with acute equine grass sickness in the United Kingdom suggested that toxin produced by the bacterium *Clostridium botulinum* type C is involved.[43] This bacterium is soil borne, gram positive, and spore forming and is capable of surviving the acidic conditions of the stomach by producing spores that, when leaving the stomach, vegetate and colonize the intestine.[44] Under favorable conditions that could be created by abrupt dietary changes, this bacterium becomes one of the predominant bacteria; it establishes a population and starts producing toxins. The type C complex toxoid toxin produced by this bacterium affects the nervous system of the horse and negatively affects the motility of the GI tract, causing intestinal dysfunction. This hypothesis is an important development that emphasizes the importance of a well-balanced microbial ecosystem in the GI tract of the horse and the need to adhere to the practice of gradually introducing horses to new types or amounts of feed. Gradual introduction allows the nonpathogenic commensal bacteria to adjust to the new environment and establish a new balance. A balanced bacterial community helps prevent pathogenic bacteria such as *C. botulinum* from colonizing the intestine and establishing an effective population.

GASTRIC ULCERS

As indicated earlier, horses maintained solely on pasture rarely develop gastric ulcers. Feeding with grain or concentrates rich in nonstructural carbohydrates, bolus feeding, and feed deprivation for prolonged periods increase the duration of exposure of the nonglandular stratified squamous epithelium to acid, potentially causing gastric ulcers.[45] The adverse effect of acid on the nonglandular part of the stomach can be prevented by administering ranitidine, an antagonist that binds to histamine type-2 receptors on parietal cells and thus inhibits acid secretion,[45] and omeprazole, a proton-pump inhibitor,[46] demonstrating that acid and low pH are implicated in the development of stomach ulcers. The use of acid-suppressing agents does not alter the abundance of micro-organisms that colonize the lesions or those responsible for production of VFAs and lactic acid in the nonglandular part of the stomach. Recent work showed a synergistic effect of VFAs and hydrochloric acid in causing damage to the nonglandular mucosa.[47,48] Lactic acid is a stronger acid than VFA, and its concentration in the stomach can be as high as 40 mmol/L 2 to 6 hours after ingestion of a starch-rich diet,[7] indicating that it may damage the lining of the nonglandular region of the stomach. Lactic acid, at a low pH, could be taken up by nonglandular mucosal cells and disrupt cellular metabolism or could work synergistically with hydrochloric acid to disrupt the tight junctions of mucosal cells and increase gastric permeability. The effect of lactic acid on the mucosa of the nonglandular stomach has not been evaluated, and little is known about stomach bacteria that produce lactic acid. Recently a joint project between investigators at the University of Queensland, Australia and the University of Tennessee provided evidence for the damaging effect of lactic acid on the mucosa of the nonglandular region of the stomach and provided information about the bacterial diversity of the stomach.[44] The combination of a high concentration of lactic acid (40 mM) and low pH (1.5) resulted in an increase in conductance and increased permeability of [^{14}C]mannitol over an incubation period of 4 hours in Ringer's solution in an Ussing chamber, as compared with exposure to the same level of lactate at pH 4.0 and 7.0. The lactic acid concentrations used are typical of those in the stomachs of horses fed diets high in soluble or nonstructural carbohydrates[7,49] and therefore provide important evidence about the negative impact of feeding such diets to horses. The greater permeability to [^{14}C]mannitol than seen in tissues exposed to the same level of lactic acid at pH 4.0 or pH 7.0 may indicate that exposure to lactic acid at a low pH (1.5) causes damage to the paracellular spaces and enables acid to leak between the cells, causing ulcers. Lactic acid may act synergistically with hydrochloric acid, VFAs, and other acids found in gastric fluid.

SUMMARY

Horses are important herbivore animals that have a unique GI tract especially suited for the digestion and utilization of fiber-rich diets. To maintain health and derive adequate nutrients to meet their requirements, horses need to graze continually and to feed on pastures that are not too rich in nonstructural carbohydrates and water-soluble carbohydrates that ferment in the GI tract, alter the GI conditions, and adversely affect the balanced microbial population. The practice of feeding concentrate diets high in energy in less frequent meals leads to complications and diseases such as acidosis, laminitis, colic, and stomach ulcers. Just as in other living things, violation the laws of nature that are a products of a complex and a very long evolutionary process inevitably leads to complications and problems that may not be easily solved.

REFERENCES

1. Bongianni M. Introduction: origins of the species. In: Simon and Schuster's guide to horses and ponies of the world. New York: Simon and Schuster/ Fireside Books; 1987. p. 10.
2. Merry RJ, Lee MR, Davies DR, et al. Effects of high-sugar ryegrass silage and mixtures with red clover silage on ruminant digestion. 1. In vitro and in vivo studies of nitrogen utilization. J Anim Sci 2006;84:3049–60.
3. Miller LA, Moorby JM, Davies DR, et al. Increased concentration of water-soluble carbohydrate in perennial ryegrass (*Lolium perenne L.*): milk production from late-lactation dairy cows. Grass and Forage Science 2001;56:383–94.
4. Longland AC, Byrd BM. Pasture nonstructural carbohydrates and equine laminitis. Proceedings of the Waltham International Nutritional Sciences Symposia. J Nutr 2006;136(7S):2099S–102S.
5. Frape D. Equine nutrition and feeding. 2nd edition. London: Blackwell Science Ltd.; 1998.
6. Kohnke J, Kelleher F, Trevor–Jones P. Feeding horses in Australia, a guide for horse owners and managers. Canberra, ACT, Australia: Union Offset; 1999.
7. Al Jassim RAM. Supplementary feeding of horses with processed sorghum grains and oats. Anim Feed Sci Technol 2006;125:33–44.
8. Sjaastad ØV, Hove K, Sand O. The digestive system. In: Sjaastad ØV, Hove K, Sand O, editors. Physiology in domestic animals. Oslo: Scandinavian Veterinary Press; 2003. p. 490–563.
9. Reece WO. Digestion and absorption. In: Reece WO, editor. Physiology of domestic animals. 2nd edition. Philadelphia: Lippincott Williams & Wilkins; 1997. p. 270–311.
10. Mackie RI, Wilkins CA. Enumeration of anaerobic bacterial microflora of the equine gastrointestinal tract. Appl Environ Microbiol 1988;54:2155–60.
11. Jackson SG. The digestive tract of the horse; practical consideration. In: Pagan ID, editor. Advances in equine nutrition. Nottingham (UK): Nottingham University Press; 1998.

12. Al Jassim RAM, Scott PT, Krause D, et al. The diversity of cellulolytic and lactic acid bacteria of the gastro-intestinal tract of the horse. Recent Advances in Animal Nutrition in Australia 2005a;15:155–63.

13. Daly K, Stewart CS, Flint HJ, et al. Bacterial diversity within the equine large intestine as revealed by molecular analysis of cloned 16S rRNA genes. FEMS Microbiol Ecol 2001;38:141–51.

14. Julliand V, Vaux AD, Millet L, et al. Identification of Ruminococcus flavefaciens as the predominant cellulolytic bacterial species of the equine caecum. Appl Environ Microbiol 1999;65:3738–41.

15. Lin C, Stahl DA. Taxon-specific probes for the cellulolytic genus Fibrobacter reveal abundant and novel equine-associated populations. Appl Environ Microbiol 1995;61:1348–51.

16. Al Jassim RAM, Rowe JB. Better understanding of acidosis and its control. Recent Advances in Animal Nutrition in Australia 1999;12:91–7.

17. Al Jassim RAM, Scott PT, Trebbin AL, et al. The genetic diversity of lactic acid producing bacteria in the equine gastrointestinal tract. FEMS Microbiol Lett 2005b;248:75–81.

18. Milinovich GJ, Trott DJ, Burrell PC, et al. Changes in equine hindgut bacterial populations during oligofructose-induced laminitis. Environ Microbiol 2006;8:885–98.

19. Milinovich GJ, Trott DJ, Burrell, PC, et al. Fluorescence in situ hybridization analysis of hindgut bacteria associated with the development of equine laminitis. Environ Microbiol 2007;9(8):2090–100.

20. Lan GQ, Ho YW, Abdullah N. Mitsuokella jalaludinii sp. nov., from the rumens of cattle in Malaysia. Int J Syst Evol Microbiol 2002;52:713–8.

21. National Research Council. Nutrients requirements of horses. 6th revised edition. Committee on Nutrient Requirements of Horses, National Research Council. Washington, DC: National Academy Press; 2007.

22. National Research Council. Nutrients requirements of horses. 5th revised edition. Committee on Animal Nutrition, Subcommittee on Horse Nutrition, National Board on Agriculture and Natural resources, National Research Council, Washington, DC: National Academy Press; 1989.

23. Pagan JD. Measuring the digestible energy content of horse feeds. In: Pagan JD, editor. Advances in equine nutrition. Nottingham, UK: Nottingham University Press; 1998. p. 71–6.

24. Zeyner A, Kienzle E. A method to estimate digestible energy in horse feed. J Nutr 2002;132:1771S–3S.

25. Ministry of Agriculture, Fisheries and Food. Energy allowances and feeding systems for ruminants. Reference book 433. Her Majesty's Stationery Office, London; 1987. p. 13.

26. Chatterton NJ, Watta KA, Jensen KB, et al. Nonstructural carbohydrates in oat forage. Proceedings of the Waltham International Nutritional Sciences Symposia. J Nutr 2006;136(7S):2111S–3S.

27. Coumbe K. Equine veterinary nursing manual. Oxford (UK): Blackwell Science Ltd; 2001.

28. Potter GD, Arnold FF, Householder DD, et al. Digestion of starch in the small or large intestine of the equine. In: Sonderheft, editor. Europäische Konferenz über die Ernährung des Pferdes. Hannover, Germany: Pferdeheilkunde; 1992. p. 107–11.

29. Kienzle E. Small intestinal digestion of starch in the horse. Revue de Médecine Véterinaire 1994;145:199–204.

30. Medina B, Girard ID, Jacotot E, et al. Effect of preparation of Saccharomyces cerevisiae on microbial profiles and fermentation pattern in the large intestine of horses fed high fiber or high starch diets. J Anim Sci 2002;80:2600–9.
31. Hussein HS, Vogedes LA, Fernandez GCJ, et al. Effect of cereal grain supplementation on apparent digestibility of nutrients and concentrations of fermentation end-products in the feces and serum of horses consuming alfalfa cubes. J Anim Sci 2004;82:1986–96.
32. Meyer H, Radicke S, Kienzle E, et al. Investigations on preileal digestion of oats, corn, and barley starch in relation to grain processing. Proceedings of the 13th Equine Nutrition and Physiology Symposium 1993;92–7.
33. Mclean BML, Hyslop JJ, Longland AC, et al. Physical processing of barley and its effect on the intra-caecal fermentation parameters in ponies. Anim Feed Sci Technol 2000;85:79–87.
34. McCracken TO, Kainer RA, Spurgeon TL. The horse. In: McCracken TO, Kainer RA, Spurgeon T, editors. Spurgeon's color atlas of large animal anatomy: the essentials. Philadelphia: Lippincott Williams & Wilkins; 1999. p. 16.
35. de Fombelle A, Varloud M, Goachet AG, et al. Characterization of the microbial and biochemical profile of the different segments of the digestive tract in horses given two distinct diets. Anim Sci 2003;77:293–304.
36. Garner HE, Hutcheson DP, Coffman JR, et al. Lactic acidosis: a factor associated with equine laminitis. J Anim Sci 1977;45:1037–41.
37. Pollitt CC, Davies CT. Equine laminitis: its development coincides with increased sublamellar blood flow. Equine Vet J Suppl 1998;26:125–32.
38. Rowe JB, Lees MJ, Pethick DW. Prevention of acidosis and laminitis associated with grain feeding in horses. J Nutr 1994;124:2742S–4S.
39. Archer DC, Proudman CJ. Epidemiological clues to preventing colic [review article]. Vet J 2006;172:29–39.
40. Chatterton NJ, Harrison PA. Fructan oligomers in Poa ampla. New Phtologist 1997;136:3–10.
41. Proudman CJ. A two year, prospective survey of equine colic in general practice. Equine Veterinary Journal 1991;24(2): 90–33.
42. Nieto J. Colic—some bright views on the horizon. Vet J 2006;172:6–7.
43. McCarthy HE, French NP, Edwards GB, et al. Equine grass sickness is associated with low antibody levels to Clostridium botulinum: a matched case-control study. Equine Veterinary journal 2004;36(2):123–9.
44. Al Jassim RAM, Denman S, Hernandez JD, et al. The bacterial community of the horse stomach. Presented at the Proceedings of the 5th RRI-INRA Gut Microbiology joint meeting. Aberdeen, UK, June 21–23, 2006.
45. Murray MJ, Eichorn ES. Effect of intermittent feed deprivation, intermittent feed deprivation with ranitidine administration, and stall confinement with ad libitum access to hay on gastric ulceration in horses. Am J Vet Res 1996;57:1599–603.
46. Andrews FM, Sifferman RL, Bernard W. Efficacy of omeprazole paste d in the treatment and prevention on gastric ulcers in horses. Equine Vet J Suppl 1999;29:81–6.
47. Nadeau JA, Andrews FM, Patton CS. Effects of hydrochloric, acetic, butyric, and propionic acids on pathogenesis of ulcers in the non-glandular portion of the stomach of horses. Am J Vet Res 2003a;64:404–12.
48. Nadeau JA, Andrews FM, Patton CS. Effects of hydrochloric, valeric and other volatile fatty acids on pathogenesis of ulcers in the non-glandular portion of the stomach of horses. Am J Vet Res 2003b;64:413–7.
49. Nadeau JA, Andrews FM, Mathew AG. Evaluation of diet as a cause of gastric ulcers in horses. Am J Vet Res 2000;61:784–90.

Prognosticating Equine Colic

Sarah Dukti, DVM*, Nathaniel A. White, DVM

KEYWORDS

• Horse • Colic • Laparotomy • Surgery • Prognosis • Fatality

Prognosticating survival in horses with colic is challenging because of the number of diseases and pathophysiologic processes that can cause the behavior. Although the treatment of horses with colic has improved dramatically over the years, case fatality can still be high because of the delay in recognizing the problem, the time delay inherent in receiving veterinary care, and the lack of effective treatment for the more severe diseases. Intensive case management and surgery for these horses may be expensive and emotionally draining for owners; therefore, providing an accurate prognosis is key to decisions needed for case management. This article is dedicated to recent advances in applying a prognosis for survival in horses at higher risk for a fatal outcome.

INCIDENCE

Colic is one of the most prevalent and challenging diseases faced by equine veterinarians. The annual number of colic cases has been reported to be as high as 4 to 10 cases per 100 horses.[1,2] This number may vary greatly between farms, ranging from 0 to 30 cases per 100 horses per year.[3–5] Most colic (80%–85%) responds to medical therapy or spontaneously resolves with no specific diagnosis identified. The prognosis for these horses with colic that has no specific signs and resolves with minimal medical care is excellent.[1,6,7] Some 10% to 15% of horses having previous colic will experience future episodes of abdominal pain.[1] Obstructing or strangulating disease requiring surgical intervention represents approximately 2% to 4% of colic cases and has been reported to be as high as 10% in some populations.[7,8] In horses, fatality due to colic is greater than any other cause of death except old age and musculoskeletal injury.[9]

MODELS

Several studies have attempted to create models that could predict the prognosis for survival. These models were developed by identifying variables that provided the best

Marion duPont Scott Equine Medical Center, Virginia-Maryland Regional College of Veterinary Medicine, Virginia Tech, P.O. Box 1938, Leesburg, VA 20177, USA
* Corresponding author.
E-mail address: sdukti@vt.edu (S. Dukti).

Vet Clin Equine 25 (2009) 217–231
doi:10.1016/j.cveq.2009.04.004
0749-0739/09/$ – see front matter. Published by Elsevier Inc.

vetequine.theclinics.com

predictive value.[10–15] One such study recorded 32 physical examination and laboratory variables during examination of 165 horses admitted for colic. This study identified four variables (heart rate [HR], peritoneal fluid total protein concentration, blood lactate concentration, and abnormal mucous membranes) that were significant and entered into the model to calculate a colic severity score (CSS). The overall accuracy of the CSS was 93% with 100% positive predictive value, 91.8% negative predictive value, and sensitivity and specificity of 66.7% and 100%, respectively.[11] Although these numbers seemed promising, the model is limited to one hospital population and has not been validated at other equine hospitals. Another study evaluated 1965 cases of equine colic from 10 equine referral hospitals. A total of 1336 cases were used for model development and the remaining 629 cases were used for validation of the model. Variables in the model included peripheral pulse (normal or weak), pulse rate, surgical or medical treatment, packed cell volume (PCV), self-inflicted trauma (absent or present), and capillary refill time. The model showed good fit with the model data set; however, it performed poorly on the validation set,[12] again illustrating the difficulty involved in model development, including population variability and standardization of model variables. In 2001 a study reported on 200 horses presented for surgical colic. The horses were placed into three categories of gravity score based on rectal palpation, frequency of borborygmi, abdominal distention, and severity of pain. The horses were also categorized into three categories of shock score based on HR, respiratory rate, arterial blood pressure, PCV, lactate, and blood urea nitrogen. Both gravity and shock score were associated with mortality.[16]

FACTORS ASSOCIATED WITH SURVIVAL
Signalment, History, and Examination

Signalment, historical information, physical examination, hematologic, and other diagnostic modalities have all been evaluated as prognostic indicators. Several studies have identified advanced age to be negatively associated with survival, including a study evaluating 774 surgical colics.[17–20] A recent study comparing geriatric (≥ 16 years of age) with control horses did not show a difference in survival.[21] Furthermore, in a recent retrospective study of 300 horses old age was not a risk factor for fatality.[22] Although colic is reported in all breeds, one study identified draft horses, thoroughbreds, and thoroughbred cross horses at increased risk for mortality.[19] A recent study found that draft horses weighing greater than 680 kg that went to surgery because of colic had longer durations of anesthesia, more postoperative complications, and a higher mortality rate than lighter draft horses (less than 680 kg). The short-term survival rate was 60%, which is lower than survival rate in many retrospective studies involving light breed horses.[23]

Several studies have demonstrated an increased mortality with decreased surgical experience,[24–26] whereas one study found surgical experience was not a factor in outcome, suggesting that with appropriate training this effect may be minimized.[27] In this same study and others survival was decreased with increased surgical time[22,27,28] and may be correlated to the severity of the lesion or surgical experience. A study evaluating 774 surgical colics found an association of the referring veterinarian with survival.[27] This finding is also most likely due to veterinarian experience and duration of time until referral.

Numerous studies have attempted to evaluate the association between physical examination findings and survival. Many studies have identified cardiovascular status and pain as associated with case fatality.[10,11,13,14,18–20,22,26,27,29–31] Proudman and colleagues[27] reported on a population of 321 horses undergoing surgery for colic and found an elevated PCV was associated with increased mortality. Subsequently, in 2005 Proudman and colleagues[20] evaluated 275 horses requiring colic surgery for large intestinal disease and reported decreased survival in horses with an elevated PCV and HR. In 2006 Proudman and coworkers[19] reported cardiovascular status and pain were associated with mortality in a population of horses undergoing surgery for colic. HR, PCV, and severity of pain affected intraoperative survival, and PCV at admission was associated with postoperative survival. Similar results were reported by Braun and colleagues,[31] who found an association between cardiovascular status (capillary refill time, PCV) and pain and mortality in 152 horses. Although the association between PCV and survival was not significant, the case fatality rate was higher (69%) in horses with a PCV greater than 54%.[31] In 2003 Van der Linden and colleagues[29] found cardiovascular status (HR, skin tent) and severity of pain were significantly associated with survival in 649 surgical cases. More recently Mair and Smith[22] reported on 300 horses undergoing surgery for colic and found cardiovascular status (HR) and severity of pain were associated with survival. Also in 2005 Garcia-Seco and colleagues[26] reported on horses with strangulating small intestinal lesions from pedunculated lipomas and found increased HR (>80) associated with increased fatality.

Other physical examination findings that have been associated with mortality include borborygmi, mucous membrane character, and temperature.[29,31] These studies are not always consistent; for instance, Proudman and colleagues[27] found no association between HR and survival, whereas Van der Linden and coworkers[29] found no association between PCV and survival. Duration until admission has been found in several studies to negatively affect survival[27,29] but was not a factor in the recent study by Mair and Smith (**Table 1**).[22]

Clinicopathologic Values

Studies have attempted to identify other laboratory variables that may be useful in determining prognosis. When cortisol, epinephrine, norepinephrine, lactate, electrolyte concentrations, acid-base variables, and HR were examined in 35 horses presented for colic by Hinchcliff and colleagues[32] higher plasma epinephrine, plasma lactate, and serum cortisol concentrations were significantly associated with fatality; however, plasma norepinephrine concentration was not. Increased HR and epinephrine indicate increased sympathetic activity and are associated with increased fatality.[31] Further research is warranted to determine the sensitivity and specificity of these biochemical variables with survival.

Electrolytes are routinely measured and renewed interest has been shown in their prognostic value. In 1982 Bristol reported that anion gap was useful as a prognostic indicator. The probability of survival decreased from 81% survival with an anion gap less than 20 mEq/L, to 47% survival with an anion gap 20 to 24.9 mEq/L, to 0% survival in horses with anion gap greater than or equal to 25 mEq/L.[33] In 35 horses admitted for surgical colic 54% had low preoperative serum ionized magnesium concentrations and 86% had subnormal serum ionized calcium concentrations.[34] Furthermore, although neither serum calcium nor magnesium were associated with survival, low ionized calcium and magnesium were associated with strangulating lesions,[34,35] and low ionized magnesium was associated with postoperative ileus.[34] A study reporting on hypomagnesemia found no association between hypomagnesemia and fatality in the hospitalized horses; however, in horses with colic and hypomagnesemia the survival rate was increased compared with horses with colic and normal or hypermagnesemia.[36] In 2005 Delesalle and colleagues[37] found that hypocalcemia was of prognostic relevance in regard to survival and to the probability

Table 1
Factors associated with survival

Factors	No Effect	Effect
Age		
	Southwood, 2008[21]	Pascoe, 1983[17]
	Phillips, 1993[28]	Reeves, 1986[18]
	Mair, 2005[22]	Proudman, 2005[20]
		Proudman, 2006[19]
Breed	Phillips, 1993[28]	Proudman, 2006[19]
	Mair, 2005[22]	Rothenbuhler, 2006[23]
Surgical Experience	Proudman, 2002[27]	Shires, 1985[24]
		Freeman, 2000[25]
		Garcia-Seco, 2005[26]
Cardiovascular/Pain		Braun, 2002[31] (PCV/CRT/pain)
		Proudman, 2002[27] (PCV)
		Van der Linden, 2003[29]
		(HR, skin tent, pain)
		Proudman, 2005[20] (PCV/HR)
		Mair, 2005[22] (HR, CRT, pain)
		Garcia-Seco, 2005[26] (HR)
		Proudman, 2006[19] (PCV/HR/pain)
Clinicopathologic	Hinchcliff, 2005[32] NE)	Bristol, 1982[33] (anion gap)
	Garcia-Lopez, 2001[34] Ca/MG)	Hinchcliff, 2005[32] (E, lactate, cortisol)
	Johansson, 2003[35] Ca/MG)	Garcia-Lopez, 2001[34] (str-Ca+/Mg+)
		Johansson, 2003[35] (str-Ca+/Mg+)
		Delesalle, 2005[37] (Ca)
		Groover, 2006[40] (Cr)
		Hollis, 2007[41] (Glu)
		Hassel, 2008[42] (Glu)
Coagulopathy	Prasse, 1993[45]	Johnstone, 1986[43] (coag panel)
	(hypercoag, FDP)	Welch, 1992[44] (coag panel)
	Johnstone, 1986[43]	Collatos, 1995[46] (fibrinolysis, AT-3)
	(PTT, FDP)	Dallap, 2004[48] (LCV-coag panel,
	Welch, 1992[44] (PTT)	thrombocytopenia, PT, Low fib,TAT)
	Dolente, 2002[47] (FDP)	Johnstone, 1986[43] (PT, AT-3)
	Dallap, 2004[48] (D-dimer)	Welch, 1992[44] (PT)
		Stokol, 2005[51] (PTT)
		Prasse, 1993[45] (AT-3)
		Dolente, 2002[47] (AT-3, low fib)
		Sandholm, 1995[54] (D-dimer)
Abdominocentesis		Freden, 1998[56] (color)
		Swanwick, 1976[57] (color)
		Reeves, 1987[58] (color)
		Ducharme, 1983[77] (color)
		Garcia-Seco, 2005[26] (color)
		Weimann, 2002[60] (PCV)
		Barton, 1999[61] (TNF, IL-6)
		Saulez, 2004[62] (ALP)
		Latson, 2005[63] (lactate)

Abbreviations: AT-3, antithrombin III; ALP, alkaline phosphatase; coag, coagulation; CRT, capillary refill time; FDP, fibrinogen degradion product; HR, heart rate; low fib, low fiblow fibrinogen; NE, norepinephrine; PCV, packed cell volume; PT, prothrombin time; PTT, partial thromboplastin time; TAT, thrombin antithrombin complexes; TNF, tumor necrosis factor.

of development of ileus during hospitalization of horses with colic. Furthermore, correction of hypocalcemia improved clinical outcome, highlighting the value of routine ionized calcium measurement and correction of hypocalcemia.[37]

Alterations in serum potassium, chloride, phosphorus, and sodium abnormalities are also reported in horses with colic. One study found that 50% of horses following colic surgery were hypokalemic, 12% hypochloremic (54% hyperchloremic), 44% hypophosphatemic (12% hyperphosphatemic), and 30% hyponatremic (12% hypernatremic).[38] Furthermore, increased phosphate concentrations in peritoneal fluid and serum suggested a need for bowel resection.[39]

Other authors have evaluated the association between renal insufficiency during colic and prognosis. In 2006, Groover[40] reported that horses that had elevated serum creatinine due to colic or colitis that failed to normalize within 72 hours of fluid therapy were three times as likely to die or be euthanized. Studies have also evaluated the role of blood glucose in horses with acute abdominal disease.[41,42] Hollis and colleagues[41] reported that hyperglycemia in the first 48 hours of hospitalization is associated with a worse prognosis for survival to discharge.

Coagulopathy

Recently several studies have attempted to elucidate the role of coagulation abnormalities and their association with fatality during colic. In 1986 Johnstone and Crane[43] reported on the coagulation status of 24 horses presented for colic, including platelet count, fibrinogen, antithrombin III (AT-3), partial thromboplastin time (PTT), prothrombin time, thrombin clotting time, soluble fibrin monomer, and fibrinogen degradation products. All horses had at least one abnormality and horses in the non-survival group had an average of five coagulation abnormalities, whereas horses in the survival group had an average of two coagulation abnormalities. In 1992 Welch reported on the prevalence and consequence of DIC in horses with colic. A total of 3.5% (23) of the horses in the study developed signs of DIC with 22 requiring surgery for correction of the lesion; significantly more of the horses within this group had strangulated small intestine associated with a 66% fatality.[44] A study evaluating a larger number of horses with colic for hypercoagulability found evidence of hypercoagulability most evident at 24 and 48 hours and fibrinolytic activity was present in all horses and was not associated with increased fatality or severity of lesion.[45] Fibrinolysis was also evaluated in a study that examined tissue plasminogen activator and plasminogen activator inhibitor type-1 (PAI-1); increased PAI-1 (inhibiting fibrinolysis) is associated with increased mortality.[46] Furthermore, Dolente and colleagues[47] reported that horses with subclinical DIC were eight times more likely to die or be euthanized when subclinical DIC was defined as three or more out of six abnormal coagulation tests. Evaluation of horses with large colon volvulus determined that 70% had abnormal results in three or more of the six coagulation tests performed. Horses with abnormal results in four or more of the six tests were significantly more likely to be euthanized.[48]

Coagulation tests vary in their correlation to prognosis. Thrombocytopenia is a frequent feature of DIC[49] and was reported in ponies with strangulating small intestinal lesions and in horses with colitis.[47,50] Furthermore, Dallap and colleagues[48] reported that in horses with large colon volvulus there was a significant association between thrombocytopenia and fatality. Prothrombin time has been reported to be abnormal in horses with colic and associated with survival.[43,44,48] PTT was reported to be common in horses with colic, but not associated with prognosis.[43,44] One study evaluating 20 horses with colic reported increased PTT to be significantly associated with nonsurvival, however.[51] Decreased AT-3 has been reported in horses with colic and associated with nonsurvival.[43,45–47,52]

Hypofibrinogenemia is not common in horses with DIC possibly because horses are able to generate large amounts of fibrinogen as an acute phase protein in response to inflammation.[53] Several studies have reported significantly lower fibrinogen levels in horses with fatal colic, however, and have suggested that the lack of an increase in fibrinogen may be suggestive of coagulation abnormalities.[47,48]

Fibrin degradation products have been reported to increase in horses with colic; however, the test has been shown to be nonspecific because it is found elevated in both survivors and nonsurvivors.[43,45,47] One study reported on 105 horses with colic and found increased D-dimer to be useful as a prognostic indicator of nonsurvival in horses with colic.[54] When horses with large colon volvulus were examined, however, all patients had increased levels and thus it was not associated with prognosis.[48] This study also reported a strong association with increased thrombin–antithrombin complexes and coagulopathy and fatality in horses with large colon volvulus.[48] A significant increase in peritoneal fibrin degradation products was identified in horses with peritonitis compared with strangulating or obstructive diseases.[55]

Abdominocentesis

Several studies examining abdominocentesis have reported that the gross color of peritoneal fluid is useful in distinguishing medical verse surgical colic (**Table 2**).[56–59] A recent study reported that measuring the hematocrit was more sensitive than visual assessment of peritoneal fluid for selecting surgical versus medical treatment.[60] In 1998 Freden and colleagues[56] reported that abdominal fluid color was useful in predicting the type of lesion and patient outcome and all variables evaluated except nucleated cell count were significantly different between horses with nonstrangulating and strangulating lesions. Garcia-Seco and coworkers[26] also reported on the association between the gross appearance of abdominal fluid and survival when reporting on 102 horses with pedunculated lipomas. When reporting the diagnostic and prognostic significance of tumor necrosis factor-α and interleukin-6 activities and endotoxin concentration in peritoneal fluid of 155 adult horses with colic Barton and Collatos[61] found an association with nonsurvival, although negative values were more useful in the prediction of survival than abnormal values in predicting fatal disease.

Saulez and colleagues[62] found that increased alkaline phosphatase was significantly associated with greater intestinal damage, increased probability of surgery, and a worse prognosis for survival. Latson and coworkers[63] reported lactate concentration in the peritoneal fluid was a better predictor of strangulating obstruction that blood plasma.

Prognosis also varies with lesion type. Several authors have reported that horses with small intestinal disease have a worse prognosis than horses with large intestinal lesions.[12,16,20,26]

Small Intestine

In the last 10 years the short-term survival reported with small intestinal lesions has been reported to be from 50% to 85%.[22,25,26,64–69] In a large recent study of 300 horses with colic, horses with simple obstruction of the small intestine were shown to have a higher short-term survival (79.6%) versus horses with strangulating lesions of the small intestine (54.8%).[22] This difference has been found in other studies,[15] but still others have not shown a significant difference.[25,28]

In 2000 Freeman and colleagues[25] found 63% of 74 horses with small intestinal disease had strangulating lesions, and of these 43 (48%) required resection and

Table 2 Survival statistics for diseases		
Small Intestine	**Type**	**Survival (%)**
Freeman, 2000[25]	Simple versus strang	Simple (91) Strang (84) Long-term (68)
Fugaro, 2001[64]	R&A SI	Short-term (65) Long-term (47)
Van der Boom, 2001[65]	Staple anastomosis	Short term (50) Long-term (61)
Semevolos, 2002[66]	SI	Short term (88) Long-term (57)
Freeman, 2005[68]	Strang SI	Short-term 64)
Mair, 2005[22]	SI	Short-term (75.2)
Stephen, 2004[67]	SI volvulus	Short-term (80)
Archer, 2004[69]	Epiploic foramen	Short-term (69)
Garcia-Seco, 2005[26]	Lipoma	Short-term (60) Long-term (64)
Freeman, 2005[68]	Epiploic foramen	Short-term (95)
Cecum		
Plummer, 2007[75]	Cecal impaction	Medical Tx short-term (81) Surgical Tx short-term (95)
Martin, 1999[76]	Cecal intussusception	(83)
Large Colon		
Ducharme, 1983[77]	LI LI impaction LI impaction	(56.7) Surgery (58) Medical (95)
Phillips, 1993[28]	LI	(80)
Mair, 2005[22]	LI	(89)
Hassel, 1999[79]	Enterolith	Short-term (96.2) Long-term (92.5)
Granot, 2008[81]	Sand	Short-term (100)
Hardy, 2000[82]	Nephrosplenic	Short-term (92.5)
Huskamp, 1983[83]	RDD	Short-term (100)
Harrison, 1988[84]	LCV	Short-term (34.7)
Snyder, 1989[85]	LCV	Short-term (36) Short-term 270 deg (71)
Southwood, 2002[86]	LCV	Short-term (68) (1998–1999)
Embertson[87]	LCV	Short-term (83)
Small Colon		
Ruggles, 1991[102]	SC impaction	Long-term medical (100) Long-term surgical (39)
Frederico, 2006[104]	SC impaction	Short-term medical (91) Short-term surgical (95)
Dart, 1992[35]	SC R&A	Short-term (100) (4 horses)

Abbreviations: LCV, large colon volvulus; LI, large intestine; R&A, resection and anastomosis; RDD, right dorsal displacement; SC, small colon; SI, small intestine; strang, strangulating; Tx, treatment.

anastomosis. Overall, short-term survival was 85%. Horses with simple small intestinal obstructions had a survival rate of 91% and horses with strangulating lesions had a survival rate of 84%. Long-term survival was reported to be 68%.

In 2001 Fugaro and Cote[64] reported on 84 horses requiring resection and anastomosis for small intestinal lesions with a short-term survival rate of 65% and long-term survival rate of 47%. All horses in the study had stapled anastomosis, including jejunojejunostomy (n = 27), jejunoileostomy (11), jejunoileocecostomy with small intestinal resection (20), and jejunoileocecostomy without small intestinal resection (26). In 2001 Van der Boom and Van der Velden[65] reported that horses with jejunojejunostomy (n = 27), jejunoileostomy (11), jejunoileocecostomy with small intestinal resection (20), and jejunoileocecostomy without small intestinal resection (26) for strangulating small intestinal lesions had a short-term survival of 50% and long-term survival of 61%. In 2002 Semevolos and colleagues[66] reported on 59 horses with small intestinal lesions and reported an 88% short-term and 57% long-term survival. In 2005 Freeman and Schaeffer[68] reported on 157 horses with strangulating lesions of the small intestine and reported short-term survival to be 64%. In 2005 Mair and Smith[22] reported on 300 horses with colic, 125 of which had small intestinal lesions. Short-term survival for horses with small intestinal lesions was found to be 75.2%.

Other reports have focused on specific small intestinal lesions. In 2004 Stephan[67] reported on 115 horses with small intestinal volvulus and reported a short-term survival rate of 80%. In 2004 Archer and colleagues[69] reported on 70 horses with epiploic foramen entrapment with a short-term survival of 69%. In 2005 Garcia-Seco and colleagues[26] reported on 102 horses with pedunculated lipomas strangulating the small intestine and found short- and long-term survival of 60% and 64%, respectively. Several studies have reported a decreased survival for horses with epiploic foramen entrapment.[27,70,71] This finding has been disputed in a recent article reporting a 95% short-term survival in horses with epiploic foramen entrapment, which was significantly higher than horses with other small intestinal lesions.[68] Horses with a diaphragmatic hernia were more likely to survive if there was normal peritoneal fluid at admission, less than 50% of the small intestine affected, and a hernia in the ventral portion of the diaphragm.[72] Younger horses with a diaphragmatic hernia and requiring a shorter duration of anesthesia were significantly more likely to survive.[72]

Decreased survival has been reported with jejunocecostomy versus jejunojejunostomy.[22,25,26,55,67,73] Recently Rendle and colleagues[74] reported that horses requiring jejunoileostomy have similar survival rates to horses requiring jejunojejunostomy, which reinforces that if the ileum is viable jejunoileostomy should be performed preferentially over jejunocecostomy.

Cecum

Cecal disease is reported to have a worse prognosis than large or small colon disease (66.7%, 89%, and 100%, respectively).[22] A recent retrospective article evaluated 114 horses with cecal impactions. Forty-four of the 54 (81%) horses treated medically were discharged from the hospital. Twelve of 49 horses treated surgically were euthanized because of cecal rupture and 35 of 37 (95%) of horses allowed to recover from surgery were discharged from the hospital.[75] In 1999 Martin and colleagues[76] reported on 30 horses with either cecocolic or cecocecal intussusception. Six horses died or were euthanized without surgery. Twenty-four were treated surgically. Six were euthanized because of peritonitis, rupture, or irreducible intussusception. Eighteen recovered from general anesthesia and 15 survived long term. Surgical treatments were reduction with or without partial typhlectomy (6 horses), partial typhlectomy through a colostomy facilitating reduction (6), reduction through a colostomy and partial typhlectomy (3), partial typhlectomy for cecocecal intussusception (1), and ileocolostomy (2).

Large Colon

Several studies have reported a higher survival rate in horses with large intestinal verse small intestinal disease.[13,17,22,28,77] In 1983 Ducharme and colleagues[77] reported on 181 horses and found short-term survival to be 56.7% and 33.8% for large and small intestinal lesions, respectively. In 1993 Phillips and Walmsley[28] reported on 151 horses requiring colic surgery and found short-term survival to be 80% and 52%, respectively. Furthermore, they reported that the prognosis for strangulating lesions of the large colon (52%) was significantly lower than simple obstructions 90%. Recently Mair and Smith[22] reported survival rates of 75.2%, 66.7%, 89%, and 100% for small intestinal, cecal, large colon, and small colon lesions in 300 horses. The survival for horses with large and small colon lesion was significantly greater than for those with small intestinal or cecal lesions. Few studies have reported prognosis with specific large intestinal lesions. Horses with large colon impactions are reported to have a survival rate of 95% if they respond to medical therapy and 58% if they require surgery.[78] A study reporting on 900 horses with enterolithiasis found 15% of horses had ruptured; however, horses undergoing surgical therapy had an excellent prognosis with 96.2% and 92.5% short- and long-term survival.[79] In 1989 Ragle and colleagues[80] reported on 40 horses undergoing surgery for sand impaction and reported short- and long-term survival of 88% and 80%, respectively. More recently Granot and colleagues[81] reported on 41 horses requiring surgery for sand colic. Four were euthanized at surgery; however, all horses recovering from anesthesia survived to discharge. Of 174 horses with nephrosplenic entrapment of the large colon, 107 horses were treated by surgery alone, 25 horses were successfully corrected by rolling under general anesthesia, and 9 required surgery after rolling, with an overall survival rate of 92.5%.[82] In 1983 Huskamp and Kopf[83] reported on 48 horses with right dorsal displacement; 47 were taken to surgery and all recovered.

The prognosis for horses with large colon volvulus has been reported to be 30% to 60%.[84–86] Recently a study reported a survival rate of 83%; however, this study was performed in a region of the United States with early referral and surgery.[87] A recent study reported that horses with large colon volvulus and plasma lactate less than 6.0 mmol/L can be predicted to survive based on a sensitivity and specificity of 84% and 83%.[88]

Determination of the viability of the large colon is most often made by clinical observation; however, many techniques have been reported in the hope of improving the accuracy of assessment. Techniques that have been reported include clinical assessment, fluorescein dye, surface oximetry, Doppler ultrasonography, luminal pressure, and histopathology.[89–99] None is 100% accurate at predicting survival. Nonsurvival was associated with a prolonged involution of the large colon after surgical volvulus reduction as determined by ultrasound.[100]

Small Colon

Small colon obstructions that respond to medical therapy are reported to have survival rates of 72% to 100%; however, those requiring surgery have survival rates reported between 47% and 75%.[101–103] More recently, in 2006 Frederico and colleagues[104] reported on 44 horses with small colon impactions and found 21 of 23 (91%) horses treated medically and 20 of 21 (95%) horses treated surgically survived to discharge.

A report on 4 horses requiring resection and anastomosis for small colon lesions had 100% short-term survival.[105]

Complications

Others have tried to identify complications in the short term that may affect survival. Mair and Smith[106] reported that 34.2% of horses with small intestinal lesions had postoperative ileus, 43.1% exhibited pain, and 21.1% exhibited signs of shock. Horses with ileus or endotoxic shock had a decreased survival rate and pain was the primary reason for euthanasia. Postoperative ileus was also reported by Morton and Blikslager to decrease survival.[71] Multiple studies have reported decreased survival with relaparotomy.[27,67,71,76] In 2005 Mair and Smith[107] reported the short-term survival for horses requiring relaparotomy was approximately 50% and the long-term survival rate was 22%. Indications for relaparotomy included persistent pain, persistent ileus, peritonitis, and wound breakdown.

Given the high cost and emotional toll that can be involved in colic surgery, providing owners with an accurate prognosis is crucial to the decision-making process. Reviewing the literature and continuing to focus on future diagnostics and prognostics indicators should improve the ability to educate clients on the likelihood of survival.

REFERENCES

1. Tinker MK, White NA, Lessard P, et al. Prospective study of equine colic incidence and mortality. Equine Vet J 1997;29:448–53.
2. Kaneene JB, Ross WA, Miller R. The Michigan equine monitoring system II. Frequencies and impact of selected health problems. Prev Vet Med 1997;29: 277–92.
3. Traub-Dargatz JL, Kopral CA, Seitzinger AH, et al. Estimate of the national incidence of and operation-level risk factors for colic among horses in the United States, spring 1998 to spring 1999. J Am Vet Med Assoc 2001;219:67–71.
4. Hillyer MH, Talor FG, French NP. A cross-sectional study of colic in horses on thoroughbred training premises in the British Isles in 1994. Equine Vet J 1997; 33:380–5.
5. Uhlinger C. Investigations into the incidence of field colic. Equine Vet J 1992;13: 11–8.
6. Proudman CJ. A two year, prospective survey of equine colic in general practice. Equine Vet J 1992;24:90–3.
7. White NA. Epidemiology and etiology of colic. In: White NA, editor. The equine acute abdomen. Philadelphia: Lea and Febiger; 1990. p. 50–64.
8. Hillyer MH, Taylor FGR, French NP. A cross-sectional study of colic in horses on thoroughbred training premises in the British Isles in 1997. Equine Vet J 2002;33: 380–5.
9. USDA 2005. Available at: http://www.usda.gov/wps/porta/usdahome. Accessed December 2008.
10. Orsini JA, Else A, Galligan D, et al. Prognostic indices used to predict survival in equine acute abdominal crisis. Vet Surg 1987;16(1):98.
11. Furr MO, Lessard P, White NA. Development of a colic severity score for predicting the outcome of equine colic. Vet Surg 1995;24(2):97–101.
12. Reeves MJ, Curtis CR, Salman MD, et al. A multivariable prognostic model for equine colic patients. Prev Vet Med 1990;9(4):241–57.

13. Parry BW, Anderson GA, Gay CC. Prognosis in equine colic: a study of individual variables used in case assessment. Equine Vet J 1983;15:337–44.
14. Puotunen-Reinert A. Study of variables commonly used in examination of equine colic cases to assess prognostic value. Equine Vet J 1986;18:275–7.
15. Pascoe PF, Ducharme NG, Ducahrme GR, et al. A computer-derived protocol using recursive partitioning to aid in estimating prognosis of horses with abdominal pain in referral hospitals. Can J Vet Res 1990;54:373–8.
16. Grulke S, Olle E, Detilleux J, et al. Determination of a gravity and shock score for prognosis in equine surgical colic. J Vet Med A Physiol Pathol Clin Med 2001;48: 465–73.
17. Pascoe PJ, McDonell WN, Trim CM, et al. Mortality rates and associated factors in equine colic operations—a retrospective study of 341 operations. Can Vet J 1983;24:76–85.
18. Reeves MF, Hilbert BJ, Morris RS. A retrospective study of 320 colic cases referred to a veterinary teaching hospital. Proceedings of the 2nd Equine Colic Research Symposium 1986;2:242–50.
19. Proudman CJ, Dugdale AH, Senior JM, et al. Pre-operative and anaesthesia-related risk factors for mortality in equine colic cases. Vet J 2006;171:89–97.
20. Proudman CJ, Edwards GA, Barnes J, et al. Modelling long-term survival of horses following surgery for large intestinal disease. Equine Vet J 2005;37(4):366–70.
21. Southwood LL, Gassert T, Lindborg S. Survival and complications rates in geriatric horses with colic, Proceedings 9th International Equine Colic Research Symposium, 2008:87–8.
22. Mair TS, Smith LJ. Survival and complication rates of 300 horses undergoing surgical treatment of colic. Part 1. Short-term survival following a single laparotomy. Equine Vet J 2005;37:296–302.
23. Rothenbuhler R, Hawkins JF, Adams SB, et al. Evaluation of surgical treatment for signs of acute abdominal pain in draft horses: 72 cases (1983–2002). J Am Vet Med Assoc 2006;228(10):1546–50.
24. Shires GM, Kaneps AJ, Wagner PC, et al. A retrospective review of 219 cases of equine colic. Proceedings of the 2nd Equine colic Research Symposium 1985;2:239–41.
25. Freeman DE, Hammock P, Baker GJ, et al. Short- and long-term survival and prevalence of post-operative ileus after small intestinal surgery in the horse. Equine Vet J Suppl 2000;32:42–51.
26. Garcia-Seco E, Wilson DA, Kramer J, et al. Prevalence and risk factors associated with outcome of surgical removal of pedunculated lipomas in horses: 102 cases (1987–2002). J Am Vet Med Assoc 2005;226:1529–37.
27. Proudman CJ, Smith JE, Edwards GB, et al. Long-term survival of equine surgical colic cases. Part1: patterns of mortality and morbidity. Equine Vet J 2002;34:432–7.
28. Phillips TJ, Walmsley JP. Retrospective analysis of the results of 151 exploratory laparotomies in horses with gastrointestinal disease. Equine Vet J 1993;25:427–31.
29. Van der Linden MA, Laffont CM, Sloet van Oldruitenborgh-Oosterbaan MM. Prognosis in equine medical and surgical colic. J Vet Intern Med 2003;17:343–8.
30. Thoefner MB, Ersboll AK, Hesselholt M. Prognostic indicators in the Danish hospital-based population of colic horses. Equine Vet J Suppl 2000;32:11–8.
31. Braun U, Schoberl M, Bracher V, et al. Prognostic factors in equine colic. Tierarztl Umsch 2002;57(1):15–22.
32. Hinchcliff KW, Rush BR, Farris JW. Evaluation of plasma catecholamine and serum cortisol concentrations in horses with colic. JAVMA 2005;227(2):276–80.

33. Bristol DG. The anion gap as a prognostic indicator in horses with abdominal pain. J Am Vet Med Assoc 1982;181(1):63–5.
34. Garcia-Lopez JM, Provost PJ, Rush JE, et al. Prevalence and prognostic importance of hypomagnesemia and hypocalcemia in horses that have colic surgery. Am J Vet Res 2001;62:7–12.
35. Johansson AM, Gardner SY, Jones SL, et al. Hypomagnesemia in hospitalized horses. J Vet Intern Med 2003;17(6):860–7.
36. Dart AJ, Snyder JR, Spier SJ, et al. Ionized calcium concentration in horses with surgically managed gastrointestinal disease: 147 cases (1988–1990). J Am Vet Med Assoc 1992;201:1244–8.
37. Delesalle C, Dewulf J, Lefebvre RA, et al. Use of plasma ionized calcium levels and ionized calcium substitution response patterns as prognostic parameters for ileus and survival in colic horses. Vet Q 2005;27(4):157–72.
38. Protopapas K. Studies on metabolic disturbance and other post-operative complications following equine surgery. DVetMed Thesis. Royal Veterinary College, University of London.
39. Arden VA, Stick JA. Serum and peritoneal fluid phosphate concentrations as predictors of major intestinal injury associated with equine colic. J Am Vet Med Assoc 1988;193:927–31.
40. Groover ES, Woolums AR, Cole DJ, et al. Risk factors associated with renal insufficiency in horses with primary gastrointestinal disease: 26 cases (2000–2003). J Am Vet Med Assoc 2006;228(4):572–7.
41. Hollis AR, Boston RC, Corley KT. Blood glucose in horses with acute abdominal disease. J Vet Intern Med 2007;21(5):1099–103.
42. Hassel DM, Hill AE, Rorabeck RA. The effect of hyperglycemia on survival in 300 horses with acute gastrointestinal disease: a retrospective study, 2003–2005. Proceedings 9th International Equine colic Research Symposium; 2008. p. 183–4.
43. Johnstone I, Crane S. Haemostatic abnormalities in horses with colic-their prognostic value. Equine Vet J 1986;18(4):271–4.
44. Welch R, Watkins J, Taylor T, et al. Disseminated intravascular coagulation associated with colic in 23 horses (1984–1989). J Vet Intern Med 1992;6(1):29–35.
45. Prasse K, Topper M, Moore J, et al. Analysis of hemostasis in horses with colic. J Am Vet Med Assoc 1993;5(1):685–93.
46. Collatos C, Barton M, Moore J. Fibrinolytic activity in plasma from horses with gastrointestinal disease: changes associated with diagnosis, surgery, and outcome. J Vet Intern Med 1995;9(1):18–23.
47. Dolente B, Wilkins P, Boston R. Clinicopathologic evidence of disseminated intravascular coagulation in horses with acute colitis. J Am Vet Med Assoc 2002;220(7):1034–8.
48. Dallap B, Dolente B, Boston R. Coagulation profiles in 27 horses with large colon volvulus. In: Proceedings of the 11th Annual Veterinary Meeting of the American College of Veterinary Surgeons. Chicago; 2004. p. 4.
49. Bick R. Disseminated intravascular coagulation. Objective critieria for diagnosis and management. Med clin North Am 1994;78(3):511–43.
50. Pablo L, Purohit R, Teer P, et al. Disseminated intravascular strangulation obstruction in ponies. Am J Vet Res 1983;44(1):2115–22.
51. Stokol T, Erb HN, De Wilde L, et al. Evaluation of latex agglutination kits for detection of fibrin(ogen) degradation products and D-dimer in healthy horses and horses with severe colic. Vet clin Pathol 2005;34:371–82.

52. Holland M, Kelly A, Snyder J, et al. Antithrombin III activity in horses with large colon torsion. Am J Vet Res 1986;47(4):897–900.
53. Morris D. Recognition and management of disseminated intravascular coagulation in horses. Vet clin North Am Equine Pract 1988;4(1):115–43.
54. Sandholm M, Vidovic A, Puotunen-Reinert A, et al. D-dimer improves the prognostic value of combined clinical and laboratory data in equine gastrointestinal colic. Acta Vet Scand 1995;36(2):255–72.
55. Delgado MA, Monreal L, Tarncon I, et al. D-Dimer concentrations in peritoneal fluid of horses with colic. Proceedings 9th International Equine colic Research Symposium; 2008. p. 78–9.
56. Freden GO, Provost PJ, Rand WM. Reliability of using results of abdominal fluid analysis to determine treatment and predict lesion type and outcome for horses with colic: 218 cases (1991–1994). J Am Vet Med Assoc 1998; 213(7):1012–5.
57. Swanwick RA, Wilkinson JS. A clinical evaluation of abdominal paracentesis in the horse. Aust Vet J 1976;52:109–17.
58. Reeves MJ, Curtis CR, Salman MD, et al. Descriptive epidemiology and risk factors indicating the need for surgery and evaluation of prognosis. The Morris Animal Foundation colic study. Proc Am Assoc Equine Pract 1987;33:83–94.
59. Ducharme NG, Pascoe PJ, Lumsden JH. A computer-derived protocol to aid in selecting medical versus surgical treatment of horses with abdominal pain. Equine Vet J 1989;21:447–50.
60. Weimann CD, Thoefner MB, Jensen AL. Spectrophotometric assessment of peritoneal fluid haemoglobin in colic horses: an aid to selecting medical versus surgical treatment. Equine Vet J 2002;34(5):523–7.
61. Barton MH, Collatos C. Tumor necrosis factor and interleukino-6 activity and endotoxin concentration in peritoneal fluid and blood of horses with acute abdominal disease. J Vet Intern Med 1999;13(5):457–64.
62. Saulez MN, Cebra CK, Tornquist SJ. The diagnostic and prognostic value of alkaline phosphatase activity in serum and peritoneal fluid from horses with acute colic. J Vet Intern Med 2004;18:564–7.
63. Latson KM, Nieto JE, Beldomenico PM, et al. Evaluation of peritoneal fluid lactate as a marker of intestinal ischaemia in equine colic. Equine Vet J 2005; 37(4):342–6.
64. Fugaro MN, Cote NM. Survival rates for horses undergoing stapled small intestinal anastomosis: 84 cases (1988–1997). J Am Vet Med Assoc 2001;218: 1603–7.
65. Van der Boom R, Van der Velden MA. Short- and long-term evaluation of surgical treatment of strangulating obstructions of the small intestine in horses: a review of 224 cases. Vet Q 2001;23:109–15.
66. Semevolos SA, Ducharme NG, Hackett RP. Clinical assessment and outcome of three techniques for jejunal resection and anastomosis in horse: 59 cases (1989–2000). J Am Vet Med Assoc 2002;220:215–8.
67. Stephen JO, Corley KT, Johnston JK, et al. Factors associated with mortality and morbidity in small intestinal volvulus in horses. Vet Surg 2004;33:340–8.
68. Freeman DE, Schaeffer DJ. Short-term survival after surgery for epiploic foramen entrapment compared with other strangulating diseases of the small intestine in horses. Equine Vet J 2005;37:292–5.
69. Archer DC, Proudman CJ, Pinchbeck G, et al. Entrapment of the small intestine in the epiploic foramen in horses: a retrospective analysis of 71 cases recorded between 1991 and 2001. Vet Rec 2004;155:793–7.

70. Huskamp B. Diagnosis and treatment of acute abdominal conditions in the horse: various types and frequency as seen at the animal hospital in Hochmoor. In: Proceedings of the 1st Equine Colic Research Symposium, University of Georgia Press, Athens, Georgia; 1982. p. 261–72.

71. Morton AJ, Blikslager AT. Surgical and post operative factors influencing short-term survival of horses following small intestinal resection: 92 cases (1994–2001). Equine Vet J 2002;34:450–4.

72. Hart SK, Brown, JA. Diaphragmatic hernia in the horse: 44 cases (1986–2006). Proceedings 9th International Equine Colic Research Symposium; 2008. p. 102–3.

73. MacDonald MH, Pascoe JR, Stover SM, et al. Survival after small intestinal resection and anastomosis in horses. Vet Surg 1989;18:415–23.

74. Rendle DI, Wood JLN, Summerhays GES, et al. End-to-end jejuno-ileal anasto-mosis following resection of strangulated small intestine in horses: a comparative study. Equine Vet J 2005;37:356–9.

75. Plummer AE, Rakestraw PC, Hardy J. Outcome of medical and surgical treat-ment of cecal impaction in horses: 114 cases (1994–2004). J Am Vet Med Assoc 2007;231(9):1378–85.

76. Martin BB, Freeman DE, Ross MW, et al. Cecocolic and cecocecal intussuscep-tion in horse: 30 cases (1976–1996). J Am Vet Med Assoc 1999;214(1):80–4.

77. Ducharme NG, Hackett RP, Ducharme GR, et al. Surgical treatment of colic results in 181 horses. Vet Surg 1983;12(4):206–9.

78. Dabareiner RM, White NA. Large colon impaction in horses: 147 cases (1985–1991). J Am Vet Med Assoc 1995;206:679–85.

79. Hassel DM, Langer DL, Snyder JR, et al. Evaluation of enterolithiasis in equieds: 900 cases (1973–1996). J Am Vet Med Assoc 1999;214(2):233–7.

80. Ragle CA, Meagher DM, Lacroix CA. Surgical treatment of sand colic. Results in 40 horses. Vet Surg 1989;18(1):48–51.

81. Granot N, Milgram J, Bdolah-Abram T. Surgical management of sand colic impactions in horses: a retrospective study of 41 cases. Aust Vet J 2008; 86(10):404–7.

82. Hardy J, Minton M, Robertson JT, et al. Nephrosplenic entrapment in the horse: a retrospective study of 174 cases. Equine Vet J 2000;(Suppl 32):95–7.

83. Huskamp B, Kopf N. Right dorsal displacement of the large colon in the horse. Equine Practice 1983;5(1):24–9.

84. Harrison IW. Equine large intestinal volvulus: a review of 124 cases. Vet Surg 1988;17(2):77–81.

85. Snyder JR, Pascoe JR, Olander HJ, et al. Strangulating volvulus of the ascending colon in horses. J Am Vet Med Assoc 1989;195(6):757–64.

86. Southwood LL, Bergslien K, Jacobi A, et al. Large colon displacement and volvulus in horses: 495 cases (1987–1999). In: Proceedings of the Seventh Inter-national Equine colic Research Symposium. Manchester, UK; 2002. p. 32–33.

87. Embertson RM, cook G, Hance SR, et al. Large colon volvulus: surgical treat-ment of 204 horses 1986–1995. In: Proceedings of the 42nd Annual Convention of the American Association of Equine Practitioners. Denver;1996. p. 254–5.

88. Johnston K, Holcombe SJ, Hauptman JG. Plasma lactate as a predictor of colonic viability and survival after 360 degree volvulus of the ascending colon in horses. Vet Surg 2007;36:563–7.

89. Snyder JR, Pascoe JR, Olander HF, et al. Vascular injury associated with natu-rally occurring strangulating obstructions of the equine large colon. Vet Surg 1990;19:446–55.

90. Freeman DE, Gentile DG, Richardon DW, et al. Comparison of clinical judgment, Doppler ultrasound, and fluorescein fluorescence as methods for predicting intestinal viability in the pony. Am J Vet Res 1988;49:895–900.
91. Sullins KE. Deterimination of intestinal viability and the decision to resect. In: White NA, Moore JN, editors. The equine acute abdomen. 1st edition. Philadelphia: WB Saunders; 1990. p. 238–44.
92. Snyder JR, Pascoe JR, Holland M, et al. Surface oximetry of healthy and ischemic equine intestine. Am J Vet Res 1986;47:2530–5.
93. Snyder JR, Pascoe JR, Meagher DM, et al. Surface oximetry for intraoperative assessment of colonic viability in horses. J Am Vet Med Assoc 1994;204:1786–9.
94. Moore RM, Hance SR, Hardy J, et al. Colonic luminal pressure in horses with strangulating and nonstrangulating obstruction of the large colon. Vet Surg 1996;25:134–41.
95. Mathis SC, Slone ED, Lynch TM, et al. Use of colonic luminal pressure to predict outcome after surgical treatment of strangulating large colon volvulus in horses. Vet Surg 2006;35(4):356–60.
96. Van Hoogmoed L, Snyder JR, Pascoe JR, et al. Use of pelvic flexure biopsies to predict survival after large colon torsion in horses. Vet Surg 2000;29:572–7.
97. Van Hoogmoed L, Snyder JR, Pascoe JR, et al. Evaluation of uniformity of morphological injury of the large colon following severe colonic torsion. Equine Vet J Suppl 2000;32:98–100.
98. Snyder JR, Olander HJ, Pascoe JR, et al. Morphologic alterations observed during experimental ischemia of the equine large colon. Am J Vet Res 1988; 49(6):801–9.
99. Dabareiner RM, Sullins KE, White NA, et al. Serosal injury in the equine jejunum and ascending colon after ischemia-reperfusion or intraluminal distention and decompression. Vet Surg 2001;30:114–25.
100. Sheats MK, Cook VL, Jones SL, et al. Use of ultrasound to evaluate outcome following colic surgery for equine large colon volvulus. Proceedings 9th International Equine colic Research Symposium; 2008. p. 82–3.
101. Dart AJ, Snyder JR, Pascoe JR, et al. Abnormal conditions of the equine descending (small) colon: 102 cases (1979–1989). J Am Vet Med Assoc 1992; 200:971–8.
102. Ruggles AJ, Ross M. Medical and surgical management of small-colon impaction in horses: 28 cases 1984–1989. J Am Vet Med Assoc 1991;199:1762–6.
103. Rhoads W. Small colon impactions in adult horses. Comp Cont Ed Pract Vet 1999;21:770–5.
104. Frederico LM, Jones SL, Blikslager AT. Predisposing factors for small colon impaction in horses and outcome of medical and surgical treatment: 44 cases (1999–2004). J Am Vet Med Assoc 2006;229(10):1612–6.
105. Dart AJ, Snyder JR, Pascoe JR. Resection and anastomosis of the small colon in four horses. Aust Vet J 1992;69(1):5–7.
106. Mair TS, Smith LJ. Survival and complication rates in 300 horses undergoing surgical treatment of colic. Part 2: short-term complications. Equine Vet J 2005;37(4):303–9.
107. Mair TS, Smith LJ. Survival and complication rates in 300 horses undergoing surgical treatment of colic. Part 4: early (acute) relaparotomy. Equine Vet J 2005;37(4):315–8.

Parasitism and Colic

Craig R. Reinemeyer, DVM, PhD[a],*, Martin Krarup Nielsen, DVM, PhD[b]

KEYWORDS
• Equine • Parasitism • Colic • Nematodes • Cestodes

Equids are the hosts of dozens of species of internal parasites that infect no other domestic animals. Virtually all horses, especially those exposed to pasture, experience some level of parasitism continuously, but in most cases, host and parasite coexist amicably at the organism level. Few parasitisms are manifested systemically in well-managed horses, despite pathologic evidence of parasitic damage in various organs and tissues.

Unlike bacterial and viral pathogens, parasitic helminths cannot amplify their numbers within the host. One nematode infective unit results in only one mature parasite. Accordingly, most parasitic disease is a consequence of the sheer numbers of parasites present, although clinical severity can be modulated by malnutrition, coexisting disease, or other concomitant stressors. Large parasite populations are invariably a consequence of exposure to high numbers of infective units, so parasitic disease generally reflects concurrent or historical management standards. Some individual horses are exquisitely susceptible to parasitism,[1] however, and may not demonstrate typical immunologic responses to an infective challenge. Such unique susceptibility is likely to have a genetic basis.

Although equine parasites cause a wide range of clinical signs, some manifestations are unique to specific parasites. Pertinent to this article, only three parasitisms can be regarded as potentially significant agents of colic in the horse, and these will be addressed in detail. Other common parasites of equids, and their propensity to cause colic, will be discussed individually, albeit briefly.

PARASITISMS ASSOCIATED WITH COLIC

Colic is a clinical manifestation of visceral abdominal pain. Of the five basic causes of colic proposed by Magdesian and Smith,[2] three mechanisms are relevant to common parasitisms of the horse, specifically (1) ischemia or infarction, (2) distention of the gut caused by fluid, gas, or ingesta, and (3) deep ulcers in the bowel.

[a] East Tennessee Clinical Research, Inc., 80 Copper Ridge Farm Road, Rockwood, TN 37854, USA
[b] Department of Large Animal Sciences, Faculty of Life Sciences, University of Copenhagen, 5 Højbakkegård Allé, DK-2630 Taastrup, Denmark
* Corresponding author.
E-mail address: crr@easttenncr.com (C.R. Reinemeyer).

Strongylus Vulgaris

Life cycle

Strongylus vulgaris is the best-known of the strongylid, or large strongyle, parasites of equids. Horses become infected with this nematode by way of ingestion of infective, third-stage larvae from the environment. The larvae exsheath after passing through the stomach and invade the submucosa of the small intestine, where they molt to the fourth larval stage (L_4).[3] The L_4 larvae then penetrate local arterioles, burrow beneath the intima, and migrate proximally to the root of the cranial mesenteric artery (CMA). Although this anatomic locale is not the exclusive destination of migrating *S vulgaris* larvae, it is the site of the greatest larval accumulations and the most dramatic intravascular lesions. The larvae dwell there for about four months, during which time they undergo another molting to reach the L_5 stage. The L_5 larvae ultimately return to the cecum by way of the bloodstream and form large nodules in the submucosa. Eventually, these nodules rupture, and the larvae return to the gastrointestinal tract as young adults. After about 6 weeks of further maturation, they become sexually mature and the females begin to shed eggs. Altogether, the parasitic phase of the *S vulgaris* life cycle takes 6 to 7 months.[4]

Pathophysiology

Larvae within the intima and lumen of the CMA cause severe local arteritis, characterized by extensive thrombi within the lumen, hypertrophy of the medial layer, and external enlargement of the root of the CMA. Although this lesion is often described as a verminous aneurysm, the arterial walls are neither thin nor dilated. "Verminous arteritis" is a more accurate term.

The presence of arterial lesions caused by *S vulgaris* larvae is clearly associated with an increased incidence of ischemic colic, but no studies have yet been done to evaluate infection with this parasite as a risk factor for colics in horses. Experimental infection with third-stage larvae produces a disease complex known as thromboembolic colic.[5,6] The mechanism behind this condition involves active coagulation while larvae are present within the artery. Platelet aggregation results in thrombus formation, and the blood supply can be reduced by 50% or more before the gut is affected.[7] Chemical mediators of vasoconstriction and ischemia have been proposed as an alternative mechanism to mechanical blockage.[7] Other explanations for *S vulgaris*–induced colic include primary changes in gut motility[8] and alterations of local neurologic control.[9]

Manifestations and clinical findings

Manifestations of thromboembolism and arteritis are well described.[10,11] The most consistent sign is intermittent colic, often horses show sweating and rolling as clear manifestations of abdominal pain.[3,12,13] Horses are often febrile and depressed, with elevated heart rates and hypermotility of the intestines. Death is a common outcome in many cases,[12,14,15] and infection with more than 750 infective larvae is invariably fatal.

Verminous arteritis has no pathognomonic clinical signs, and sensitive and definitive techniques for antemortem diagnosis have not been developed. The enlarged root of the CMA can be palpated during a rectal examination, but this may only be feasible in small horses.[13] Contrast arteriography has been used to demonstrate the vascular compromise associated with active larval infections and the return of perfusion following successful therapy, but this technique has no application for clinical cases.[16] Transrectal ultrasonography has been evaluated as a technique for detection of verminous arteritis.[17–20] Although technically possible and potentially more reliable than rectal palpation, this method suffers from similar limitations, such as problems in reaching the CMA in larger horses and risks for both person and horse when rectally inserting an ultrasound probe in a standing horse.

Substantial effort has been invested in developing serologic assays to detect IgG(T) antibodies that are specific against S vulgaris.[21–24] Unfortunately, cross-reactivity with other nematode species seems to confound specificity,[21–23] and no satisfactory serologic assay for detecting S vulgaris infection has been developed to date. A PCR technique is currently being evaluated to detect the presence of S vulgaris DNA in blood samples of horses with larval infections. This technique can potentially avoid the problems with cross-reactivity and can be designed to be highly sensitive. When fully developed, such an assay would have wide applications in a clinical setting.

Treatment

Acute management of gut infarction is beyond the scope of this article, but there are no rapid solutions for the underlying parasitic problem. Of the anthelmintics currently marketed for use in horses, only three have recognized larvicidal efficacy against S vulgaris (**Table 1**). However, the nematocidal activity of these regimens may not be complete until several days or weeks after treatment. The author (CRR) has observed viable S vulgaris larvae in active aneurysms 2 weeks after ivermectin treatment, but full efficacy (>99%) was evident by 5 weeks posttreatment.[25]

It is remarkable to the authors that anthelmintic resistance by S vulgaris has not been reported to date.

Management

A larvicidal regimen using an anthelmintic (see **Table 1**) should remove nearly all manifestations of adult and immature S vulgaris from infected horses. Thereafter, if the treated animals become reinfected, it will be 6 months before they might again pass large strongyle eggs in the feces. Therefore, future, patent S vulgaris infections could be precluded by repeating larvicidal treatments at intervals not to exceed 6 months. Because the maximum duration of survival for infective stages of S vulgaris living in the environment is approximately 1 year, no source of reinfection would exist on any farm where this regimen had been implemented for all resident equids for a period of 18 months or longer.[26] Indeed, large strongyles have been eradicated from most well-managed herds in North America[27] because the typical horse owner uses macrocyclic lactone anthelmintics (ivermectin or moxidectin) far more frequently than just once every 6 months.

One possible disadvantage to eradication of any infectious agent is that naïve hosts may be exquisitely susceptible to disease if the organism is reintroduced through alteration of the existing management program or transfer of the animals to a new premise.

Table 1			
Anthelmintic regimens with efficacy against larval stages of S vulgaris in the CMA			
Generic Name	**Brand Name**	**Dose**	**Regimen**
Fenbendazole	Panacur PowerPak	10 mg/kg	Once daily for five consecutive days
Ivermectin	Eqvalan, Zimecterin, numerous generics	200 µg/kg	Once
Moxidectin	Quest, Quest Plus	400 µg/kg	Once

Parascaris Equorum

Life cycle
Parascaris equorum is the largest nematode parasite of equids; adult parasites are found in the small intestines of juvenile horses. Horses acquire ascarid infections through ingestion of larvated eggs from the environment. The eggs hatch in the small intestine, and the larvae are carried by the portal circulation to the liver. After 1 week of intrahepatic migration, the larvae re-enter the circulation and travel to the lungs. There, they leave the circulation, penetrate the alveoli, migrate up the airways, and are swallowed. Back in the small intestine yet again, the larvae molt into adults and reproduce. Eggs first appear in the feces approximately 75 to 80 days postinfection.[28,29] Horses develop excellent acquired immunity to *P equorum*, so infections are limited to sucklings, weanlings, and yearlings, and are observed only occasionally in horses older than 2 years of age.

Pathophysiology
P equorum infection causes a host of clinical signs, but only impaction colic is relevant to this article. Mature *P equorum* are very large worms, approximately 4 mm in diameter and 25 cm long, and a typical infection might involve several hundred individuals. Viable ascarids generally avoid serious "traffic jams," but when large numbers of ascarids are killed by the use of an effective anthelmintic, the resulting tangle of dead worms may be sufficient to mechanically obstruct the small intestine. In one retrospective study of surgical colic cases,[30] slightly more than 50% of all foals presenting with ascarid impactions had been dewormed less than 6 days previously. A more recent study reported that in 72% of the cases under consideration, the horses had been treated with an anthelmintic within 24 hours before the onset of colic.[31]

Manifestations and clinical findings
Foals with ascarid impaction colic often present with gastric reflux and shock. Two retrospective studies both reported that the median age at presentation was 5 months, male foals were twice as likely to be represented as females, and the majority of cases occurred during late summer through autumn.[30,31]

Treatment
Horses with suspected ascarid impactions should be treated initially by the passage of a nasogastric tube for alimentary decompression and administration of mineral oil. Supportive therapy should maintain hydration, treat shock, and manage pain. Because ascarid impactions are often precipitated by anthelmintic treatment, deworming is contraindicated in the face of obstructive colic in a foal. If medical management fails to relieve the obstruction, enterotomy may be attempted. In one retrospective study cited previously in this article,[30] postoperative complications included adhesions, colic, fever, endotoxemia, peritonitis, intestinal perforation, and infection of the incision site. Survival in cases of ascarid impaction that went to surgery was less than 10%.

Residual ascarid populations should be removed chemically after successful resolution of an obstructive crisis. The anthelmintics presented in **Table 2** are labeled as effective against luminal stages of *P equorum*, but some local ascarid populations have recently developed resistance to one or more of these compounds. Beginning in 2002, *P equorum* isolates in six countries apparently developed resistance to the macrocyclic lactones ivermectin[32–38] and moxidectin.[32,38] These studies all reported inadequate reductions in *P equorum* fecal egg counts at 10 to 14 days posttreatment. In a model using naïve foals infected with a Canadian ascarid isolate, unequivocal

Table 2
Anthelmintics with efficacy against luminal stages of *P equorum*

Generic Name	Brand Name	Dose	Regimen
Fenbendazole	Panacur PowerPak, Safeguard	10 mg/kg	Once
Ivermectin[a]	Eqvalan, Zimecterin, numerous generics	200 µg/kg	Once
Moxidectin[a]	Quest, Quest Plus	400 µg/kg	Once
Oxibendazole	Anthelcide EQ	10 mg/kg	Once
Piperazine	Various	88 mg/kg	Once
Pyrantel pamoate[b]	Strongid, various generics	6.6 mg/kg	Once
Pyrantel tartrate	Strongid C, Continuex 2X	2.64 mg/kg/day	Top-dressed daily

[a] Some populations of *P equorum* are known to be resistant to the macrocyclic lactone anthelmintics ivermectin and moxidectin.
[b] Although relatively uncommon, *P equorum* populations with resistance to pyrantel pamoate have been reported.[35,41]

resistance to ivermectin was demonstrated, based on only 22% reduction in worm counts.[39]

Anthelmintic treatment decisions are difficult to make for foals that may be candidates for impaction (eg, no prior history of deworming, very high *P equorum* egg counts, abdominal enlargement). For such animals, the likelihood of an obstructive complication probably increases with the efficacy of the anthelmintic, so initial treatment with a less-effective deworming regimen may lessen the risk of a posttreatment impaction. Fenbendazole at the adult-horse dose of 5 mg/kg may be more predictable for this purpose than modified doses of other equine anthelmintics.

Management

Routine anthelmintic treatment of foals should not begin earlier than 60 to 70 days of age, and treatments thereafter should be repeated at the greatest interval that minimizes environmental contamination with ascarid eggs. Treating foals at bimonthly intervals (ie, approximately every 60 days) is considered the maximum dosing interval for controlling ascarids. It should be recognized, however, that bimonthly treatment might not preclude all egg contamination and that some eggs might pass in the feces between scheduled dewormings. Conversely, deworming at more frequent intervals intensifies selection for anthelmintic resistance, so practitioners are faced with a quandary. Tolerating some level of egg shedding may be the lesser of two evils in the long run, because a survey in the Netherlands (M. Eysker, personal communication, 2008) determined that macrocyclic lactone resistance was significantly less prevalent on farms where foals were dewormed at intervals greater than or equal to 8 weeks, in comparison with more frequent treatments.

If macrocyclic lactone–resistant ascarids are known to occur on a farm, acceptable efficacy usually can be achieved by treatment with benzimidazoles or pyrimidines, and rotation between effective drug classes is recommended.[38,40] It has recently been reported[35,41] that some *P equorum* isolates in Texas and Kentucky, respectively, were resistant to pyrantel pamoate in addition to macrocyclic lactones. Therefore, practitioners are encouraged to monitor the efficacy of all drug classes against *P equorum* populations on each farm and to confirm the sustained utility of effective classes at least once annually.

Anoplocephala Perfoliata

Life cycle

Anoplocephala perfoliata is the most prevalent cestode parasite of horses worldwide. This tapeworm is usually found in large congregations attached to the cecal mucosa near the ileocecal valve. Gravid segments (proglottids) break away from the body of the cestode and pass distally with the ingesta. The proglottids apparently disintegrate during this passage, and individual eggs are released into the feces. Once in the environment, *A perfoliata* eggs are ingested by various species of oribatid mites. The mites serve as intermediate hosts, and the life cycle stage found therein is termed a cysticercoid. Horses are infected inadvertently by ingesting infective mites while grazing. Adult cestodes develop within 2 to 4 months after infection.

Pathophysiology

Masses of *A perfoliata* attached near the ileocecal valve cause ulceration of the cecal mucosa, often with formation of pseudomembranes, local inflammation, and development of fibrous connective tissue. Inflammatory changes may involve the entire thickness of the cecal wall, including the serosal layer.

Although the detailed mechanisms are unknown, *A perfoliata* infection has been associated with an increased incidence of ileocecal intussusceptions and cecal rupture.[42,43] Epidemiologic studies have provided evidence of increased risk for ileocecal colic in the presence of tapeworms,[44] and of risk for ileal impaction and spasmodic colic.[45] In contrast, a recent Canadian study evaluating a large number of horses failed to demonstrate an association between tapeworm burdens and the risk of colic, but instead found a significant correlation between *A perfoliata* antibody titers and time on pasture.[46] This confirms that pastured horses experience greater exposure to tapeworms, but that grazing per se does not necessarily increase the risk of colic. The precise role of *A perfoliata* in equine colic remains unknown, and elucidation likely must await the development of a successful model for inducing artificial tapeworm infections in horses.

The mechanisms by which tapeworms contribute to colic are not understood, but one common theory holds that local inflammation interferes with gut motility, particularly the transport of ingesta from the distal small intestine into the cecum through the ileocecal orifice. Changes in motility may be manifested as spasmodic colic or intussusception. It has also been proposed that local fibrous connective tissue mechanically constricts the ileocecal valve, thus potentiating ileal impaction. A theory has also been advanced that tapeworm infection perhaps affects gut motility by way of neurologic alterations in regional ganglia.[47,48]

Manifestations and clinical findings

The impact of an average tapeworm infection in a typical horse is unknown, but subclinical effects on productivity or performance are the most likely consequences. Spasmodic colic has been associated with *A perfoliata* infection,[45] and this syndrome has been characterized as mild or moderate in severity, with hypermotility, absence of gastric reflux, and favorable response to antispasmodic and analgesic therapy. Although, spasmodic colics are generally considered mild and manageable in the field, a wide range of severity has been observed and unremitting cases may require referral.

Treatment

Praziquantel is uniformly 100% effective against *A perfoliata* infections when administered at doses that are equal to or greater than 1 mg/kg,[49] and pyrantel pamoate

(13.2 mg/kg) is more than 95% effective.[50,51] The activity of both compounds is fairly rapid, with death and detachment of the majority of the cestodes within 24 to 48 hours posttreatment. Colic has been reported after treatment with praziquantel.[51]

Management

Evidence-based recommendations for controlling tapeworm infections have not been developed in North America. The most common management program involves two therapeutic treatments per year, but the optimal seasonal timing of those treatments has not been determined.

PARASITISMS UNLIKELY TO CAUSE COLIC

Nearly every alimentary parasite of the horse has been incriminated at one time or another as a potential causative agent of colic. Many equine parasites are highly prevalent, so their presence in any horse presenting with colic is not unexpected. This association is not proof of causation, however, and recognition of this fact is useful for prioritizing differential diagnoses for any colic case with concurrent parasitism.

Gasterophilus spp

Larvae of bot flies are found seasonally within the body of the horse. Adult female bot flies attach their eggs to the hair coat of a horse. The initial parasitic stages, first- and second-instar larvae, develop in various sites of the oral cavity before they migrate to the proximal gastrointestinal tract. Second- and third-instar larvae of *Gasterophilus intestinalis* are found attached to the nonglandular mucosa of the stomach, and larvae of *G nasalis* occupy the duodenal ampulla, just distal to the pylorus. *G intestinalis* often form dense mats numbering hundreds of individuals, yet the bots are always arrayed in a single layer and any associated lumenal compromise is minimal. Several older textbooks presented the theory that bots interfere with the passage of ingesta through the stomach, but there is little evidence to support this contention. In addition, bots have been listed as potential causes of gastric rupture,[52] which is similarly unlikely. Bot infections are highly prevalent, often occurring in more than 90% of herd members during the autumn and winter months. Gastric rupture, in contrast, is a relatively rare event, and the contemporaneous juxtaposition of rare and common conditions does not prove cause and effect. Finally, there is little credible evidence that bot infestations cause visceral pain or contribute to the severity of gastric ulcers. The latter condition is often accompanied by signs of abdominal pain (See Videla and Andrews on Gastric ulcers in this issue).

Strongylus Edentatus

S edentatus is another large strongyle species that is closely related to *S vulgaris*, but one that follows a different systemic migratory pattern. After ingestion from the environment, infective larvae penetrate the gut and are carried to the liver. They migrate temporarily within hepatic tissues, but ultimately move into the retroperitoneum and the peritoneal cavity and spend several months growing and developing in those locations.[53,54] Although colic has not been associated specifically with migrating *S edentatus*, postmortem examination of infected horses frequently reveals intense local inflammation around migrating larvae, characterized by hemorrhage, edema, congestion, and swelling. Ultimately, fibrin deposits and fibrous adhesions may develop on the surface of various abdominal organs.[53,54] The previous recommendations for treatment and management of *S vulgaris* made in this article are appropriate for *S edentatus* as well.

Strongyloides Westeri

Strongyloides westeri is a fairly common nematode that is found almost exclusively in suckling foals. Infective larvae are sequestered within the somatic tissues of mares, and the hormones of pregnancy and lactation induce the larvae to migrate to the mammary glands. Infective larvae appear in the milk during the first week of lactation and are transmitted to the foals during suckling. *S westeri* adults develop within the small intestine of the foals, and eggs are passed in the feces as early as the second week of life. Although patent infections are common, *S westeri* is only occasionally pathogenic. Clinical signs are those of enteritis, including diarrhea, fever, weight loss, and dehydration. It is possible that this form of juvenile enteritis might be accompanied by cramping or abdominal pain, but that has not been reported as a common feature of *S westeri* infections.

Foals with *S westeri* infections can be treated using oxibendazole (15 mg/kg) or ivermectin (200 μg/kg). Rote treatment of foals using ivermectin during the first month of life has long been a common practice for managing *S westeri* infections. However, it is now recognized that such regimens have probably selected for populations of *P equorum* that are resistant to macrocyclic lactone anthelmintics (eg, ivermectin, moxidectin). Accordingly, rote treatment of foals younger than 1 month of age is discouraged, and anthelmintic therapy for *S westeri* should be limited to clinical cases. Horses invariably acquire excellent immunity to *S westeri* by 5 months of age, so this parasite is virtually never seen in foals after weaning. (For a review, see.[55])

Cyathostomins (Small Strongyles, Cyathostomes)

Cyathostomins are ubiquitous parasites of grazing horses. They are close relatives of the large strongyles, as represented in this article by *Strongylus vulgaris*, but their life cycles do not feature somatic migration. After infective cyathostomin larvae are ingested from the environment, they exsheath and penetrate the mucosa or submucosa of the large intestine, primarily in the cecum and ventral colon. Within the mucosal lining, each larva develops inside a fibrous capsule that sequesters it from immune or inflammatory responses of the host. Host and parasites experience a rather benign coexistence as long as the capsule remains intact. Ultimately, however, the larvae must emerge from the cyst to complete their life cycle, and excystment is accompanied by the release of the excretory and secretory products that had accumulated over a period of weeks to more than 2 years. Larval emergence results in intense, albeit focal, inflammation, characterized by congestion, edema, and leakage of plasma proteins into the intestinal lumen. Such focal damage may occur in the large intestine of the typical grazing horse at hundreds of discrete sites each day, and damage is cumulative.

A severe clinical syndrome may occur if very large numbers of cyathostomin larvae emerge synchronously. This syndrome, known as larval cyathostominosis, is characterized by diarrhea, rapid weight loss, hypoproteinemia, and the presence of numerous larval cyathostomins in the feces.[56,57] Larval cyathostominosis does not respond favorably to anthelmintic therapy, and it may be fatal. However, colic has not been reported as a prominent feature of this most severe manifestation of cyathostomin infections.

Treatment and management of cyathostomin infections is beyond the scope of this paper. Practical management in North America has become much more difficult in recent years as the result of the nearly ubiquitous resistance of cyathostomin populations to benzimidazole anthelmintics and an expanding resistance to pyrimidine products.[58,59] Little relief is in sight because it appears unlikely that any new classes of nematocides will be approved for equine use within the next few years.

Oxyuris Equi *(Pinworms)*

Following ingestion of larvated eggs from the environment, third-stage *Oxyuris equi* larvae develop within mucosal crypts of the cecum and ventral colon. Although larval pinworms are reputed to cause local mucosal irritation, it would be extremely difficult to differentiate this effect from the ubiquitous inflammatory changes caused by cyathostomin larvae infecting the same organs. Regardless, any potential pathogenicity of larval pinworms is unlikely to be clinically significant. Adult *O equi* do not feed on the colonic mucosa, so the clinical impact of pinworm infection is apparently limited to perianal irritation resulting from the egg-laying activities of gravid females.

No anthelmintics are 100% effective against adult or larval pinworms, but anthelmintic resistance by this nematode has not been demonstrated to date. Daily use of pyrantel tartrate may be a useful adjunct for clinical management of persistent *O equi* problems. (For a review, see.[55])

Draschia Megastoma *(Stomach Worm)*

Draschia megastoma and *Habronema* spp are related nematodes that reside in the equine stomach and share a common requirement for dipteran intermediate hosts. Both parasites are better known for causing dramatic, granulomatous lesions when they are deposited in dermal or mucocutaneous sites in their larval stages. *D megastoma* is unique because nematodes in the adult stages are found within large granulomas in the gastric mucosa. These granulomas may reach up to 10 cm in diameter and reputedly can interfere with the passage of ingesta through the stomach.[60] Regardless of this pathogenic footnote, *D megastoma* has become an extremely rare parasite. The prevalence of *D megastoma* was 47% in a postmortem survey of 55 horses conducted 25 years ago.[61] However, the first author of this article has not observed a single infection with this worm during the past 20 years, despite performing necropsies of several hundred horses that had no history of prior anthelmintic treatment. The presence of a *D megastoma* granuloma in the stomach can be diagnosed easily using gastroscopy. Macrocyclic lactone anthelmintics (eg, ivermectin, moxidectin) are effective, and the widespread use of this drug class is the most likely explanation for the dramatic decline in prevalence.

Triodontophorus Tenuicollis

Triodontophorus tenuicollis is a large strongyle, but one that does not migrate within the host. Populations of *T tenuicollis* occasionally congregate within deep ulcers in the dorsal colon. These so-called "worm nests" may harbor several dozen adult specimens, and the ulcers become packed with dark concretions of exudate, blood, and ingesta. Infected horses usually harbor only one or two ulcers, which can be as large as 1 cm to 4 cm across and from 4 mm to 5 mm deep. *T tenuicollis* nests are fairly rare lesions and have not been associated with colic, but they are mentioned in this article because of their tendency to induce the formation of deep ulcers. All of the anthelmintics listed in **Table 2**, with the exception of piperazine, would likely be effective against *T tenuicollis.*

SUMMARY

Despite common notions to the contrary, only three common parasitisms of horses are likely to be manifested as colic: *S vulgaris*, *P equorum*, and *A perfoliata*.

Excellent control recommendations for the long-term management, indeed, eradication, of *S vulgaris* have been developed, but complacency arising from a perceived, perpetual solution is dangerous. Horses remain highly susceptible to infection if management programs are altered, if the horse is transferred to a different premise where the standards of parasite control have been less rigorous, or if large strongyles should ever develop resistance to anthelmintic larvicidal regimens. Occasional monitoring of herds for the presence of large strongyles is prudent, and new tools for detecting larval infections may be available in the near future.

A perfoliata undoubtedly plays a role in certain types of colic, and highly effective drugs are currently marketed. However, evidence-based control recommendations for this parasite have not been proposed in North America. Because overuse of cestocides could conceivably result in anthelmintic-resistant populations of tapeworms, administering a few strategically timed treatments during the year is preferable to the use of frequent, rote deworming.

The most severe threat for parasitic colic in the future is posed by anthelmintic-resistant strains of *P equorum*. The prevalence of populations that are no longer susceptible to macrocyclic lactone dewormers is expanding among breeding operations, and recent evidence suggests that pyrantel products may also have limited utility on certain premises. Fortunately, ascarid resistance can be detected by diligent monitoring using commonly available techniques, and alternative, effective dewormers are still available.

REFERENCES

1. Nielsen MK, Haaning N, Olsen SN. Strongyle egg shedding consistency in horses on farms using selective therapy in Denmark. Vet Parasitol 2006;135:333–5.
2. Magdesian KG, Smith BP. Colic. In: Smith BP, editor. Large animal internal medicine. Philadelphia: Mosby; 2002. p. 108.
3. Duncan JL, Pirie HM. The life cycle of *Strongylus vulgaris* in the horse. Res Vet Sci 1972;13:374–9.
4. Wetzel R. Über die Entwicklungsdauer der Palisadenwurmer im Körper des Pferdes und ihre praktische Auswertung. (*On the duration of development of large strongyles in the body of the horse and its practical evaluation.*) Dtsch Tierarztl 1942;50:443–4 [in German].
5. Duncan JL, Pirie HM. The pathogenesis of single experimental infections with *Strongylus vulgaris* in foals. Res Vet Sci 1975;18:82–93.
6. Enigk K. Die Pathogenese der thrombotisch-embolische Kolik des Pferdes. (*The pathogenesis of thromboembolic colic of the horse.*) Monatsh Tierheilk 1951;3: 65–74 [in German].
7. White NA. Intestinal infarction associated with mesenteric vascular thrombotic disease in the horse. J Am Vet Med Assoc 1981;178(3):259–62.
8. Sellers AF, Lowe JE, Drost CJ, et al. Retropulsion-propulsion in equine large colon. Am J Vet Res 1982;43:390–6.
9. Wright AI. Verminous arteritis as a cause of colic in the horse. Equine Vet J 1972; 4:169.
10. Duncan JL. *Strongylus vulgaris* infection in the horse. Vet Rec 1974;95:34–7.
11. Drudge JH. Clinical aspects of *Strongylus vulgaris* infection in the horse. Emphasis on diagnosis, chemotherapy, and prophylaxis. Vet Clin North Am Large Anim Pract 1979;1:251–65.
12. Drudge JH, Lyons ET, Szanto J. Pathogenesis of migrating stages of helmimths, with special reference to *Strongylus vulgaris*. In: Soulsby EJL, editor. Biology of

parasites. Emphasis on veterinary parasites. New York and London: Academic Press Inc.; 1966. p. 199–214.

13. Greatorex JC. Diagnosis and treatment of "verminous aneurysm" formation in the horse. Vet Rec 1977;101:184–7.

14. Enigk K. Zur Entwicklung von Strongylus vulgaris (Nematodes) im Wirtstier. (On the development of Strongylus vulgaris (Nematodes) in the host animal.) Z Tropenmed Parasitol 1950;2:287–306 [in German].

15. Kester WO. Strongylus vulgaris - the horse killer. Mod Vet Pract 1975;56:569–72.

16. Slocombe JOD, Rendano VT, Owen RAR, et al. Arteriography in ponies with Strongylus vulgaris arteritis. Can J Comp Med 1977;41:137–45.

17. Bueno L, Dorchies P, Franc M, et al. Détection ultrasonore des anéurismes mésentériques dus à Strongylus vulgaris chez le cheval. (Ultrasonic detection of mesenteric aneurysms due to Strongylus vulgaris in the horse.) Pratique Vétérinaire Équine 1978;10:153–5 [in French].

18. Wallace KD, Selcer BA, Becht JL. Technique for transrectal ultrasonography of the cranial mesenteric artery of the horse. Am J Vet Res 1989a;50:1695–8.

19. Wallace KD, Selcer BA, Tyler DE, et al. Transrectal ultrasonography of the cranial mesenteric artery of the horse. Am J Vet Res 1989b;50:1699–703.

20. Wallace KD, Selcer BA, Tyler DE, et al. In vitro ultrasonographic appearance of the normal and verminous equine aorta, cranial mesenteric artery and its branches. Am J Vet Res 1989c;50:1774–8.

21. Klei TR, Chapman MR, Torbert BJ, et al. Antibody responses of ponies to initial and challenge infections of Strongylus vulgaris. Vet Parasitol 1983;12:187–98.

22. Nichol C, Masterson WJ. Characterisation of surface antigens of Strongylus vulgaris of potential immunodiagnostic importance. Mol Biochem Parasitol 1987;25: 29–38.

23. von Weiland G, Hasslinger MA, Mezger S, et al. Möglichkeiten und Grenzen der Immundiagnostik des Strongylidenbefalles beim Pferd. (Possibilities and limitations for immunodiagnosis of strongylid infections of the horse.) Berl Munch Tierartzl Wochenschr 1991;104(1):149–53 [in German].

24. Adeyefa CAO. Precipitin response of the mitogen produced by Strongylus vulgaris arterial larvae. Vet Parasitol 1992;43(3–4):243–7.

25. Slocombe JOD, McCraw BM, Pennock PW, et al. Strongylus vulgaris in the tunica media of arteries of ponies and treatment with ivermectin. Can J Vet Res 1987;51: 232–5.

26. Dunsmore JD. Integrated control of Strongylus vulgaris infection in horses using ivermectin. Equine Vet J 1985;17:191.

27. Herd RP. The changing world of worms: the rise of the cyathostomes and the decline of Strongylus vulgaris. Compend Contin Educ Vet 1990;12:732.

28. Clayton HM, Duncan JL. The migration and development of Parascaris equorum in the horse. Int J Parasitol 1979a;9:285–92.

29. Clayton HM, Duncan JL. The migration and development of Parascaris equorum in the foal. Res Vet Sci 1979b;26:383–4.

30. Southwood LL, Ragle CA, Snyder JR, et al. Surgical treatment of ascarid impactions in horses and foals. Proceedings of the American Association of Equine Practitioners 1966;42:258.

31. Cribb NC, Coté NM, Bouré LP, et al. Acute small intestinal obstruction associated with Parascaris equorum infection in young horses: 25 cases (1985–2004). N Z Vet J 2006;54:338–43.

32. Boersema JH, Eysker M, Nas JW. Apparent resistance of Parascaris equorum to macrocyclic lactones. Vet Rec 2002;150:279–81.

33. Hearn FP, Peregrine AS. Identification of foals infected with *Parascaris equorum* apparently resistant to ivermectin. J Am Vet Med Assoc 2003;223:482–5.
34. Stoneham S, Coles GC. Ivermectin resistance in *Parascaris equorum*. Vet Rec 2006;158:572.
35. Craig TM, Diamond PL, Ferwerda NS, et al. Evidence of ivermectin resistance by *Parascaris equorum* on a Texas horse farm. J Equine Vet Sci 2007;27:67–71.
36. von Samson Himmelstjerna G, Fritzen B, Demeler J, et al. Cases of reduced cyathostomin egg-reappearance period and failure of *Parascaris equorum* egg count reduction following ivermectin treatment as well as survey on pyrantel efficacy on German horse farms. Vet Parasitol 2007;144:74–80.
37. Schougaard H, Nielsen MK. Apparent ivermectin resistance of *Parascaris equorum* in foals in Denmark. Vet Rec 2007;160:439–40.
38. Slocombe JOD, de Gannes RV, Lake MC. Macrocyclic lactone-resistant *Parascaris equorum* on stud farms in Canada and effectiveness of fenbendazole and pyrantel pamoate. Vet Parasitol 2007;145:371–6.
39. Kaplan RM, Reinemeyer CR, Slocombe JO, et al. Confirmation of ivermectin resistance in a purportedly resistant Canadian isolate of *Parascaris equorum* in foals. Proceedings of the American Association of Veterinary Parasitologists. Proceedings of the American Association of Veterinary Parasitologists 2006;51:69–70.
40. Reinemeyer CR, Marchiondo AA. Efficacy of pyrantel pamoate in horses against a macrocyclic lactone-resistant isolate of *Parascaris equorum*. Proceedings of the American Association of Veterinary Parasitologists. Proceedings of the American Association of Veterinary Parasitologists 2007;52:78.
41. Lyons ET, Tolliver SC, Ionita M, et al. Evaluation of parasiticidal activity of fenbendazole, ivermectin, oxibendazole, and pyrantel pamoate in horse foals with emphasis on ascarids (*Parascaris equorum*) in field studies on five farms in Central Kentucky in 2007. Parasitol Res 2008;103:287–91.
42. Barclay WP, Phillips TN, Foerner JJ. Intussusception associated with *Anoplocephala perfoliata* infection in five horses. J Am Vet Med Res 1982;180:752–3.
43. Owen R, Jagger DW, Quan-Taylor R. Caecal intussusceptions in horses and the significance of *Anoplocephala perfoliata*. Vet Rec 1989;124:34–7.
44. Proudman C, Edwards G. Are tapeworms associated with equine colic? A case control study. Equine Vet J 1993;25(3):224–6.
45. Proudman CJ, French NP, Trees AJ. Tapeworm infection is a significant risk factor for spasmodic colic and ileal impaction colic in the horse. Equine Vet J 1998;30:194–9.
46. Trotz-Williams L, Physick-Sheard P, McFarlane H, et al. Occurrence of *Anoplocephala perfoliata* infection in horses in Ontario, Canada and associations with colic and management practices. Vet Parasitol 2008;153(1/2):73–84.
47. Bain SA, Kelly JD. Prevalence and pathogenicity of *Anoplocephala perfoliata* in a horse population in South Auckland. N Z Vet J 1977;25:27–8.
48. Lee DL, Tatchell RJ. Studies on the tapeworm *Anoplocephala perfoliata* (Goeze, 1782). Parasitol 1964;54:467–79.
49. Marchiondo AA, Reinemeyer CR. Equine Cestodiasis: Biology and Treatment of *Anoplocephala perfoliata*. Japanese J Vet Parasitol 2006;4:1–8.
50. Reinemeyer CR, Hutchens DE, Eckblad WP, et al. Dose-confirmation studies of the cestocidal activity of pyrantel pamaote paste in horses. Vet Parasitol 2006;138:234–9.
51. Barret EJ, Blair CW, Farlam J, et al. Postdosing colic and diarrhoea in horses with serological evidence of tapeworm infection. Vet Rec 2005;156:252–3.

52. Dart AJ, Hutchins DR, Begg AP. Suppurative splenitis and peritonitis in a horse after gastric ulceration caused by larvae of *Gasterophilus intestinalis*. Aust Vet J 1987;64:155–8.
53. McCraw BM, Slocombe JOD. Early development of and pathology associated with *Strongylus edentatus*. Can J Comp Med 1974;38:124–38.
54. McCraw BM, Slocombe JOD. *Strongylus edentatus*: Development and lesions from ten weeks postinfection to patency. Can J Comp Med 1978;42:340–56.
55. Reinemeyer CR, Nielsen MK. Gastrointestinal nematodes. In: Sellon DC, Long MT, editors. Equine infectious diseases. St. Louis (MO): Saunders; 2007. p. 480–90.
56. Mair TS, Westerlaken LV, Cripps PJ, et al. Diarrhoea in adult horses: A survey of clinical cases and assessment of some prognostic indices. Vet Rec 1990;126: 479–81.
57. Love S, Murphy D, Mellor D. Pathogenicity of cyathostome infection. Vet Parasitol 1999;85:113–22.
58. Kaplan RM. Anthelmintic resistance in nematodes of horses. Vet Res 2002;33: 491–507.
59. Kaplan RM. Drug resistance in nematodes of veterinary importance: a status report. Trends Parasitol 2004;20:477–81.
60. Lyons ET, Swerzcek TW, Drudge JH, et al. A large *Draschia megastoma* related gastric lesion in a thoroughbred. Vet Med 1991;86:332–4.
61. Reinemeyer CR, Smith SA, Gabel AA, et al. The prevalence and intensity of internal parasites of horses at necropsy in the U.S.A. Vet Parasitol 1984;15:75–83.

Coagulopathies in Horses with Colic

Luis Monreal, DVM, PhD*, Carla Cesarini, DVM

KEYWORDS

- Horse • Gastrointestinal disorders • Hypercoagulation
- Disseminated intravascular coagulation • Clinical management

Historically, coagulopathies secondary to gastrointestinal disorders have been the most prevalent cause of hemostatic disorders in horses.[1] Much of the research published on equine coagulation dysfunctions has been done in horses with colic, and several studies evaluating hemostatic profiles in horses with colic obtained results indicating that coagulopathies in these patients may be a frequent finding.[2–11]

In this article coagulation dysfunctions that horses with gastrointestinal disease may develop are reviewed. Readers desiring more information about normal hemostatic function in the horse are referred to already published reviews.[1,12,13]

TYPES OF COAGULOPATHIES IN HORSES WITH COLIC

Coagulation dysfunctions are normally classified according to the pathophysiology in two processes: (1) the excessive activation of the coagulation system (hypercoagulable state), and (2) the deficient coagulation activation (hypocoagulable state) (**Box 1**). In horses with gastrointestinal disease, coagulopathies are commonly characterized by excess of activation, which may be moderate, marked, or extremely marked depending on the severity and duration of the coagulation activation associated with the gastrointestinal disease. For instance, colon obstructions/displacements usually produce a mild to moderate activation of the coagulation system, which is totally compensated by a proportional activation of the coagulation inhibitory systems (coagulation inhibitors and the fibrinolysis system), with no hemostatic consequences. Acute enteritis may produce a marked activation of the coagulation system frequently compensated by inhibitory systems. This marked hypercoagulation produces coagulation abnormalities consistent with disseminated intravascular coagulation (DIC), but mainly compensated (the subclinical form of DIC). When this hypercoagulation persists over time, marked coagulation consumption may develop and may progress to a coagulation deficiency characterized by a hemorrhagic syndrome (the bleeding form of DIC). In contrast, an extremely severe hypercoagulable state in a short period

Servei de Medicina Interna Equina, Departament de Medicina i Cirurgia Animals, Facultat de Veterinària, Universitat Autònoma de Barcelona, 08193-Bellaterra, Barcelona, Spain
* Corresponding author.
E-mail address: lluis.monreal@uab.es (L. Monreal).

Vet Clin Equine 25 (2009) 247–258
doi:10.1016/j.cveq.2009.04.001
0749-0739/09/$ – see front matter © 2009 Elsevier Inc. All rights reserved.

vetequine.theclinics.com

Box 1
Types of coagulopathies in horses with colic

Hypercoagulation and DIC (the most common)

Moderate coagulation activation (eg, obstructions, displacements)

    Compensated by the inhibitory systems (hyperfibrinolysis)

Severe coagulation activation (eg, ischemic or inflammatory problems at early stages)

    Compensated by the inhibitory systems

    Some clinicopathologic abnormalities consistent with DIC (evidence of platelet consumption, coagulation factor consumption, and hyperfibrinolysis)

    Subclinical form of DIC

Extremely severe coagulation activation (eg, severe ischemic and inflammatory disorders, severe peritonitis)

    Uncompensated form of DIC with massive fibrin deposition in different tissues

    Marked alterations in the coagulation profile, consistent with DIC (evidence of platelet consumption, coagulation factor consumption, coagulation inhibitor consumption, and hyperfibrinolysis)

    Horses may show clinical signs of DIC consistent with venous thrombosis, tissue hypoxia, and multiorgan dysfunction/failure (the MOFS form of DIC). Few cases may also show hemorrhagic clinical signs consistent with the bleeding form of DIC.

Hypocoagulation (infrequent)

Exception has to be taken for the bleeding form of DIC

Normally detected in horses without gastrointestinal disease, but showing abdominal discomfort

Normally associated with liver diseases

---

of time without subsequent inhibitory reaction may occur in intestinal volvuli or severe colitis with endotoxemia, producing massive fibrin and microthrombi formation and deposition in different tissues, which contributes to multiple organ dysfunction/failure. This severe hypercoagulable state is consistent with DIC (the multiorgan failure form of DIC, MOFS), and contributes to the high mortality rate of these severe cases.[14]

Hypocoagulable states may also be observed in some horses with clinical signs of abdominal discomfort. This coagulopathy is uncommonly seen in these patients, however, and when detected it generally corresponds to the bleeding form of DIC (if associated with a severe primary gastrointestinal disease) or is associated with liver disease.

HYPERCOAGULATION AND DISSEMINATED INTRAVASCULAR COAGULATION IN HORSES WITH COLIC
Definition

DIC is an acquired coagulopathy characterized by a marked activation of the coagulation system that is normally counteracted by a proportional activation of inhibitory systems. When the marked hypercoagulation overwhelms the inhibitory system, it may cause exaggerated intravascular fibrin formation, with widespread fibrin deposition and microvascular thrombus formation in different tissues. This fibrin deposition and thrombus formation may lead to ischemic tissue lesions and subsequent multiorgan dysfunction/failure (MODS/MOFS). Additionally, the marked activation of the coagulation system leads to a significant depletion of platelets, coagulation factors, and coagulation inhibitors, which causes clinicopathologic evidence of consumption coagulopathy and, if consumption is severe, signs of spontaneous hemorrhage.

In horses with colic, DIC is always secondary to severe gastrointestinal diseases, mainly associated with endotoxemia.[1,12]

Horses with Colic at Risk for Disseminated Intravascular Coagulation

The gastrointestinal diseases associated with DIC are the following:

- Ischemic lesions, such as small or large intestinal volvuli, large colon torsions, herniations (inguinal, epiploic foramen, and others), incarcerations, and so forth. The incidence of DIC in horses with ischemic disorders is cited around 55%,[3,6] and specifically in horses with a large colon volvulus around 70%.[9]
- Acute inflammatory conditions, such as severe colitis and duodenitis-proximal enteritis. Different studies have reported that horses with acute colitis or proximal enteritis may commonly show clinicopathologic evidence of DIC, and some of them may show hemorrhagic signs.[3,6,7] The reported incidence of DIC in horses with acute enteritis is 32% to 36%,[6,7] although this percentage was mildly higher (38%) in diarrheic horses with poor prognosis that died or were euthanized.[15] Dolente and colleagues[7] also mentioned that horses with acute colitis that had evidence of DIC were more likely to die or be euthanatized.
- Severe peritonitis, such as septic peritonitis, intestinal tears and ruptures, uterine tears, intra-abdominal abscesses, and so forth. These severe clinical conditions may also develop a marked hypercoagulation and DIC, which may contribute to the high mortality rate.[16]
- Chronic enteropathies, such as protein-losing enteropathy.[17]
- Other uncommon diseases, such as disseminated abdominal malignancies.

How to Diagnose Disseminated Intravascular Coagulation in Horses with Colic

Clinical manifestations of disseminated intravascular coagulation

Clinical signs may be observed in severe forms of DIC. Hemorrhagic diathesis due to excessive coagulation factor consumption is the most reported clinical manifestation of DIC in veterinary textbooks (the bleeding form of DIC), because prolonged bleeding is easily viewed and recognized as hemostatic disorder. This bleeding form is characterized by spontaneous hemorrhages from mucous membranes and genitourinary and gastrointestinal tracts (eg, epistaxis, hematuria) or a hemorrhagic tendency after venipuncture or minor trauma/surgery. In horses with colic, these clinical findings are not frequently seen, although they have been reported in some cases with severe inflammatory problems and surgical cases with severe ischemic lesions.[3,9] In experimentally induced ischemic lesion in ponies significant abnormalities in coagulation parameters consistent with DIC were evident after few hours of strangulation, but ponies died without showing hemorrhagic signs.[18]

Thrombotic events have rarely been reported in horses with colic, maybe because of the difficulty of recognizing them clinically, except for catheter-associated jugular thrombophlebitis or some thrombotic events found at postmortem examination.

Jugular thrombophlebitis may be a common complication in horses with severe colic (eg, inflammatory conditions). It was reported that horses with salmonellosis or clinical signs compatible with endotoxemia (eg, fever, neutropenia, and so forth) are more likely to develop jugular thrombophlebitis (the odds of developing thrombophlebitis were 68 times greater for a horse with salmonellosis and 18 times greater for a horse with endotoxemia).[19] The higher incidence of catheter-associated jugular thrombosis in these patients is mainly related to their hypercoagulable state and the development of DIC, and to drugs administered through the catheter and the type of catheter material used (eg, polyurethane is a less thrombogenic catheter material than others).[20]

Other thrombotic events have also been reported in horses with severe gastrointestinal disease at postmortem examination, such as massive fibrin deposition in capillaries of lung, kidney, and liver,[15,21] and massive pulmonary thromboembolism.[22] In human medicine, less than 5% of patients with DIC show hemorrhagic signs, whereas clinical signs consistent with thrombosis or MOFS are frequently diagnosed.

Finally, clinical signs compatible with organ dysfunction/failure (the MOFS form of DIC), such as oliguria, tachyarrhythmias, shock, and so forth, may be observed in these patients, although MOFS is more easily and frequently detected by the laboratory abnormalities that it produces.[14] Clinicians must be aware of the risk for DIC and MOFS in their patients, otherwise they rarely associate the mentioned clinical signs and clinicopathologic abnormalities with an underlying coagulopathy.

Laboratory diagnosis of disseminated intravascular coagulation

DIC is normally diagnosed based on clinicopathologic evidence of the marked activation of the coagulation system, with the subsequent evidence of coagulation consumption and activation of inhibitory systems. The reported coagulation abnormalities that horses with colic may have are the following:

Platelet consumption In horses with DIC, platelet activation and consumption normally lead to a mild to moderate thrombocytopenia (<100,000/μL). Different studies have included platelet count as one of the common tests to assess coagulation activation and DIC in horses with colic, and thrombocytopenia has been frequently detected in these patients, although the sensitivity and specificity for the diagnosis of DIC may be low.[3,6,9]

Platelet activation Platelet activation can be suspected when a decreased mean platelet component (MPC) value is found, which means that platelets are being activated and degranulated because of coagulation activation. In a recent study, a significant decrease of MPC values was observed in horses with colon obstruction (23 ± 5 g/dL), enteritis (23.6 ± 4.6 g/dL), and ischemic lesion (23.9 ± 5.1 g/dL) compared with control horses (26.2 ± 3.5 g/dL); values were much lower in those horses with thrombocytopenia compatible with DIC (20.2 ± 5.7 g/dL).[23] Because MPC is currently included by modern complete blood count analyzers, it can be easily and rapidly assessed together with platelet count, which helps to conclude when platelet activation and consumption occurs.

Coagulation factor activation Coagulation factor activation can be detected by an increase of plasma thrombin–antithrombin complexes (TAT) concentration and an increase in soluble fibrin monomers. TAT levels were assessed in horses with colic and they were found significantly increased, especially in those with severe gastrointestinal diseases (inflammatory and ischemic disorders) and in nonsurvivors.[3,9,24] Fibrin monomer concentration was also determined in different surgically treated horses with colic and it was increased after surgery and remained increased over time.[25] These tests have only been used in research and are not available in clinical settings.

Coagulation factor consumption Coagulation factor consumption causes a mild to marked prolongation of prothrombin time (PT) and activated partial thromboplastin time (aPTT), being the tests most frequently altered in horses with DIC and easily performed in any laboratory.[3–6,9,25,26] A hypofibrinogenemia may also be seen in some cases consistent with fibrinogen consumption caused by excessive coagulation activation,[6,7] but this decrease can be masked by the liver's ability to generate large amounts of fibrinogen in response to inflammatory conditions.[3,25,26]

Coagulation factor inhibitor consumption This abnormality could be detected by the decrease of plasma antithrombin (AT) or protein C activities. The decrease of AT in horses with colic and DIC has been reported by different studies, which concluded that AT is a sensitive test for the diagnosis of DIC and is of great prognostic value with respect the outcome.[2–4,6,25,27] Results of protein C in horses with severe colic were not specific, however, because it may respond as an acute-phase reaction protein.[4,5,26]

Fibrinolysis system consumption Plasminogen concentration has been evaluated in horses with colic to assess the fibrinolysis activation and subsequent plasminogen consumption, but it has limited usefulness in diagnosing DIC.[4,5,26]

Fibrinolysis system activation

Measurement of fibrinolysis activator The main activator of the fibrinolysis system is tissue plasminogen activator (t-PA). It has been evaluated in horses with colic, and no significant differences were found when compared with control horses.[5,28,29] In a recent study a significant decrease of t-PA levels has been detected in horses with colic (especially in inflammatory and ischemic conditions and peritonitis).[16] This decrease of t-PA has been associated with t-PA activation and consumption.

Measurement of fibrinolysis activator inhibitors The activation of the fibrinolytic system leads to a subsequent increase of the main fibrinolysis inhibitor, such as plasminogen activator inhibitor type-1 (PAI-1). Collatos and colleagues[5,28,29] demonstrated that PAI-1 levels were significantly increased in horses with colic during hospitalization, in nonsurvivors, in horses that underwent surgery, in horses with inflammatory conditions, and in horses with endotoxemia.

Other fibrinolysis inhibitors, such as α_2-antiplasmin, have been evaluated in horses with colic with limited usefulness.[5,26]

Products of fibrinolysis activation The measurement of plasma plasmin–antiplasmin complexes has been demonstrated to be a sensitive marker of detecting fibrinolysis system activation, but the test has not been evaluated in horses with colic. In contrast, the measurement of fibrin(ogen) degradation products (FDPs) and D-dimer concentration has been demonstrated to be useful assessing fibrinolysis activity in the clinical setting in horses with colic and DIC. FDPs have been used to evaluate fibrinolysis activation in horses with colic during the last years, but the sensitivity is low.[2–4,6,7,9,30] On the other hand, D-dimer concentration, as a specific and sensitive fibrin degradation product linked to plasmin activity, has been assessed in horses with colic and has been demonstrated to increase significantly in severe inflammatory conditions (eg, enteritis, peritonitis) and ischemic problems.[10,16,31]

Coagulation and fibrinolysis system activation It has been proposed that thromboelastography may be useful to diagnose hypercoagulability and hypocoagulability in horses with colic, but specific studies assessing its usefulness in these patients are in process.

In summary, the coagulation profile that most frequently has been used to diagnose DIC in horses with colic, including tests cost effective in clinical setting and available in most laboratories, consists of platelet count, clotting times (PT and aPTT), fibrinogen concentration, AT activity, and D-dimer concentration.[1] DIC is generally diagnosed when more than three of these tests are significantly altered.[3,6,9,14] Different studies have assessed coagulation abnormalities in horses with gastrointestinal disease using these tests. The conclusion is that horses with colon obstructions rarely have coagulation abnormalities, whereas inflammatory and ischemic intestinal lesions may show some abnormalities on admission, consistent with DIC in the most severe cases (**Box 2**).[3–7,9,27] These coagulation alterations normally increase during the first days of hospitalization (medical cases) and after surgery (ischemic cases), but they usually return to reference ranges when discharged.[9,11,25]

In addition to the coagulation abnormalities, a serum biochemical study should be included in the clinicopathologic investigation of severe cases, to detect tissue hypoxia, organ dysfunction, and organ failure when present. Biochemistry abnormalities (such as increased serum concentration of creatinine and blood urea nitrogen) can be found in colic cases with renal failure related to coagulopathy.

Treatment of Disseminated Intravascular Coagulation in Horses with Colic

The first objective of DIC treatment is to control the underlying gastrointestinal disease that is causing the severe hypercoagulable state. In ischemic disorders surgical resolution of the situation decreasing blood supply is paramount, including, if necessary, removal of the affected intestine and the administration of antibiotics in horses with septic peritonitis, the administration of those treatments to reduce endotoxemia (such as fluid therapy, low-dose flunixin meglumine, polymyxin B), and so forth.[32]

The second objective of DIC treatment (for both compensated and uncompensated forms) is to stop the severe hypercoagulable state and subsequent consumptive coagulopathy. The administration of heparin in horses with colic at risk for DIC from the beginning is considered the most effective and safe treatment for reducing the severe hypercoagulable state and DIC.[32,33] Other anticoagulants (such as aspirin and warfarin) are not recommended in horses because of their low effectiveness and high incidence of adverse effects.

Two types of heparin are recommended in horses with colic at risk for DIC:

- Unfractioned heparin (UFH): Its efficacy in horses as antithrombotic is controversial, and different detrimental effects have been reported when using this kind of heparin. The main detrimental effects are a dose-dependent erythrocyte agglutination effect that can produce an extravascular hemolysis and moderate anemia, and a thrombocytopenic effect that can increase the risk for hemorrhage.[33,34] When used, the recommended dosage is 40 to 100 U/kg every 12 hours subcutaneously or intravenously.

Box 2
Hemostatic profile recommended in clinical settings for the diagnosis of disseminated intravascular coagulation in a horse with colic

Platelet count

Mean platelet component

Clotting times (PT and aPTT)

Fibrinogen concentration

D-dimer concentration

- Low molecular weight heparin (LMWH): This heparin is more effective and safer than UFH and does not have reported detrimental effects, such as the erythrocyte agglutination and the secondary hemolysis and anemia.[33–35] Depending on the LMWH used, recommended dosages of the most effective marketed LMWHs are the following:
- Dalteparin (Kabi Pharmacia AB, Stockholm, Sweden): 50 IU/kg subcutaneously every 24 hours for 3 to 4 days
- Enoxaparin (Sanofi-Aventis US, Bridgewater, NJ): 0.5 mg/kg subcutaneously every 24 hours for 3 to 4 days

In horses with colic with clinicopathologic evidence of coagulation abnormalities and without clinical signs consistent with organ failure or bleeding (subclinical form of DIC), the early administration of LMWH helps to reduce (1) excessive fibrin deposition that might progress to multiorgan dysfunction/failure, and (2) excessive coagulation consumption that might progress to the hemorrhagic form of DIC. Horses with inflammatory disorders receiving LMWH from the first day of hospitalization and horses with ischemic lesions receiving LMWH after surgery rapidly normalize their coagulation abnormalities, as observed by Cesarini and colleagues[11] and Cotovio and colleagues.[15]

When horses with colic show the uncompensated forms of DIC (the MOFS or the bleeding form of DIC), additional treatments should complement those previously cited for DIC in general.[32] In these cases, however, the primary gastrointestinal problem and the treatment decided has to be reassessed regularly/frequently to detect bad progression leading to poor prognosis. These other treatments are the following:

- The MOFS form of DIC: In horses showing evidence of organ failure, adequate fluid therapy (crystalloids and colloids) reduces the effects of fibrin deposition in tissues and therefore improves blood supply. When a specific organ dysfunction/failure is diagnosed, supportive therapy is needed depending on the organ affected. For instance, in cases with hypoxia and respiratory failure, intranasal oxygen administration is recommended; in cases with renal failure, dobutamine, dopamine (to improve renal blood flow), furosemide, and adequate fluid therapy are recommended.
- The bleeding form of DIC: When horses with colic show spontaneous hemorrhages, transfusion of fresh plasma (15–30 mL/kg) is the most recommended treatment to replace the platelets, coagulation factors, and coagulation inhibitors that have been consumed. If only hemorrhagic tendency is detected after minor trauma/surgery or venipunctures, fresh-frozen plasma transfusion can be used. In both cases, the LMWH therapy is recommended, although treatment is controversial.

Why Any Horse with Compensated or Uncompensated Disseminated Intravascular Coagulation Should Be Treated: Consequences of Disseminated Intravascular Coagulation

The main consequence of hypercoagulation and DIC is the formation and deposition of fibrin microthrombi in capillaries of different organs, which may cause tissue hypoxia, organ dysfunction/failure, and death. Using specific histochemical and immunohistochemical stainings for visualizing fibrin in equine tissue specimens, Cotovio and colleagues[15,21] demonstrated that fibrin deposition is observed in capillaries of different organs (lungs, kidneys, and liver) in horses with different gastrointestinal diseases (such as inflammatory/ischemic conditions and peritonitis). But this fibrin deposition may occur not only in horses with DIC of poor prognosis (uncompensated forms of DIC) but also in less severe forms of DIC (compensated form of DIC). The administration of antithrombotic drugs should be considered in any horse with colic at risk for DIC, to control the hypercoagulable state, to reduce the amount of fibrin deposition from the beginning, and to avoid the subsequent development of MOFS. The control of fibrin deposition may help to improve prognosis in horses with colic at risk for DIC.

Other Nonintravascular Coagulopathies Observed in Horses with Colic

In horses with colic, it has also been reported that severe gastrointestinal disorders produce significant changes in intraperitoneal coagulation and fibrinolysis activities. The formation of fibrin in the peritoneal cavity is a physiologic response of the mesothelial cells after visceral trauma, to produce a matrix covering the damaged area before the cellular regeneration is performed.[36,37] This peritoneal hypercoagulation produces a secondary increase of the peritoneal fibrinolysis activity, to control fibrin formation and deposition in the serosa and peritoneal cavity, and, consequently, to avoid the risk for adhesions.

In horses suffering from gastrointestinal disorders, those diseases producing more damage of the intestinal wall (such as inflammatory and ischemic disorders) are expected to induce greater increases in fibrin formation, thus increasing the risk for adhesions. Collatos and colleagues[5,28] demonstrated that in horses with colic, especially those horses with endotoxins in peritoneal fluid and those horses that did not survive, the peritoneal hyperfibrinolysis was significantly higher compared with other horses with colic without endotoxemia (such as obstructions), based on the measurement of peritoneal FDPs and t-PA.

More recently, the measurement of D-dimer concentration in peritoneal fluid by the authors' group has been demonstrated to be a useful test for the assessment of peritoneal fibrinolysis activity in horses with colic, and for the diagnosis and outcome of horses with different acute gastrointestinal diseases.[16] Particularly, in this study it has been observed that peritoneal D-dimer concentration was significantly higher in all colic groups compared with control horses and significantly higher in horses suffering severe GI diseases (such as enteritis, peritonitis, and ischemic lesions) compared with horses with large intestinal obstructions.[16] The peritoneal D-dimer concentration in control horses was low (median, 25th–75th; 36 ng/mL, 4–88), much lower than that observed in plasma, whereas it was significantly higher in horses with colon obstructions (2022.8 ng/mL, 576.8–7198), and markedly higher in horses with enteritis (8028 ng/mL, 3185.1–13,720), ischemic lesions (16,181 ng/mL, 3946–31,844), and severe peritonitis (24,301 ng/mL, 1682–82,208). The increase of D-dimer concentration in peritoneal fluid was significantly correlated with a decrease in peritoneal t-PA activity, which was consistent with t-PA consumption.[16] Results of this study also showed that the peritoneal coagulopathy observed in horses with colic (increase of the coagulation and fibrinolysis activities) is totally independent of changes in coagulation and fibrinolysis occurring in blood.[16] Regarding the outcome, peritoneal D-dimer values also were significantly higher in nonsurvivors. Finally, blood contamination of peritoneal fluid occurring during routine sampling did not affect peritoneal D-dimer concentration evaluation.[38]

HYPOCOAGULATION IN HORSES WITH COLIC

Hypocoagulable state is uncommon in horses showing clinical signs of colic. When this coagulopathy is detected in horses with a primary gastrointestinal disease (generally in horses with a clinical history of diarrhea and with a severe inflammatory disorder and endotoxemia diagnosed), it normally corresponds to the bleeding form of DIC. But hypocoagulation can also be diagnosed in horses showing clinical signs of abdominal discomfort without having a primary gastrointestinal problem, such as in liver diseases.

The coagulopathy is mainly characterized by a defect in coagulation due to a decrease in coagulation factor synthesis (eg, hepatopathies), or excessive coagulation consumption (bleeding form of DIC), although other defects in coagulation might occur (eg, platelet destruction due to an immune-mediated reaction secondary to bacterial or viral infections).

The coagulation deficiency leads to a hemorrhagic syndrome, with petechiation in mucous membranes; prolonged bleeding following minor surgery, wounds, or venipunctures; or spontaneous bleeding from mucous membranes, genitourinary tract, and gastrointestinal tract (ie, epistaxis, hematuria).[39] These clinical signs are easily detected, and clinicians can rapidly associate them with a coagulation dysfunction.

From a clinical point of view, in horses with colic with a severe gastrointestinal disease that suddenly show a hemorrhagic syndrome, the bleeding form of DIC should first be considered. On the other hand, if horses show abdominal discomfort with bleeding signs and DIC can be ruled out, few other causes can be associated with a coagulation defect. These other clinical conditions are the following:

Hepatopathy

It is known that horses with liver disease may show clinical signs suggestive of intestinal disease, such as colic and diarrhea,[40–43] and some primary gastrointestinal disorders may affect the liver (eg, biliary obstruction and ischemia in severe distended colon, high concentrations of endotoxins in inflammatory and ischemic lesions, and so forth).[44,45] Liver damage must be severe to cause coagulation dysfunction and failure.[39]

Horses with liver disease commonly may have abnormalities of the coagulation system consistent with a hypocoagulable state. Hepatic failure is mainly associated with a decrease in the majority of coagulation factor function and synthesis that produces the coagulation defect. Hemostasis may also be impaired in these patients by other alterations, however, such as platelet dysfunction, anticoagulant dysfunction, abnormal clearance of fibrinolytic activators, and so forth.[46,47] Although an abnormal hemostatic panel consistent with a hypocoagulable state can be commonly observed in horses with hepatic failure, clinical bleeding signs are rarely observed. In a recent study, the frequency of abnormalities in the coagulation panel performed in horses with histopathologically confirmed liver disease was high (58%), although no association was observed between abnormalities in hemostatic parameters and bleeding complications after liver biopsy.[48]

Clinical management

- Diagnosis is based on the laboratory evidence of liver damage and dysfunction (altered serum concentration of liver enzymes, bilirubins, bile acids, and so forth) and the coagulation defect (prolongation of clotting times, and so forth), with no evidence of hyperfibrinolysis (normal to mildly increased plasma D-dimer concentration).[33,43]
- Treatment should focus on first resolving the liver disease whenever possible, although antihemorrhagic drugs (eg, ε-aminocaproic acid) and fresh plasma transfusion should be added when the horse shows spontaneous bleeding.[33,43]

Other Clinical Conditions

There are other clinical conditions with which horses may show clinical signs consistent with a coagulation defect and uncommonly might show abdominal discomfort:

- Some viral or bacterial diseases (eg, *Streptococcus equi* infection). In these cases, the coagulation defect frequently is secondary to immune-mediated vasculitis or thrombocytopenia.
- Vitamin K deficiency (eg, dicumarol and warfarin intoxication).

SUMMARY

The most common coagulopathy in horses with colic is a hypercoagulable state associated with DIC. The intensity of this coagulopathy depends on the severity and duration of the gastrointestinal lesion, with the ischemic and inflammatory problems and peritonitis being the most frequently affected by coagulopathies. DIC can be related to severe complications, such as fibrin deposition in the microvasculature, tissue ischemia, multiorgan failure, bleeding diathesis, and death. Early initiation of prophylactic therapy in horses with intestinal conditions recognized at high risk for DIC significantly reduces the severe hypercoagulable state, decreasing the amount of fibrin formation, fibrin deposition, and consequently a bad progression of DIC.

In addition to the systemic coagulopathy observed in horses with colic, a peritoneal coagulopathy independent from that occurring in blood has been observed, and its recognition and assessment may have clinical usefulness in the diagnosis of the gastrointestinal diseases and outcome.

REFERENCES

1. Dallap BL. Coagulopathy in the equine critical patient. Vet Clin North Am Equine Pract 2004;20(1):231–51.
2. Johnstone I, Crane S. Haemostatic abnormalities in horses with colic—their prognostic value. Equine Vet J 1986;18(4):271–4.
3. Welch R, Watkins J, Taylor T, et al. Disseminated intravascular coagulation associated with colic in 23 horses (1984–1989). J Vet Intern Med 1992;6(1):29–35.
4. Prasse K, Topper M, Moore J, et al. Analysis of hemostasis in horses with colic. J Am Vet Med Assoc 1993;5(1):685–93.
5. Collatos C, Barton MH, Prasse KW, et al. Intravascular and peritoneal coagulation and fibrinolysis in horses with acute gastrointestinal tract disease. J Am Vet Med Assoc 1995;207(4):465–70.
6. Monreal L, Anglés A, Espada Y, et al. Hypercoagulation and hypofibrinolysis in horses with colic and DIC. Equine Vet J 2000;32(Suppl):19–25.
7. Dolente BA, Wilkins PA, Boston RC. Clinicopathologic evidence of disseminated intravascular coagulation in horses with acute colitis. J Am Vet Med Assoc 2002; 220(7):1034–8.
8. Yilmaz Z, Şentürk S, İçöl Y. Analysis of hemostasis in horses with colic. Israel J Vet Med 2002;57(2):19–25.
9. Dallap BL, Dolente B, Boston R. Coagulation profiles in 27 horses with large colon volvulus. J Vet Emerg Crit Care 2003;13(4):215–25.
10. Armengou L, Monreal L, Segura D, et al. Plasma D-dimers in horses with colic. In: Proceeding of the 8th Equine Colic Research Symposium. Quebec (Canada), 2004.
11. Cesarini C, Monreal L, Segura D, et al. Hemostatic follow up of horses with medical and surgical colic. J Vet Intern Med 2009;23(2):434.

12. Lassen ED, Swardson CJ. Hematology and hemostasis in the horse: normal functions and common abnormalities. Vet Clin North Am Equine Pract 1995;11(3): 351–89.

13. Brooks MB. Equine coagulopathies. Vet Clin North Am Equine Pract 2008;24(2): 335–55.

14. Monreal L. Disseminated intravascular coagulation. In: Hinchkliff KN, Couëtil L, editors. Blackwell's five-minute veterinary consult. 2nd edition. Oxford (UK): Blackwell Publishing; 2009, in press.

15. Cotovio M, Monreal L, Navarro M, et al. Detection of fibrin deposits in tissues from horses with severe gastrointestinal disorders. J Vet Intern Med 2007;21(2):308–13.

16. Delgado MA, Monreal L, Armengou L, et al. Peritoneal D-dimer concentration for assessing peritoneal fibrinolytic activity in horses with colic. J Vet Intern Med 2009;23, in press.

17. Morris DD, Vaala WE, Sartin E. Protein-losing enteropathy in a yearling filly with subclinical disseminated intravascular coagulation and autoimmune hemolytic disease. Comp Cont Educ Pract Vet 1982;4(12):542–6.

18. Pablo L, Purohit R, Teer P, et al. Disseminated intravascular coagulation in experimental intestinal strangulation obstruction in ponies. Am J Vet Res 1983;44(11): 2115–22.

19. Dolente BA, Beech J, Lindborg S, et al. Evaluation of risk factors for the development of catheter-associated jugular thrombophlebitis in horses: 50 cases (1993–1998). J Am Vet Med Assoc 2005;227(7):1134–41.

20. Divers TJ. Prevention and treatment of thrombosis, phlebitis, and laminitis in horses with gastrointestinal diseases. Vet Clin North Am Equine Pract 2003; 19(3):779–90.

21. Cotovio M, Monreal L, Navarro M, et al. Detection of fibrin deposits in horse tissues by immunohistochemistry. J Vet Intern Med 2007;21(5):1083–9.

22. Norman TE, Chaffin MK, Perris EE, et al. Massive pulmonary thromboembolism in six horses. Equine Vet J 2008;40(5):514–7.

23. Segura D, Monreal L, Armengou L, et al. Mean platelet component as an indicator of platelet activation in foals and adult horses. J Vet Intern Med 2007;21(5): 1076–82.

24. Topper M, Prasse K. Use of enzyme-linked immunosorbent assay to measure thrombin-antithrombin III complexes in horses with colic. Am J Vet Res 1996; 57(4):456–62.

25. Feige K, Kästner SBR, Dempfle CE, et al. Changes in coagulation and markers of fibrinolysis in horses undergoing colic surgery. J Vet Med A Physiol Pathol Clin Med 2003;50(1):30–6.

26. Topper MJ, Prasse KW. Analysis of coagulation proteins as acute-phase reactants in horses with colic. Am J Vet Res 1998;59(5):542–5.

27. Holland M, Kelly A, Snyder J, et al. Antithrombin III activity in horses with large colon torsion. Am J Vet Res 1986;47(4):897–900.

28. Collatos C, Barton MH, Schleef R, et al. Regulation of equine fibrinolysis in blood and peritoneal fluid based on a study of colic cases and induced endotoxaemia. Equine Vet J 1994;26(6):474–81.

29. Collatos C, Barton MH, Moore JN. Fibrinolytic activity in plasma from horses with gastrointestinal diseases: Changes associated with diagnosis, surgery, and outcome. J Vet Intern Med 1995;9(1):18–23.

30. Stokol T, Erb HN, De Wilde L, et al. Evaluation of latex agglutination kits for detection of fibrin(ogen) degradation products and D-dimer in healthy horses and horses with severe colic. Vet Clin Pathol 2005;3(4):375–82.

31. Sandholm M, Vidovic A, Puotunen-Reinert A, et al. D-dimer improves the prognostic value of combined clinical and laboratory data in equine gastrointestinal colic. Acta Vet Scand 1995;36(2):255–72.

32. Monreal L. Treating disseminated intravascular coagulation. Comp Cont Educ Vet Equine 2008;3(6):326–30.

33. Monreal L, Aguilera E. Management of horses with coagulopathies. In: Corley K, Stephen J, editors. The equine hospital manual. Oxford (UK): Blackwell Publishing; 2008. p. 409–16.

34. Monreal L, Villatoro AJ, Monreal M, et al. Comparison of the effects of low-molecular-weight and unfractioned heparin in horses. Am J Vet Res 1995;56(10): 1281–5.

35. Feige K, Schwarzwald CC, Bombeli T. Comparison of unfractioned and low molecular weight heparin for prophylaxis of coagulopathies in 52 horses with colic: a randomised double-blind clinical trial. Equine Vet J 2003;35(5):506–13.

36. diZerega GS, Campeau JD. Peritoneal repair and post-surgical adhesion formation. Hum Reprod Uptake 2001;7(6):547–55.

37. Cheong YC, Laird SM, Li TC, et al. Peritoneal healing and adhesion formation/reformation. Hum Reprod Uptake 2001;7(6):556–66.

38. Delgado MA, Monreal L, Tarancón I, et al. Effects of blood contamination on peritoneal D-dimer concentration in horses with colic. In: Proceedings of the 9th International Equine Colic Research Symposium. Liverpool (UK), 2008.

39. Monreal L. Monitoring the coagulation system. In: Corley K, Stephen J, editors. The equine hospital manual. Oxford (UK): Blackwell Publishing; 2008. p. 401–9.

40. Turner TA, Brown CA, Wilson JH, et al. Hepatic lobe torsion as a cause of colic in a horse. Vet Surg 1993;22(4):301–4.

41. Durando MM, MacKay RJ, Staller GS, et al. Septic cholangiohepatitis and cholangiocarcinoma in a horse. J Am Vet Med Assoc 1995;206(7):1018–21.

42. Ryu SH, Bak UB, Lee CW, et al. Cholelithiasis associated with recurrent colic in a thoroughbred mare. J Vet Sci 2004;5(1):79–82.

43. Durham A. Monitoring and treating the liver. In: Corley K, Stephen J, editors. The equine hospital manual. Oxford (UK): Blackwell Publishing; 2008. p. 520–32.

44. Vachon AM, Fisher AT. Small intestinal herniation through the epiploic foramen: 53 cases (1987–1993). Equine Vet J 1995;27(5):373–80.

45. Davis JL, Blikslager AT, Catto K, et al. A retrospective analysis of hepatic injury in horses with proximal enteritis (1984–2002). J Vet Intern Med 2003;17(6):896–901.

46. Lisman T, Leebeek FWG, de Groot PG. Haemostatic abnormalities in patients with liver disease. J Hepatol 2002;37(2):280–7.

47. Tripodi A, Manucci PM. Abnormalities of hemostasis in chronic liver disease: reappraisal of their clinical significance and need for clinical and laboratory research. J Hepatol 2007;46(4):727–33.

48. Johns IC, Sweeney RW. Coagulation abnormalities and complications after percutaneous liver biopsy in horses. J Vet Intern Med 2008;22(1):185–9.

Update on Treatments for Endotoxemia

Gal Kelmer, DVM, MS[a,b,]*

KEYWORDS

- Horses • Endotoxemia • Colic
- Lipopolysaccharide • Polymyxin B

ENDOTOXEMIA BACKGROUND

Endotoxemia is a leading cause of morbidity, mortality, and economic loss to the equine industry.[1] Colic, specifically intestinal strangulation, is the most common cause of endotoxemia in horses. Lipopolysaccharide (LPS), a component of the outer cell membrane of Gram-negative bacteria, stimulates the release of mediators of inflammation, including prostaglandins, histamine, serotonin, kinins, platelet-activating factors and others.[2] Initially, LPS binds to a soluble cell membrane binding protein (LPS-BP), which transfers LPS to the macrophage cell wall receptor CD14-MD2 complex, and in turn transfers the signal through a transduction toll-like-receptor (TLR4) into the cell. The stimulation of TLR4 activates the genes responsible for stimulating production of proinflammatory mediators. Massive inflammation results, which in turn is responsible for cardiovascular depression, pulmonary hypertension, and arterial hypoxemia, which lead to decreased tissue perfusion and peripheral hypoxia and, eventually, if unchecked, multiple organ dysfunction and death.

TREATMENT APPROACH FOR ENDOTOXEMIA

Over the years, many treatment modalities have been used to treat and prevent endotoxemia, but only a few have been proved to be effective therapies. This article reviews treatments that have been proved to be efficacious in the treatment and prevention of endotoxemia in horses. Newer treatment options that show promise and may be clinically useful in the near future are also reviewed. The signal transduction pathway of LPS is complicated, and treatments to block the effects of LPS focus on several targets along this cascade. The first level of treatment intervention focuses on elimination of the source of LPS. Initial treatment for endotoxemia in horses with colic involves

[a] Large Animal Department, Koret Veterinary Teaching Hospital, Hebrew University of Jerusalem, Rehovot, Israel
[b] Department of Large Animal Clinical Sciences, The University of Tennessee College of Veterinary Medicine, 2407 River Drive, Knoxville, TN 37996, USA
* Large Animal Department, Koret Veterinary Teaching Hospital, Hebrew University of Jerusalem, Rehovot, Israel
E-mail address: kelmerg@agri.huji.ac.il

Vet Clin Equine 25 (2009) 259–270
doi:10.1016/j.cveq.2009.04.012
0749-0739/09/$ – see front matter © 2009 Elsevier Inc. All rights reserved.

vetequine.theclinics.com

treating the underlying cause. A strangulating intestinal lesion should be removed in a timely manner, which entails quick decisions on referral, and efficient evaluation and diagnosis to provide rapid surgical exploration and removal.

The second level of treatment intervention involves elimination of LPS before it interacts with the host's receptors sites. This can be achieved by neutralizing LPS, either by administering intravenous polymyxin B or using hemofiltration with polymyxin B as the binding agent. In both techniques, polymixin B binds LPS and thus prevents its contact with receptor sites on mononuclear cells, which in turn prevents the initiation of the inflammatory cascade. The use of antibodies against the CD14 receptor on the macrophages (ie, those responsible for binding the LPS-BP complex) represents another therapeutic avenue aimed at limiting LPS interaction with the body's immune system.

When the inflammatory cascade has been initiated, the use of nonsteroidal anti-inflammatory agents (NSAIDs), specifically flunixin meglumine, may be beneficial. NSAIDs block cyclooxygenase, which prevents the release of prostaglandins, which are important in causing inflammation.

Also, when LPS binds to mononuclear cells, there is a release of proinflammatory cytokines, including tumor necrosis factor (TNF) and others. When these proinflammatory mediators are released, they can be inhibited or blocked by administering antibodies against these cytokines. Antibodies to TNF can potentially block the detrimental effect of these cytokines.

When the inflammatory cascade has been activated, the main effort uses supportive fluid therapy to ameliorate the cardiovascular shock that occurs. Also, laminitis is a common sequel to endotoxemia, so the use of cryotherapy may be helpful in horses with endotoxemia to prevent laminitis. However, covering laminitis prophylaxis is beyond the scope of this article, and the interested reader is referred to an excellent review by van Eps and Pollitt.[3]

TREATMENT MODALITIES
Fluid Therapy

Fluid therapy is the mainstay basic, nonspecific, supportive therapeutic strategy to combat the hemodynamic effects of LPS. This article is limited to a brief discussion of fluid therapy in the endotoxemic patient because a complete discussion of all available fluid therapy is beyond its scope. Nearly all endotoxemic patients are at least moderately, if not severely dehydrated, and thus the use of balanced crystalloid solutions are an essential part of the initial stabilization therapy. Endotoxemia leads to an alternation in vascular and mucosal permeability, leading to protein loss and reduced colloidal oncotic pressure. The use of colloid therapy, including synthetic and natural colloids, is indicated to increase the colloidal oncotic pressure and arrest the vicious cycle of protein loss.

The use of hypertonic saline (7%–7.5% Na-Cl at 4 mL/kg) is indicated initially in horses presenting with endotoxemia, and it provides immediate improvement in tissue perfusion and has been shown to exert some antiendotoxemic effects.[4,5]

Hetastarch (HES; hydroxyethyl starch at 10–20 mL/kg) is an effective colloidal solution in the horse, increasing the colloidal oncotic pressure and maintaining it for a 24-hour period. Studies on rat models of endotoxemia have demonstrated that the use of HES decreased production of liver inflammatory mediators, improved intestinal microcirculation, and restored pulmonary function.[6–8] Also, in a study involving induced endotoxemia in hamsters, the use of HES improved microcirculation in normotensive hamsters, even when it was given after LPS administration. However, the effects of

HES in horses have been questioned. In a controlled prospective study, hypertonic saline and HES administered to endotoxemic horses failed to abate the hemodynamic effects of LPS.[9] Clearly, further studies, ideally clinical trials, are necessary to better evaluate the role of these agents in the management of endotoxemia in horses.

Fresh-frozen plasma (2–8 L/horse, IV), a natural colloid, is often included in the treatment of endotoxemia in horses.[10] Hyperimmune plasma is typically used and provides essential proteins and natural inflammatory agents that help block the effects of endotoxemia. In addition to providing albumin, which improves the plasma's oncotic pressure, the plasma provides a variety of molecules active in the clotting cascade, such as fibronectin, antithrombin, complement, and other factors.

The addition of unfractioned heparin (100 international units/kg, body weight [bwt]) to the plasma may prime the antithrombin and improve coagulation function. Because endotoxemia often affects the coagulation system and eventually leads to disseminated coagulation, plasma therapy carries a significant added benefit and may be a highly effective treatment modality.[10] However, evidence to support these assumptions and studies evaluating the potential benefit of plasma administration in horses with endotoxemia are lacking. More information on coagulopathies in horses with colic can be found elsewhere in this issue.

Flunixin Meglumine

Flunixin meglumine (FM) is a potent NSAID that is considered one of the mainstays in antiendotoxemic treatment in horses. FM inhibits the cyclooxygenase breakdown of arachidonic acid to prostaglandins, which are important in producing the systemic effects of endotoxemia, including arterial hypoxemia, vasodilation, cardiovascular shock, and diarrhea.[11] Studies have shown that pretreatment using FM in horses administered endotoxin effectively prevents the occurrence of clinical signs related to endotoxemia.[12,13] However, in the clinical setting, pretreatment is a rare situation, whereas combating existing endotoxemia is the common scenario. In addition, there is a continuous insult of LPS in the naturally occurring disease process as the intestines become nonviable. The clinical condition of small intestinal strangulation is likely to be far more complicated than the administration of low-dose LPS in the experimental model. For these reasons, although it is helpful clinically, FM may not lead to complete amelioration of the clinical signs produced by endotoxin challenge. In addition, several studies conclusively showed that FM has detrimental effects on the small intestine by decreasing the transepithelial electric resistance and increasing the influx of endotoxin from the intestine, and that it may paradoxically exacerbate existing endotoxemia.[14,15] Other studies showed that the decrease in transepithelial electric resistance and recovery of large colon mucosa were not affected by FM administration.[16,17] Therefore, for horses suffering from large colon ischemia such as large colon volvulus, administration of FM (1.1 mg/kg, IV) is safe and effective. Because detrimental effects were demonstrated in horses administered FM (1.1 mg/kg, IV), administration of a lower dose (0.25 mg/kg, IV) has been shown to be effective. In horses suffering from small intestinal ischemia, a lower dose of FM (0.25 mg/kg, IV) may be used, because it has been shown to be effective in experimentally induced endotoxemia in horses[18] and has been used extensively in the clinical setting.[10] Administration of FM in this lower dose may eliminate side effects such as gastrointestinal ulceration and nephrotoxicity. Furthermore, because the lower dose may not prevent the clinical signs of endotoxemia in horses, an intermediate dose (0.55 mg/kg, IV) may be helpful in ameliorating endotoxemia-induced clinical signs such has abdominal pain, fever, and depression,[1] while being less likely to cause detrimental side effects. Clinically, this dose seems useful when given three to four times each day in the postoperative period, but further studies are needed to examine its efficacy and side effects.

Alternatively, specific Cox-2 inhibitors such as firocoxib may be useful in the treatment of endotoxemia in horses. An initial study by Cook and colleagues[19] demonstrated the visceral analgesic effects of firocoxib, whereas there was no deleterious effect on small intestinal mucosal permeability. Currently, firocoxib is only available as an oral formulation, and its safety and efficacy in horses presenting for colic has not been clinically evaluated. Thus, taking its limitations into account, FM is still currently the anti-inflammatory drug of choice for perioperative colic cases.

Antibiotics

The use of antibiotic therapy in the management of endotoxemia is controversal.[1] Administration of antibiotics to horses with endotoxemia may exacerbate the condition by further killing Gram-negative bacteria and releasing more endotoxin. This is a concern in septic human patients and can cause clinical deterioration.[20] However, because the immune system in endotoxemic patients is overwhelmed and dysfunctional, antibiotic administration during cases of acute endotoxemia may protect against opportunistic infections.[1] This scenario occurs in neonatal foals with failure of passive transfer, in which administration of antibiotics is indicated to prevent opportunistic infection.[21]

Antibiotics are routinely used in horses with perioperative colic, but horses with nonsurgical lesions such as colitis or long-standing impactions may be treated using antibiotics depending on their clinical status and complete blood count. In a survey of equine medicine and surgery specialists, a majority used antibiotics for treatment of endotoxemia in their patients, and it was the third most chosen treatment modality.[10]

An in vitro septicemia model in neonatal foals showed that the use of β-lactam antimicrobials, including ampicillin and ceftiofur, caused an increase in endotoxin release and TNF-α activity, whereas concurrent administration of amikacin significantly decreased endotoxin activity.[21] It previously had been shown that antimicrobials such as aminoglycosides and carbapenems cause minimal LPS release because of their rapid kill and their ability to inhibit protein synthesis without disrupting the bacteria's cell wall. In addition, aminoglycosides neutralize LPS and inhibit its synthesis, minimizing endotoxemia.[22,23] In conclusion, when antibiotic use in the endotoxemic patient is indicated, the choice of antibiotic should be made carefully.

Dimethyl Sulfoxide

Dimethyl sufoxide (DMSO), an oxygen–free radical scavenger and potent anti-inflammatory agent, was one of the most commonly used drugs against endotoxemia in a recent survey of clinical equine specialists.[10] Interestingly, despite its ubiquitous use, evidence to support its alleged antiendotoxic effect in the horse is lacking.[24] The justification for its use is that endotoxin induces oxidative damage, which leads to the clinical signs.[25] In mice, high-dose DMSO totally prevented intestinal injury subsequent to experimentally induced endotoxemia.[26] In humans and rats, DMSO inhibits IL-8 production[27] and prevents adhesion of neutrophils to the endothelium, respectively;[28] DMSO also effectively scavenges free radical oxygen species and reduces platelet aggregation in humans and rats.[29,30] In mice, DMSO inhibits LPS-induced TNF-α production and formation of intercellular adhesion molecules, reduces activation of the nuclear transcription factor kappa B (NF-kappa B), and markedly reduces LPS-induced liver damage.[31] Although high-dose DMSO (1 g/kg bwt, IV) is used clinically in horses with compromised gastrointestinal tracts, there is no study indicating its efficacy. Low-dose DMSO (20 mg/kg bwt) has antiadhesive properties in foals and protects against experimentally induced small intestinal ischemia in adult horses.[32,33] In a recent study performed in the author's laboratory, horses administered endotoxin were pretreated using a high dose (1 mg/kg, IV) or low dose (20 mg/kg, IV) of DMSO, and the high dose produced mild changes in clinical parameters.[34] In two studies, the use of high-dose DMSO failed to provide benefits to horses with ischemic large colon, and to some degree it worsened mucosal damage and caused increased levels of oxidized glutathione.[35,36] Because high concentrations of DMSO (1 gm/kg, IV) paradoxically cause lipid peroxidation and potentially exacerbate the injury to the ischemic intestine, it should not be used in horses with large intestinal lesions, and probably it should be altogether avoided in horses with gastrointestinal lesions until there is evidence to the contrary.[35] Because the use of low-dose DMSO showed beneficial effects in an ischemic small intestine model, despite its lack of efficacy as a specific antiendotoxic drug, its can be recommended at this dose for clinical use. However, further investigation, including prospective clinical trials, is needed to determine its role in the treatment of horses with colic.

Lidocaine

Lidocaine is a local anesthetic drug that exerts this effect by blocking sodium channels, which prevents action-potential propagation. Lidocaine has been reported to be the most commonly used postoperative prokinetic drug (1.3 mg/kg bolus IV, followed by CRI 0.05 mg/kg/min) in horses;[37] however, studies evaluating its prokinetic effects yielded mixed results. A thorough, systematic review in 2008 of the medical literature concerning its use in humans revealed that lidocaine did have some positive prokinetic effects, but the evidence was not conclusive.[38] In recent reports of its use in postoperative clinical human patients, lidocaine that was administered intraoperatively and continued postoperatively as a constant rate infusion (CRI) resulted in decreased length of postoperative ileus (POI), shorter hospitalization stays, and decreased postoperative small intestinal distension, as determined using ultrasonograms.[39,40] However, reports from one of the latter studies support the ineffectiveness of lidocaine as a prokinetic because it failed to decrease the length of POI and did not affect the presence of gastric reflux and gastrointestinal sounds and the passage of feces in the first postoperative day.[39] A study of healthy horses failed to demonstrate any effect of lidocaine on motility, duration of migrating myoelectric complexes, and spiking activity in the instrumented jejunum.[41] Also, in an in vitro study, lidocaine failed to induce contractility in isolated small intestinal smooth muscle.[42] Similarly, in a recent study of healthy horses, the use of lidocaine had no effect on jejunal motility and gastric and cecal emptying.[43] In another study, CRI of lidocaine decreased motility, as shown by longer fecal transit time.[44] Thus, in healthy horses, lidocaine does not produce prokinetic effects. However, in a recent clinical study of horses, lidocaine improved the survival rate in postoperative cases; however, it did not decrease the duration of POI.[45] This interesting clinical finding supports the use of lidocaine postoperatively; however, the mode of action of lidocaine in these cases may be unrelated to its prokinetic effects. Although lidocaine is an effective and commonly used analgesic, it does not seem to have an effect on visceral pain in the horse.[46]

One possible mechanism for POI is traumatic manipulation of the intestine during surgery leading to inflammation and ileus. In this model, lidocaine has been shown to have anti-inflammatory properties. Because in clinical cases inflammation is likely to be at least partially responsible for causing POI,[47] this is a plausible explanation as to why lidocaine may be effective as a prokinetic agent in postoperative colic patients and not in normal horses. Further evidence of this in other species has been established. In a research study using rabbits, lidocaine administered intravenously after injection of LPS showed profound anti-inflammatory effects and completely abolished clinical signs of endotoxemia.[48]

Lidocaine has been shown to attenuate intestinal ischemia in an experimental model.[45] In that study, lidocaine decreased LPS influx after ischemia was induced in the jejunum. Lidocaine also negated the deleterious effects of FM on transepithelial electric resistance and LPS influx. Thus, lidocaine has anti-ischemic effects on different organs in multiple species.[47] Because FM is routinely used in the perioperative period in horses with surgical colic for its useful analgesic and anti-inflammatory properties, concurrent routine use of lidocaine with CRI seems to have a justifiable indication. For further reading on the use of lidocaine in equine gastrointestinal lesions, the reader is referred to the 2008 comprehensive review by Cook and Blikslager.[47]

Polymyxin B

Polymyxin B is a cationic cyclic polypeptide antimicrobial drug that is effective against Gram-negative bacteria; however, at antibacterial doses it has severe nephrotoxicity and neurotoxicity-limiting side effects.[49] It is interesting that as a result of the rapid development of multidrug-resistant bacterial strains, there is a renewed interest in polymyxin B as an effective antibiotic for human sepsis, and recent evidence suggests that it is far less toxic than previously considered.[50] At lower doses, polymyxin B acts as a chelating agent by binding to the lipid-A moiety of LPS, which removes endotoxin from the vascular system, and by that action prevents the development of the proinflammatory cascade of endotoxemia.[49] The lipid-A portion of LPS is highly conserved in Gram-negative bacteria, and thus polymyxin B is effective regardless of which Gram-negative bacteria is isolated.[51] In a study of foals administered endotoxin, polymyxin B ameliorated clinical signs such as fever and tachycardia and decreased concentrations of TNF-α and IL-6.[52] Other studies have established safety and dose regimens of polymyxin B (5000 units/kg, IV) in horses and have further elucidated its ability to bind to LPS and its antiendotoxic effects in ex vivo and in vivo models at this effective dose.[49,53,54] In a more recent in vivo study, polymyxin B (5000 units/kg, IV, given over 30 minutes) was found to be effective in lessening clinical signs of endotoxemia such as fever, tachycardia, and tachypnea and in reducing serum TNF-α concentrations, without adverse effects.[53] Another recent study of polymyxin B (6000 units/kg, IV, in a liter of saline solution, given over 15 minutes, every 8 hours, for five doses) showed that it was safe and effective in treating endotoxemia in horses.[49] Although polymyxin B was found safe in these studies in healthy horses with mild, experimentally induced endotoxemia, in the clinical setting, horses are often dehydrated and have compromised renal function; thus, polymyxin B should be used cautiously. In horses with clinical evidence of endotoxemia, the use of aggressive IV fluid therapy is indicated before the use of polymyxin B, and a lower initial dose of polymyxin B (1000–2000 units/kg bwt, IV, over 30 minutes) can be given until hemodynamic status is achieved and azotemia is resolved.[55] In the author's clinical experience, the use of polymyxin B for treatment of endotoxemia following gastrointestinal insult and other causes is safe and effective. However, there is need for clinical trials to further evaluate the efficacy of polymyxin B as a treatment for endotoxemia.

Ketamine

Ketamine is a dissociative anesthetic that blocks the N-methyl-D-aspartate receptors. It is used extensively in horses with other pharmacologic agents to induce general anesthesia. Also, ketamine is a potent analgesic, and a recent review reported that its use as part of a multimodal analgesia protocol markedly reduced acute postoperative pain in human patients.[56] In horses, ketamine (0.6 mg/kg bwt, followed by

0.02 mg/kg bwt/hour as CRI) provided some somatic analgesia and was found to be as effective as lidocaine as a local anesthetic and an epidural analgesic.[57–59] Ketamine's analgesic properties can potentially aid in the management of postoperative colic. Multiple studies in which ketamine was administered to rodents reported it to be highly effective as an antiendotoxic agent. In models of endotoxemia in rats, ketamine effectively prevented the deleterious effects of LPS on the liver and the gastrointestinal and respiratory tracts.[60–62] In rats, ketamine blocked activation of NF-kappa B and TLR4 and arrested TNF-α, among other proinflammatory mediators. Ketamine also completely abolished endotoxic shock when given before administration of LPS.[62–64] Similar effects were found when ketamine was incubated with equine mononuclear cells.[65] Ketamine can be safely administered to horses at a CRI (see above dosage) without causing visible sedation or other side effects. However, further studies to evaluate the antiendotoxic effects of ketamine in horses are indicated.

Detergent (Tyloxapol)

Tyloxapol is a nonionic liquid alkyl aryl polyether alcohol that is used as a surfactant to aid in the liquification and removal of mucus and exudate from bronchopulmonary secretions. Tyloxapol also blocks the lipolytic activity of plasma and the breakdown of triglyceride-rich lipoproteins. The use of a detergent to treat endotoxemia has proved highly effective in experimental models using rats and rabbits.[66] In a study of sheep, tyloxapol blocked nearly 80% of the systemic and pulmonary responses to intravenous LPS administration.[67] Also, in a study of horses administered endotoxin, pretreatment using intravenous tyloxapol was effective in preventing fever, leucopenia, and pulmonary hypertension in horses.[68] Tyloxapol has a chemical structure similar to that of bile acids, and like bile acids, acts as a detergent. Bile acids play a critical role in the body's defense mechanism against infection by binding to LPS, thereby preventing LPS from exerting its deleterious effects.[69] Similar to bile acids, amphipathic molecules like tyloxapol bind to the macrophage membrane, directly to the LPS-BP, or to LPS, and interfere with the physiologic response to LPS.[67] Results in horses suggest that tyloxapol may have a place in the treatment of endotoxemia; however, further studies on safety, effective doses, and pharmacokinetic and pharmacodynamics properties are necessary before this or other detergents should be used in the clinical setting.

Phospholipid Emulsion

Protein-free phospholipid emulsion (PLE) has been shown to bind and neutralize endotoxin in humans. When PLE was administrated intravenously to healthy male volunteers before administration of endotoxin, it prevented increases in rectal temperature, heart rate, and pulmonary artery pressure.[70] Also, the use of PLE prevented the development of leucopenia, and TNF-α concentration was significantly lower in the treated group.[70] The concentration of high-density lipoprotein is lower in people with sepsis, and the phospholipid portion of the high-density lipoprotein is the active part, which is capable of binding and neutralizing LPS.[70,71] The administration of PLE showed promise in ameliorating the effects of endotoxin in an induced peritonitis model in pigs and in humans.[72,73] Hemolysis was observed in horses treated with PLE;[70] thus, the clinical application of PLE may be limited or it should be administered more rapidly or at a lower total dose.[74] Rapid PLE infusion before LPS administration yielded similarly positive results by preventing the majority of the detrimental effects of LPS; however, hemolysis still occurred. In the initial PLE study[70], hemolysis was only grossly evaluated and was not described quantitatively; thus, comparing the hemolysis levels between the two studies is impossible. In the later study,[74] hemolysis was examined using light spectrometry; only three of six horses showed hemolysis, and in two of those three the hemolysis was mild. Thus, the results in this later study are encouraging, but further studies are needed before this treatment can be recommended.

Hemofiltration

One novel treatment approach to sepsis in human medicine involves circulating the patient's blood through an external filter, thereby adsorbing the proinflammatory cytokines, ameliorating the uncontrolled inflammatory response, and improving survival rates.[75] The use of hemofiltration was reported in horses and yielded no significant improvement in clinical and hematological response to LPS challenge.[76] A more specific hemofiltration method involves filtration of the blood through a column containing bound polymixin B, removing LPS by adsorption. A recent systematic literature review found this method effective in improving hemodynamic and oxygenation status and, even more importantly, in increasing survival rates in septic human patients.[77] Hemofiltration using a polymixin B column depends on the high affinity of polymixin B to LPS and completely avoids all concerns about toxicity because the drug does not enter the patient. This highly effective, elegant, technologically advanced method may have an important role in the future of equine endotoxemia therapy. However, no trials have been reported in horses to date.

SUMMARY

Endotoxemia is common in horses with colic and contributes to the morbidity and mortality. Endotoxin is intimately associated with the cell walls of Gram-negative bacteria, and the LPS component stimulates the release of inflammatory mediators and produces the clinical signs of shock that are seen in equine patients with colic. Pretreatment using pharmacologic agents and prevention of the effect of endotoxin on the inflammatory cascade is ideal. At the time that a veterinarian evaluates a horse, endotoxin likely has already been released and has produced clinical signs characteristic of shock. However, many of the pharmacologic agents mentioned in this article can, to some degree, block the effects of endotoxin after the cascade has been initiated and block further release of endotoxin. In the clinical situation, this may be the difference between survival and nonsurvival in colic patients, because cardiovascular status is most likely the determinant of survival in horses with colic. It must be emphasized that good scientific data is lacking on many of the treatment modalities presented in this article. However, many of these treatments have been used for years, and this article presents the author's current knowledge of these agents in hopes that more information will be forthcoming.

REFERENCES

1. Sykes BW, Furr MO. Equine endotoxaemia—a state-of-the-art review of therapy. Aust Vet J 2005;83:45–50.
2. Werners AH, Bull S, Fink-Gremmels J. Endotoxaemia: a review with implications for the horse. Equine Vet J 2005;37:371–83.
3. van Eps AW, Pollitt CC. Equine laminitis: cryotherapy reduces the severity of the acute lesion. Equine Vet J 2004;36:255–60.
4. Bertone JJ, Gossett KA, Shoemaker KE, et al. Effect of hypertonic vs. isotonic saline solution on responses to sublethal Escherichia coli endotoxemia in horses. Am J Vet Res 1990;51:999–1007.

5. Kreimeier U, Messmer K. [Use of hypertonic saline solutions in intensive care and emergency medicine—developments and perspectives]. Klin Wochenschr 1991; 69(Suppl 26):134–42.

6. Kupper S, Mees ST, Gassmann P, et al. Hydroxyethyl starch normalizes platelet and leukocyte adhesion within pulmonary microcirculation during LPS-induced endotoxemia. Shock 2007;28:300–8.

7. Lv R, Zhou W, Zhang LD, et al. Effects of hydroxyethyl starch on hepatic production of cytokines and activation of transcription factors in lipopolysaccharide-administered rats. Acta Anaesthesiol Scand 2005;49:635–42.

8. Schaper J, Ahmed R, Schafer T, et al. Volume therapy with colloid solutions preserves intestinal microvascular perfusion in endotoxaemia. Resuscitation 2008;76:120–8.

9. Pantaleon LG, Furr MO, McKenzie HC 2nd, et al. Cardiovascular and pulmonary effects of hetastarch plus hypertonic saline solutions during experimental endotoxemia in anesthetized horses. J Vet Intern Med 2006;20:1422–8.

10. Shuster R, Traub-Dargatz J, Baxter G. Survey of diplomates of the American College of Veterinary Internal Medicine and the American College of Veterinary Surgeons regarding clinical aspects and treatment of endotoxemia in horses. J Am Vet Med Assoc 1997;210:87–92.

11. Moore JN, Garner HE, Shapland JE, et al. Prevention of endotoxin-induced arterial hypoxaemia and lactic acidosis with flunixin meglumine in the conscious pony. Equine Vet J 1981;13:95–8.

12. Moore JN, Hardee MM, Hardee GE. Modulation of arachidonic acid metabolism in endotoxic horses: comparison of flunixin meglumine, phenylbutazone, and a selective thromboxane synthetase inhibitor. Am J Vet Res 1986;47:110–3.

13. Moore JN, Morris DD. Endotoxemia and septicemia in horses: experimental and clinical correlates. J Am Vet Med Assoc 1992;200:1903–14.

14. Tomlinson JE, Blikslager AT. Effects of cyclooxygenase inhibitors flunixin and deracoxib on permeability of ischaemic-injured equine jejunum. Equine Vet J 2005;37: 75–80.

15. Tomlinson JE, Wilder BO, Young KM, et al. Effects of flunixin meglumine or etodolac treatment on mucosal recovery of equine jejunum after ischemia. Am J Vet Res 2004;65:761–9.

16. Matyjaszek S, Morton A, Freeman D, et al. Effects of flunixin meglumine on recovery of colonic mucosa from ischemia in horses. Am J Vet Res 2009;70: 236–46.

17. Morton A, Grosche A, Polyak M, et al. Effects of flunixin meglumine on permeability of ischaemic-injured equine large colon. Presented at the: Ninth International Equine Colic Research Symposium. Liverpool, UK, June 15–18, 2008.

18. Semrad SD, Hardee GE, Hardee MM, et al. Low dose flunixin meglumine: effects on eicosanoid production and clinical signs induced by experimental endotoxaemia in horses. Equine Vet J 1987;19:201–6.

19. Cook V, Meyer C, Campbell N, et al. Effect of firocoxib or flunixin meglumine on recovery of ischaemic-injured equine jejunum. In: Ninth International Equine Colic Research Symposium, Liverpool UK, p. 68.

20. Lepper PM, Held TK, Schneider EM, et al. Clinical implications of antibiotic-induced endotoxin release in septic shock. Intensive Care Med 2002;28: 824–33.

21. Bentley AP, Barton MH, Lee MD, et al. Antimicrobial-induced endotoxin and cytokine activity in an in vitro model of septicemia in foals. Am J Vet Res 2002;63: 660–8.

22. Kusser WC, Ishiguro EE. Effects of aminoglycosides and spectinomycin on the synthesis and release of lipopolysaccharide by *Escherichia coli*. Antimicrobial Agents Chemother 1988;32:1247–50.

23. Lamp KC, Rybak MJ, McGrath BJ, et al. Influence of antibiotic and E5 monoclonal immunoglobulin M interactions on endotoxin release from *Escherichia coli* and *Pseudomonas aeruginosa*. Antimicrobial Agents Chemother 1996;40: 247–52.

24. Schleining JA, Reinertson EL. Evidence for dimethyl sulphoxide (DMSO) use in horses. Part 2: DMSO as a parenteral anti-inflammatory agent and as a pharmacological carrier. Equine Vet Educ 2007;19:598–9.

25. Hammond RA, Hannon R, Frean SP, et al. Endotoxin induction of nitric oxide synthase and cyclooxygenase-2 in equine alveolar macrophages. Am J Vet Res 1999;60:426–31.

26. Brackett DJ, Lerner MR, Wilson MF. Dimethyl sulfoxide antagonizes hypotensive, metabolic, and pathologic responses induced by endotoxin. Circ Shock 1991;33: 156–63.

27. DeForge LE, Fantone JC, Kenney JS, et al. Oxygen radical scavengers selectively inhibit interleukin 8 production in human whole blood. J Clin Invest 1992; 90:2123–9.

28. Sekizuka E, Benoit JN, Grisham MB, et al. Dimethylsulfoxide prevents chemoattractant-induced leukocyte adherence. Am J Physiol 1989;256:H594–7.

29. Cetin M, Eser B, Er O, et al. Effects of DMSO on platelet functions and P-selectin expression during storage. Transfus Apheresis Sci 2001;24:261–7.

30. Rosenblum W. Dimethyl sulfoxide effects on platelet aggregation and vascular reactivity in pial microcirculation. Ann N Y Acad Sci 1983;411:110–9.

31. Essani NA, Fisher MA, Jaeschke H. Inhibition of NF-kappa B activation by dimethyl sulfoxide correlates with suppression of TNF-alpha formation, reduced ICAM-1 gene transcription, and protection against endotoxin-induced liver injury. Shock 1997;7:90–6.

32. Dabareiner RM, White NA, Snyder JR, et al. Effects of Carolina rinse solution, dimethyl sulfoxide, and the 21-aminosteroid, U-74389G, on microvascular permeability and morphology of the equine jejunum after low-flow ischemia and reperfusion. Am J Vet Res 2005;66:525–36.

33. Sullins KE, White NA, Lundin CS, et al. Prevention of ischaemia-induced small intestinal adhesions in foals. Equine Vet J 2004;36:370–5.

34. Kelmer G, Doherty TJ, Elliott S, et al. Evaluation of dimethyl sulphoxide effects on initial response to endotoxin in the horse. Equine Vet J 2008;40:358–63.

35. Moore RM, Muir WW, Bertone AL, et al. Effects of dimethyl sulfoxide, allopurinol, 21-aminosteroid U-74389G, and manganese chloride on low-flow ischemia and reperfusion of the large colon in horses. Am J Vet Res 1995;56:671–87.

36. Reeves MJ, Vansteenhouse J, Stashak TS, et al. Failure to demonstrate reperfusion injury following ischaemia of the equine large colon using dimethyl sulphoxide. Equine Vet J 1990;22:126–32.

37. Van Hoogmoed LM, Nieto JE, Snyder JR, et al. Survey of prokinetic use in horses with gastrointestinal injury. Vet Surg 2004;33:279–85.

38. Traut U, Brugger L, Kunz R, et al. Systemic prokinetic pharmacologic treatment for postoperative adynamic ileus following abdominal surgery in adults. Cochrane Database Syst Rev 2008;CD004930.

39. Brianceau P, Chevalier H, Karas A, et al. Intravenous lidocaine and small-intestinal size, abdominal fluid, and outcome after colic surgery in horses. J Vet Intern Med 2002;16(1):736–41.

40. Malone E, Ensink J, Turner T, et al. Intravenous continuous infusion of lidocaine for treatment of equine ileus. Vet Surg 2006;35:60–6.
41. Milligan M, Beard W, Kukanich B, et al. The effect of lidocaine on postoperative jejunal motility in normal horses. Vet Surg 2007;36:214–20.
42. Nieto JE, Rakestraw PC, Snyder JR, et al. In vitro effects of erythromycin, lidocaine, and metoclopramide on smooth muscle from the pyloric antrum, proximal portion of the duodenum, and middle portion of the jejunum of horses. Am J Vet Res 2000;61:413–9.
43. Okamura K, Sasaki N, Yamada M, et al. Effects of mosapride citrate, metoclopramide hydrochloride, lidocaine hydrochloride, and cisapride citrate on equine gastric emptying, small intestinal and caecal motility. Res Vet Sci 2009;86:302–8.
44. Rusiecki K, Nieto J, Puchalski S, et al. Evaluation of continuous infusion of lidocaine on gastrointestinal tract function in normal horses. Vet Surg 2008; 37:564–70.
45. Wiemer P, Laan T, Lashley M: Equine post operative ileus: comparison between continuous lidocaine infusion and other prokinetic medications. In: The International Equine Colic Research Symposium, Liverpool, p. 57.
46. Robertson SA, Sanchez LC, Merritt AM, et al. Effect of systemic lidocaine on visceral and somatic nociception in conscious horses. Equine Vet J 2005;37:122–7.
47. Cook VL, Blikslager AT. Use of systemically administered lidocaine in horses with gastrointestinal tract disease. J Am Vet Med Assoc 2008;232:1144–8.
48. Taniguchi T, Shibata K, Yamamoto K, et al. Effects of lidocaine administration on hemodynamics and cytokine responses to endotoxemia in rabbits. Crit Care Med 2000;28:755–9.
49. Morresey PR, Mackay RJ. Endotoxin-neutralizing activity of polymyxin B in blood after IV administration in horses. Am J Vet Res 2006;67:642–7.
50. Falagas ME, Kasiakou SK. Toxicity of polymyxins: a systematic review of the evidence from old and recent studies. Crit Care 2006;10:R27.
51. Coyne CP, Fenwick BW. Inhibition of lipopolysaccharide-induced macrophage tumor necrosis factor-alpha synthesis by polymyxin B sulfate. Am J Vet Res 1993;54:305–14.
52. Durando MM, MacKay RJ, Linda S, et al. Effects of polymyxin B and Salmonella typhimurium antiserum on horses given endotoxin intravenously. Am J Vet Res 1994;55:921–7.
53. Barton MH, Parviainen A, Norton N. Polymyxin B protects horses against induced endotoxaemia in vivo. Equine Vet J 2004;36:397–401.
54. Parviainen AK, Barton MH, Norton NN. Evaluation of polymyxin B in an ex vivo model of endotoxemia in horses. Am J Vet Res 2001;62:72–6.
55. Barton M. Use of polymyxin B for treatment of endotoxemia in horses. Comp Cont Edu Pract Vet 2000;22:1056–9.
56. Bell RF, Dahl JB, Moore RA, et al. Peri-operative ketamine for acute post-operative pain: a quantitative and qualitative systematic review (Cochrane review). Acta Anaesthesiol Scand 2005;49:1405–28.
57. Gomez de Segura IA, De Rossi R, Santos M, et al. Epidural injection of ketamine for perineal analgesia in the horse. Vet Surg 1998;27:384–91.
58. Lopez-Sanroman FJ, Cruz JM, Santos M, et al. Evaluation of the local analgesic effect of ketamine in the palmar digital nerve block at the base of the proximal sesamoid (abaxial sesamoid block) in horses. Am J Vet Res 2003;64:475–8.
59. Peterbauer C, Larenza PM, Knobloch M, et al. Effects of a low dose infusion of racemic and S-ketamine on the nociceptive withdrawal reflex in standing ponies. Vet Anaesth Analg 2008;35:414–23.

60. Helmer KS, Suliburk JW, Mercer DW. Ketamine-induced gastroprotection during endotoxemia: role of heme-oxygenase-1. Dig Dis Sci 2006;51:1571–81.
61. Suliburk JW, Helmer KS, Gonzalez EA, et al. Ketamine attenuates liver injury attributed to endotoxemia: role of cyclooxygenase-2. Surgery 2005;138:134–40.
62. Yu M, Shao D, Feng X, et al. Effects of ketamine on pulmonary TLR4 expression and NF-kappa-B activation during endotoxemia in rats. Methods Find Exp Clin Pharmacol 2007;29:395–9.
63. Taniguchi T, Shibata K, Yamamoto K. Ketamine inhibits endotoxin-induced shock in rats. Anesthesiology 2001;95:928–32.
64. Yu Y, Zhou Z, Xu J, et al. Ketamine reduces NFkappaB activation and TNFalpha production in rat mononuclear cells induced by lipopolysaccharide in vitro. Ann Clin Lab Sci 2002;32:292–8.
65. Lankveld DP, Bull S, Van Dijk P, et al. Ketamine inhibits LPS-induced tumour necrosis factor-alpha and interleukin-6 in an equine macrophage cell line. Vet Res 2005;36:257–62.
66. Serikov VB, Glazanova TV, Jerome EH, et al. Tyloxapol attenuates the pathologic effects of endotoxin in rabbits and mortality following cecal ligation and puncture in rats by blockade of endotoxin receptor–ligand interactions. Inflammation 2003; 27:175–90.
67. Staub NC Sr, Longworth KE, Serikov V, et al. Detergent inhibits 70–90% of responses to intravenous endotoxin in awake sheep. J Appl Phys 2001;90: 1788–97.
68. Longworth KE, Smith BL, Staub NC, et al. Use of detergent to prevent initial responses to endotoxin in horses. Am J Vet Res 1996;57:1063–6.
69. Bertok L. Bile acids in physico-chemical host defence. Pathophysiology 2004;11: 139–45.
70. Winchell WW, Hardy J, Levine DM, et al. Effect of administration of a phospholipid emulsion on the initial response of horses administered endotoxin. Am J Vet Res 2002;63:1370–8.
71. Chien JY, Jerng JS, Yu CJ, et al. Low serum level of high-density lipoprotein cholesterol is a poor prognostic factor for severe sepsis. Crit Care Med 2005; 33:1688–93.
72. Goldfarb RD, Parker TS, Levine DM, et al. Protein-free phospholipid emulsion treatment improved cardiopulmonary function and survival in porcine sepsis. Am J Physiol Regul Integr Comp Physiol 2003;284:R550–7.
73. Gordon BR, Parker TS, Levine DM, et al. Neutralization of endotoxin by a phospholipid emulsion in healthy volunteers. J Infect Dis 2005;191:1515–22.
74. Moore JN, Norton N, Barton MH, et al. Rapid infusion of a phospholipid emulsion attenuates the effects of endotoxaemia in horses. Equine Vet J 2007;39:243–8.
75. Ronco C, Ricci Z, Bellomo R. Importance of increased ultrafiltration volume and impact on mortality: sepsis and cytokine story and the role of continuous veno-venous haemofiltration. Curr Opin Nephrol Hypertens 2001;10:755–61.
76. Veenman JN, Dujardint CL, Hoek A, et al. High volume continuous venovenous haemofiltration (HV-CVVH) in an equine endotoxaemic shock model. Equine Vet J 2002;34:516–22.
77. Cruz DN, Perazella MA, Bellomo R, et al. Effectiveness of polymyxin B–immobilized fiber column in sepsis: a systematic review. Crit Care 2007;11:R47.

Update on Recent Advances in Equine Abdominal Surgery

Gal Kelmer, DVM, MS[a,b],*

KEYWORDS

• Equine • Surgery • Colic • Complications • Prognosis

In recent years important advancements in colic surgery have led to improved prediction of survival rates, better survival rates, and decreased complication rates. This article describes several modalities to combat and prevent incisional hernia and intestinal adhesion formation in horses undergoing colic surgery. These modalities have had a positive impact on reducing complications in horses after surgery.

LACTATE

Prognostication in horses with strangulating large colon volvulus (LCV) can be difficult even during abdominal exploration. This severe, peracute-type colic can result in rapid colonic devitalization; therefore, a better grasp of prognosis preoperatively can be helpful. A recent study by Johnston and colleagues[1] found plasma lactate concentration to be highly accurate in predicting survival of horses with LCV. Plasma lactate less than 6 mmol/L had a positive predictive value of 96%, and no horses with lactate greater than 10 mmol/L survived. Stall-side portable lactate sampling is simple and quick and is proven to be a reliable technique for measuring plasma and peritoneal fluid lactate.[2] For LCV, specifically, plasma lactate is an accurate and invaluable preoperative prognostic tool. For other gastrointestinal lesions, plasma lactate is valuable; however, peritoneal fluid lactate has a better correlation with survival rates, and neither plasma nor peritoneal fluid lactate values predict survival once the lesion is not strangulating.[2] Because determining the strangulating nature of the lesion is often impossible preoperatively in small intestinal lesions, one must use caution when using lactate to predict survival in horses that seem to have small intestinal lesions. Peritoneal lactate can be a useful tool, however, to predict the need for surgery by determining the strangulating nature of the lesion in any horse presenting for colic.[3]

[a] Large Animal Department, Koret Veterinary Teaching Hospital, Hebrew University of Jerusalem, Rehovot, Israel
[b] Equine Surgery Section, Department of Large Animal Clinical Sciences, College of Veterinary Medicine, University of Tennessee, 2407 River Drive, Knoxville, TN 37996, USA
* Large Animal Department, Koret Veterinary Teaching Hospital, Hebrew University of Jerusalem, Rehovot, Israel
E-mail address: kelmerg@agri.huji.ac.il

Vet Clin Equine 25 (2009) 271–282
doi:10.1016/j.cveq.2009.04.007
0749-0739/09/$ – see front matter

ADHESION PREVENTION

Intestinal adhesions are one of the most common complications that limit survival rates after abdominal surgery in horses (**Fig. 1**), and the primary mode of prevention is an atraumatic surgical technique.[4] Recently, several studies have addressed the issue and found support for preoperative intravenous treatments, including dimethyl sulfoxide (20 mg/kg), potassium penicillin (22,000 IU/kg), and flunixin meglumine (Banamine, 1.1 mg/kg), and for intraoperative treatments, including intraperitoneal unfractionated heparin administration (20,000 IU) and the use of sodium carboxymethylcellulose (SCMC 7 mL/kg).[5–7] In addition, an omentectomy has been shown to significantly decrease the rate of adhesion formation according to one study,[8] and in a more recent study by Mair and Smith[6] the same trend was noted. Santschi and colleagues[9] reported an 8% rate of adhesions after colic surgery in more than 200 juvenile horses, and they attributed their relatively low adhesion rate to the routine performance of omentectomies. Several recent studies have found that adhesions involving the omentum are a significant cause for colic and for repeat celiotomy,[4,10,11] and this is consistent with our clinical experience. In addition, incarcerations of the intestine through the greater omentum have been reported.[12,13] Peritoneal lavage has been shown to decrease adhesion formation in horses.[14] Omentectomy greatly facilitates peritoneal dialysis[15] by preventing catheter occlusion, which is one of the most common complications with peritoneal lavage;[16] thus, omentectomy may also enhance the efficacy of postoperative peritoneal lavage. Removal of the omentum has multiple advantages, and it is an additional sensible, quick, and simple technique to reduce postoperative complications following equine abdominal surgery.

Highly viscous solutions, such as SCMC, have two antiadhesive properties: they act as lubricants to decrease bowel handling trauma and as surface barriers, separating serosal surfaces. Intraoperative use of SCMC has been previously shown not to interfere with healing of either small intestinal anastomosis or the abdominal incision.[5,17] In contrast to previous theories and experimental studies, clinically, adhesions seem to involve any region of the intestine (**Fig. 2**) without predilection for anastomosis or enterotomy sites, and thus the use of pan-abdominal adhesion preventative

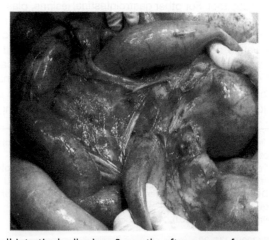

Fig. 1. Diffused small intestinal adhesions 3 months after surgery for correction of a severe large colon impaction. The adhesions in this horse were so extensive that the horse was euthanized on the table.

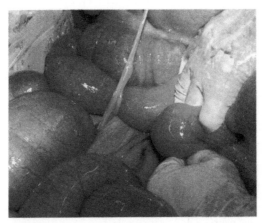

Fig. 2. Single, long stalked adhesion involving the large colon. The adhesion in this horse did not cause any obstruction and seemed to be an incidental finding on abdominal exploration.

measures, such as SCMC, is advocated in all abdominal surgeries in the horse.[4] Recently Fogle and colleagues[18] presented the strongest and most up-to-date evidence supporting routine use of SCMC by demonstrating that horses that received intraoperative SCMC were twice as likely to survive as horses not receiving SCMC. To summarize, as opposed to other techniques we commonly implement in equine surgery, the routine use of SCMC in abdominal surgeries has a strong clinical evidence basis.

ABDOMINAL BANDAGE

Incisional complications are common in equine abdominal surgery; they significantly increase the morbidity and expenses associated with the procedure and occasionally can be fatal.[19] Edema, drainage, infection, hernia formation, and dehiscence are the typical complications in decreased order of frequency. A recent study by Mair and Smith[6] has shown that an iodophor-impregnated adhesive drape (Ioban, 3M USA, St. Paul, Minnesota) applied to the incision at the end of surgery and removed once the horse recovers from general anesthesia is more effective than a sutured stent in preventing incisional complications. Edema formation can predispose the horse to further incisional complications, such as hernia.[20,21] Recently, a study by Smith and colleagues[22] found that applying an abdominal bandage immediately after recovery from abdominal surgery and maintaining it for 2 weeks post discharge significantly decreased incisional complications. In a recent study by Nieto and colleagues,[16] decreased incisional complications were attributed to in-hospital use of postoperative abdominal bandages. Two studies compiling 142 cases concluded that use of a commercially available abdominal bandage (CM Hernia Belt, CM Equine Products, Norco, California) after a complicated ventral midline incision and after a paramedian abdominal incision markedly decreased the incidence of incisional hernia formation.[23,24] Overall, abundant evidence in recent literature suggests that the use of an abdominal bandage to prevent and treat incisional complications is beneficial. Our experience parallels that; we found that the use of the same commercially available abdominal bandage (**Fig. 3**) as part of routine postoperative case management is

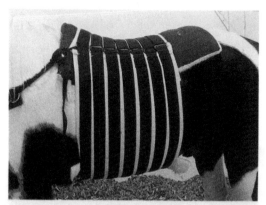

Fig. 3. Postoperative use of a commercial multiuse abdominal bandage (CM Hernia Belt, CM Equine Products, Norco, California).

highly effective in preventing edema and minimizing incisional complications, and its use is simple and economically worthwhile.

SMALL INTESTINAL ANASTOMOSIS

Small intestinal lesions are typically strangulating and often necessitate resection and anastomosis. It is interesting that although the ileum represents only about 5% of the small intestine, it is involved in about 50% of common cases of small intestinal incarceration, such as inguinal hernia and epiploic foramen entrapment.[25,26] Jejunocecostomy (JC) was the recommended procedure in cases in which the ileum was involved; connecting the jejunum to the ileum was considered undesirable because of differences in wall thickness and concerns about uncoordinated motility. Recently, multiple studies including a large number of horses have shown that JC is more likely to result in postoperative complications, including a higher rate of repeat celiotomy and an increase in mortality risk compared with jejunojejunostomy (JJ).[13,27] In addition several recent studies have shown that jejunoileostomy (JI) is highly successful[28] and results in a success rate equal to that of end-to-end JJ.[10,29] According to current information, whenever possible, creating an anastomosis between the jejunum and the ileum is definitively preferable to JC. JC remains a viable, often life-saving option, however, when not enough ileum is available for anastomosis. JC and JJ can be performed successfully hand sewn and with the aid of stapling devices. Using stapling devices can decrease surgery times, thus decreasing anesthesia and recovery-related complications. In addition, using the stapling technique may substantially decrease intraoperative contamination and decrease chances of postoperative infection.[30] All this correlates well with our recent clinical experience in having good results with stapled, closed, one-stage functional end-to-end[31] JI in all recent relevant clinical cases.

LARGE COLON RESECTION AND ANASTOMOSIS

Large colon resection and anastomosis (LCRA) has been considered a salvage procedure with poor prognosis for survival. Early studies on LCRA reported high survival rates; however, these studies included only a few cases.[32] Two recent reports, including one on a large number of horses, suggest that the prognosis for LCRA may not be as poor as once believed.[33,34] In one study including 73 horses treated with LCRA for strangulated large colon volvulus, 74% of the horses survived to discharge,[34] and in another study partially overlapping the previous one, from the same clinic, 80% short-term survival was found for horses with LCV treated with LCRA.[35] This latter study included in the survival analysis only horses recovered successfully from surgery, which artificially increased the success rate because it omitted cases that were euthanized or died during surgery and those that had catastrophic recovery. As suggested by the authors, the high survival rate in this study can be in part attributed to the short duration of clinical signs before presentation due to the close proximity of the breeding farms to the clinic.[35] In another study, Driscoll and colleagues[33] reported a similar survival rate for LCRA; however, the survival rate in these horses was less than 50% when only strangulated lesions were included, and horses with a strangulated lesion were four times less likely to survive. Heart rate (HR) at 24 hours after surgery was significantly associated with survival. Short-term survivors had a median HR of 48 beats per minute (bpm), whereas the nonsurvivors had a median HR of 80 bpm. Colonic luminal pressure was found to be an inaccurate prognostic indicator.[35] Intraoperative gross assessment of colonic viability is prone to error because of the high level of subjectivity in values such as serosal color and arterial pulse strength; however, histologic evaluation of fresh frozen sections of the pelvic flexure was found to be accurate in predicting survival in horses with large colon volvulus.[32] Unfortunately, this technique is not available in most equine surgical facilities and thus subjective assessment of colonic viability remains the mainstay method to determine if resection is indicated. Serum lactate can serve as an accurate predictor of survivability of horses with LCV,[1] but we do not have information regarding its usefulness to predict survivability following resection of a compromised colon. It is encouraging that in one study, all horses that were discharged survived at least 1 year,[33] although more than 50% of them experienced complications, of which the most common were colic and weight loss. The procedure of LCRA has been advocated not just as a treatment of LCV with a nonviable colon but also as a preventative measure against recurrence of LCV.[36] Despite the recently reported good results for LCRA, complication rates are high and occasionally may prove fatal. For this reason we believe LCRA, as a preventative measure, should be reserved for "repeat offenders" that have an athletic career. Colopexy is less invasive and carries good results as a preventative measure against LCV and displacement.[37] The procedure can be performed as an open surgery or through laparoscopy; however, it has not been proven safe for an athletic horse.[37,38] Different techniques for LCRA have been reported, and the ones recently reported to yield good results involve end-to-end anastomosis with or without the aid of staples for extending the stoma and for ligating the mesocolon.[33,39] Overall, LCRA is a viable treatment option for several large colon lesions, especially LCV, and the procedure has been recently shown to carry reasonable prognosis. Because of the high risk for complications, however, LCRA should be performed only when clinically deemed absolutely necessary.

HAND-ASSISTED LAPAROSCOPY

In recent years laparoscopy has gained much popularity in the equine world as a less invasive method for diagnostic and surgical purposes. The technique of hand-assisted laparoscopy (HAL) has been used successfully in several clinical cases lately. The procedures performed using HAL include left and right nephrectomies, splenectomy, and removal of ovarian and uterine tumors.[40-43] The technique was adopted from human medicine and adapted for use in horses under general anesthesia and under standing sedation. HAL is advantageous over open surgery and laparoscopy because it combines the excellent visibility achieved by laparoscopy with the tactile sensation, tissue handling, and maneuverability capabilities enabled by having a hand in the abdomen, while being only moderately invasive. As the procedure gains in popularity, it is reasonable to assume that additional procedures currently performed in horses by laparoscopy or open surgery, such nephrosplenic space obliteration and adhesiolysis, will also be adapted to HAL because the procedure has significant advantages over both approaches in many cases. Another option, to incorporate the visual advantage of laparoscopy, is to use it for initial assessment and exteriorization and then perform a procedure in an open fashion. Röcken and colleagues[44] reported on cystic calculi removal in this manner, and the technique combines the advantages of open surgery and laparoscopy in an elegant way. Overall, HAL seems to have an important place in the future of equine abdominal surgery.

DIAPHRAGMATIC HERNIA

Recent information suggests that diaphragmatic hernia (DH) as a cause of colic is not as rare as previously considered (**Fig. 4**). One recent review compiled 114 cases of DH, and another recent retrospective study included 44 additional cases.[45,46] An incidence of between 0.67% and 7.77% was estimated by compiling more than 1400 surgical colic cases in one study.[46] When these data are compared to two large retrospective studies including nearly 1000 surgical colic cases, this incidence level is on par with lesions such as small intestine incarceration in the gastrosplenic ligament, cecal impaction, and other lesions that are not considered that rare.[10,47] According to a recent review article, a good inquiry into the history of most cases of DH reveals a traumatic incident or other event, such as breeding, that increased the

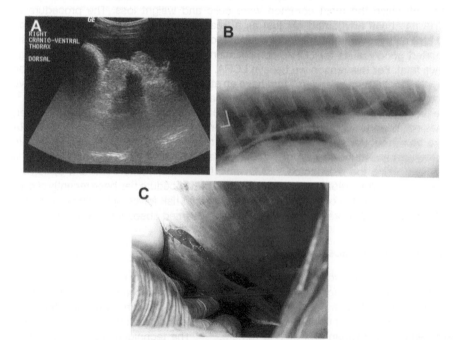

Fig. 4. (*A–C*) Diaphragmatic hernia in a weanling; after reduction of incarcerated small intestine a traumatic rent can be seen in the muscular portion of the diaphragm.

intra-abdominal pressure abruptly;[46] however, most horses in the mentioned retrospective study did not include such an event in their recorded history. Acquisition of a reliable and thorough history in each colic case cannot be overemphasized. Typically DH is diagnosed on abdominal exploration, but preoperative diagnosis, when achieved, has been established mainly using ultrasonography and radiography. Because DH is not that uncommon, it is important to include it in the differential diagnosis list in each case presenting for colic. By increasing our awareness of the problem we will improve chances of early diagnosis and a better outcome. Clinical signs accompanying DH are typically these of abdominal pain or colic, but they can also include respiratory compromise, such as tachypnea and dyspnea. According to these recent studies, most DHs, or diaphragmatic rents, are acquired, are more prevalent on the left side, and are dorsally located.[45,46] Some identical prognostic indicators were found in both recent studies; specifically, the more dorsal and larger the tear, the less likely the surgery is to succeed.[48] Diaphragmatic hernia, when presented with clinical signs, is a surgical lesion, but survival rate after surgical correction is low.[45] Although no breakthroughs were recently made in the treatment of DH, earlier diagnosis and HAL or thoracoscopy may offer an improved method to increase survival rates of DH.

INCISIONAL HERNIA—PREVENTION AND TREATMENT

An incisional hernia (**Fig. 5**) is a common complication of colic surgery in horses and, according to recent reports, occurs in 7% to 10% of cases.[6,49] Most hernias are preceded by surgical site drainage and infection (**Fig. 6**) in the first week after surgery.[50] Avoiding incisional infection substantially decreases the incidence of incisional hernia formation, and recent advances in this field were mentioned previously in the paragraph discussing abdominal bandage. Klohnen and colleagues[23,24] recently reported that once complications develop, use of an abdominal bandage (CM Hernia Belt) can effectively reduce the incidence of hernia formation after celiotomy by using ventral midline and right paramedian approaches. The same abdominal bandage may also be used effectively as a conservative treatment modality for small- to medium-sized incisional hernias, especially in the early stages of hernia formation when healing and fibrosis are still active. Large hernias are commonly repaired surgically and although most incisional hernias can be closed with sutures alone, multiple small hernias can often be palpated at the surgery site when healing is complete. In large hernia repair use of a synthetic mesh is recommended for added strength and better cosmetic results. Typically the mesh is placed external to the peritoneum

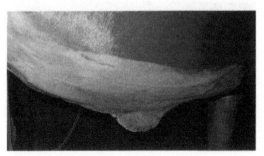

Fig. 5. Small incisional hernia in a mare 1 year after colic surgery for large colon displacement that was complicated by incisional infection.

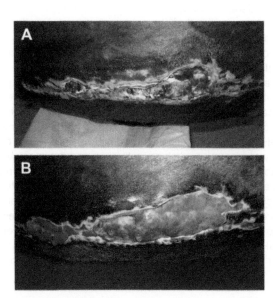

Fig. 6. Incisional infection in a gelding after surgical correction of a large colon volvulus. (*A*) The infection is progressing in the first postoperative week. (*B*) Two weeks after initial signs of infection with providing drainage and cleansing and the use of abdominal bandage the infection is resolving and healthy granulation tissue is seen.

(retroperitoneal) and the incidence of postoperative complications associated with retroperitoneal placement of mesh, such as tearing of the internal abdominal oblique muscle and incisional swelling and drainage, is relatively high.[51] Recently, an alternative technique was reported in which first the hernia ring was sutured closed with inversion of the hernia sac, and then a polypropylene mesh (Bard, Murray Hill, New Jersey) was implanted subcutaneously (**Fig. 7**).[52] Closing the hernial ring before

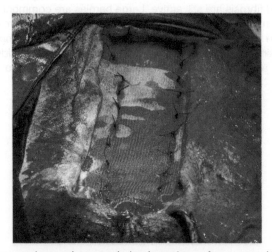

Fig. 7. Subcutaneous polypropylene mesh implantation, after suture herniorrhaphy, for repair of ventral abdominal incisional hernia in a horse.

implanting a mesh may strengthen the repair and improve postoperative appearance. Use of a hernia or kidney needle decreases the likelihood of penetrating a viscus during the repair. Based on our experience and that of others,[53] placing the mesh subcutaneously makes mesh repair less complicated, and concerns about development of subcutaneous infection around the mesh[54] seem to be unjustified. Recurrence of the hernia is a relatively common complication of herniorrhaphy and has been reported after using sutures alone[55] and after herniorrhaphy in which a mesh was implanted.[26] No hernias recurred using this combination technique on a large number of horses. Suture material used to secure the mesh should be absorbable so that if infection or an allergic reaction at the surgery site occurs, the mesh can be more easily removed. In summary, abdominal incisional hernias can be easily and successfully repaired by closing the hernia with sutures and implanting a mesh subcutaneously over the sutured hernial ring.

SUMMARY

Exciting advances have been made in certain areas of abdominal surgery in the horse. Recently developed methods to decrease the rate of complications, such as adhesions, incisional infections, and hernias, have proved effective. New approaches to abdominal surgery, such as HAL, have been adapted from human surgery and seem to show promise by decreasing morbidity and increasing the efficacy and feasibility of many procedures previously fraught with complications. Advances in supportive care and surgical techniques have brought increased success rates to small intestinal and large colon resection and anastomosis. Overall, significant advancements continue to improve the survival and decrease postoperative complication in colic surgery.

ACKNOWLEDGEMENTS

The author thanks Ms. Misty Bailey for her great help with technical writing of the manuscript.

REFERENCES

1. Johnston K, Holcombe SJ, Hauptman JG. Plasma lactate as a predictor of colonic viability and survival after 360 degrees volvulus of the ascending colon in horses. Vet Surg 2007;36(6):563–7.
2. Delesalle C, Dewulf J, Lefebvre RA, et al. Determination of lactate concentrations in blood plasma and peritoneal fluid in horses with colic by an Accusport analyzer. J Vet Intern Med 2007;21(2):293–301.
3. Latson KM, Nieto JE, Beldomenico PM, et al. Evaluation of peritoneal fluid lactate as a marker of intestinal ischaemia in equine colic. Equine Vet J 2005;37(4): 342–6.
4. Gorvy DA, Barrie Edwards G, Proudman CJ. Intra-abdominal adhesions in horses: a retrospective evaluation of repeat laparotomy in 99 horses with acute gastrointestinal disease. Vet J 2008;175(2):194–201.
5. Hay WP, Mueller PO, Harmon B, et al. One percent sodium carboxymethylcellulose prevents experimentally induced abdominal adhesions in horses. Vet Surg 2001;30(3):223–7.
6. Mair TS, Smith LJ. Survival and complication rates in 300 horses undergoing surgical treatment of colic. Part 3: long-term complications and survival. Equine Vet J 2005;37(4):310–4.

7. Sullins KE, White NA, Lundin CS, et al. Prevention of ischaemia-induced small intestinal adhesions in foals. Equine Vet J 2004;36(5):370–5.

8. Kuebelbeck KL, Slone DE, May KA. Effect of omentectomy on adhesion formation in horses. Vet Surg 1998;27(2):132–7.

9. Santschi EM, Slone DE, Embertson RM, et al. Colic surgery in 206 juvenile thoroughbreds: survival and racing results. Equine Vet J Suppl 2000;(32):32–6.

10. Mair TS, Smith LJ. Survival and complication rates in 300 horses undergoing surgical treatment of colic. Part 2: short-term complications. Equine Vet J 2005; 37(4):303–9.

11. Butson RJ, England GC, Blackmore CA. Omento-omental adhesion around the uterine horn as a cause of recurrent colic in a mare. Vet Rec 1996;139(23): 571–2.

12. Kelmer G, Holder TEC, Donnell RL. Small intestinal incarceration through an omental rent in a horse. Equine Vet Educ 2008;20(12):635–8.

13. van den Boom R, van der Velden MA. Short- and long-term evaluation of surgical treatment of strangulating obstructions of the small intestine in horses: a review of 224 cases. Vet Q 2001;23(3):109–15.

14. Hague BA, Honnas CM, Berridge BR, et al. Evaluation of postoperative peritoneal lavage in standing horses for prevention of experimentally induced abdominal adhesions. Vet Surg 1998;27(2):122–6.

15. Lee M, Donovan JF. Laparoscopic omentectomy for salvage of peritoneal dialysis catheters. J Endourol 2002;16(4):241–4.

16. Nieto JE, Snyder JR, Vatistas NJ, et al. Use of an active intra-abdominal drain in 67 horses. Vet Surg 2003;32(1):1–7.

17. Mueller PO, Harmon BG, Hay WP, et al. Effect of carboxymethylcellulose and a hyaluronate-carboxymethylcellulose membrane on healing of intestinal anastomoses in horses. Am J Vet Res 2000;61(4):369–74.

18. Fogle CA, Gerard MP, Elce YA, et al. Analysis of sodium carboxymethylcellulose administration and related factors associated with postoperative colic and survival in horses with small intestinal disease. Vet Surg 2008;37(6):558–63.

19. Mair TS, Smith LJ. Survival and complication rates in 300 horses undergoing surgical treatment of colic. Part 1: short-term survival following a single laparotomy. Equine Vet J 2005;37(4):296–302.

20. Galuppo LD, Pascoe JR, Jang SS, et al. Evaluation of iodophor skin preparation techniques and factors influencing drainage from ventral midline incisions in horses. J Am Vet Med Assoc 1999;215(7):963–9.

21. Gibson KT, Curtis CR, Turner AS, et al. Incisional hernias in the horse. Incidence and predisposing factors. Vet Surg 1989;18(5):360–6.

22. Smith LJ, Mellor DJ, Marr CM, et al. Incisional complications following exploratory celiotomy: does an abdominal bandage reduce the risk? Equine Vet J 2007;39(3): 277–83.

23. Klohnen A, Lores M, Fischer A. Management of post operative abdominal incisional complications with a hernia belt: 85 horses (2001–2005). Paper presented at the 9th International Equine Colic Research Symposium 2008, Liverpool, UK, June 15–18, 2008.

24. Klohnen A, Panizzi L. Incisional complications after right paramedian celiotomy in horses with colic: 57 cases (2002–2005). Paper presented at the 9th International Equine Colic Research Symposium, 2008, Liverpool, UK, June 15–18, 2008.

25. Archer DC, Proudman CJ, Pinchbeck G, et al. Entrapment of the small intestine in the epiploic foramen in horses: a retrospective analysis of 71 cases recorded between 1991 and 2001. Vet Rec 2004;155(25):793–7.

26. van der Velden MA. Surgical treatment of acquired inguinal hernia in the horse: a review of 51 cases. Equine Vet J 1988;20(3):173–7.

27. Proudman CJ, Edwards GB, Barnes J. Differential survival in horses requiring end-to-end jejunojejunal anastomosis compared to those requiring side-to-side jejunocaecal anastomosis. Equine Vet J 2007;39(2):181–5.

28. Loesch DA, Rodgerson DH, Haines GR, et al. Jejunoileal anastomosis following small intestinal resection in horses: seven cases (1999–2001). J Am Vet Med Assoc 2002;221(4):541–5.

29. Rendle DI, Woodt JL, Summerhays GE, et al. End-to-end jejuno-ileal anastomosis following resection of strangulated small intestine in horses: a comparative study. Equine Vet J 2005;37(4):356–9.

30. Tobias KM. Surgical stapling devices in veterinary medicine: a review. Vet Surg 2007;36(4):341–9.

31. Latimer FG, Blackford JT, Valk N, et al. Closed one-stage functional end-to-end jejunojejunostomy in horses with use of linear stapling equipment. Vet Surg 1998;27(1):17–28.

32. Van Hoogmoed L, Snyder JR, Pascoe JR, et al. Use of pelvic flexure biopsies to predict survival after large colon torsion in horses. Vet Surg 2000;29(6):572–7.

33. Driscoll N, Baia P, Fischer AT, et al. Large colon resection and anastomosis in horses: 52 cases (1996-2006). Equine Vet J 2008;40(4):342–7.

34. Ellis C, Lynch D, Slone F, et al. Survival and complications of 73 horses undergoing large colon resection and anastomosis due to strangulating large colon volvulus (1995–2005). Paper presented at the 9th International Equine Colic Research Symposium, 2008, Liverpool, UK, June 15–18, 2008.

35. Mathis SC, Slone DE, Lynch TM, et al. Use of colonic luminal pressure to predict outcome after surgical treatment of strangulating large colon volvulus in horses. Vet Surg 2006;35(4):356–60.

36. Markel MD. Prevention of large colon displacements and volvulus. Vet Clin North Am Equine Pract 1989;5(2):395–405.

37. Hance SR, Embertson RM. Colopexy in broodmares: 44 cases (1986-1990). J Am Vet Med Assoc 1992;201(5):782–7.

38. Trostle SS, White NA, Donaldson L, et al. Laparoscopic colopexy in horses. Vet Surg 1998;27(1):56–63.

39. Hughes FE, Slone DE. A modified technique for extensive large colon resection and anastomosis in horses. Vet Surg 1998;27(2):127–31.

40. Janicek JC, Rodgerson DH, Boone BL. Use of a hand-assisted laparoscopic technique for removal of a uterine leiomyoma in a standing mare. J Am Vet Med Assoc 2004;225(6):911–4.

41. Ortved K, Witte S, Fleming K, et al. Laparoscopic assisted splenectomy in a horse with splenomegaly. Equine Vet Educ 2008;20(7):357–61.

42. Rocken M, Mosel G, Stehle C, et al. Left- and right-sided laparoscopic-assisted nephrectomy in standing horses with unilateral renal disease. Vet Surg 2007; 36(6):568–72.

43. Rodgerson DH, Brown MP, Watt BC, et al. Hand-assisted laparoscopic technique for removal of ovarian tumors in standing mares. J Am Vet Med Assoc 2002; 220(10):1503–7.

44. Röcken M, Stehle C, Mosel G, et al. Laparoscopic-assisted cystotomy for urolith removal in geldings. Vet Surg 2006;35(4):394–7.

45. Hart SK, Brown JA. Diaphragmatic hernia in the horse: 44 cases (1986–2006). Paper presented at the 9th International Equine Colic Research Symposium, 2008, Liverpool, UK, June 15–18, 2008.

46. Kelmer G, Kramer J, Wilson DA. Diaphragmatic hernia: etiology, clinical presentation and diagnosis. Compendium on the Continuing Education of Equine Practice 2008;3(1):28–36.
47. Abutarbush SM, Carmalt JL, Shoemaker RW. Causes of gastrointestinal colic in horses in western Canada: 604 cases (1992 to 2002). Can Vet J 2005;46(9): 800–5.
48. Kelmer G, Kramer J, Wilson DA. Diaphragmatic hernia: treatment, complications and prognosis. Compendium on the Continuing Education of Equine Practice 2008;3:37–46.
49. French NP, Smith J, Edwards GB, et al. Equine surgical colic: risk factors for postoperative complications. Equine Vet J 2002;34(5):444–9.
50. Wilson DA, Baker GJ, Boero MJ. Complications of celiotomy incisions in horses. Vet Surg 1995;24(6):506–14.
51. Elce Y, Kraus B, Orsini J. Mesh hernioplasty for repair of incisional hernias of the ventral body wall in large horses. Equine Vet Educ 2005;17(5):252–6.
52. Kelmer G, Schumacher J. Repair of abdominal wall hernias in horses using primary closure and subcutaneous implantation of mesh. Vet Rec 2008; 163(23):677–9.
53. van der Velden MA, Klein WR. A modified technique for implantation of polypropylene mesh for the repair of external abdominal hernias in horses: a review of 21 cases. Vet Q 1994;16(Suppl 2):S108–10.
54. Freeman D, Rotting A, Inoue O. Abdominal closure and complications. Clin Tech Equine Pract 2002;1(3):174–87.
55. Cook G, Bristol D, Tate L. Ventral midline herniorrhaphy following colic surgery in the horse. Equine Vet Educ 1996;8:304–7.

New Perspectives in Equine Gastric Ulcer Syndrome

Ricardo Videla, DVM[a], Frank M. Andrews, DVM, MS[b],*

KEYWORDS

• Horse • Colic • Stomach • Equine gastric ulcer syndrome
• Treatment

EQUINE GASTRIC ULCER SYNDROME

Equine gastric ulcer syndrome (EGUS) is characterized by ulceration in the terminal esophagus, proximal (squamous) stomach, distal (glandular) stomach, and proximal duodenum.[1] Diagnosis of EGUS is based on history, clinical signs, endoscopic examination, and response to treatment. All ages and breeds of horses are susceptible to EGUS, and intermittent mild colic signs, especially during and after eating, can be a feature of this disease. Current pharmacologic agents used to control abdominal pain in horses traditionally include administration of nonsteroidal antiinflammatory agents (NSAIDs; phenylbutazone and flunixin meglumine), but these agents can cause and exacerbate gastric ulcers.[2] In horses with gastric ulcers, other pharmacologic agents can be administered to control pain associated with gastric ulcers without exacerbating already ulcerated mucosa. Controlling abdominal pain is essential until effective antiulcer agents can be administered to promote healing.

Current pharmacologic agents for treatment of gastric ulcers in horses focus on blocking gastric acid secretion and increasing stomach pH (≥ 4.0), which creates a permissive environment for ulcer healing. A sustained pH ≥ 4.0 for 24 hours has been shown to heal esophageal ulcers in people with gastroesophageal reflux disease (GERD). Also, because gastric acid is likely the cause of the pain associated with ulcers, effective acid control can decrease abdominal pain.

This chapter focuses on pain control, antiulcer treatment, and management strategies in horses with EGUS. Highlights of this chapter include basic anatomy and physiology of the equine stomach, current management practices that put the horse at risk for EGUS, treatment strategies in horses with abdominal pain, effective antiulcer

[a] Department of Large Animal Clinical Sciences, The University of Tennessee College of Veterinary Medicine, 2407 River Drive, Knoxville, TN 37996, USA
[b] Equine Health Studies Program, Department of Veterinary Clinical Sciences, School of Veterinary Medicine, Louisiana State University, Skip Bertman Drive, Baton Rouge, LA 70803, USA
* Corresponding author.
E-mail address: fandrews@lsu.edu (F.M. Andrews).

Vet Clin Equine 25 (2009) 283–301
doi:10.1016/j.cveq.2009.04.013
0749-0739/09/$ – see front matter © 2009 Elsevier Inc. All rights reserved.
vetequine.theclinics.com

therapy, and preventative measures to decrease ulcer severity and prevent recurrence.

ANATOMY, GASTRIC ACID SECRETION

Horses are predisposed to gastric ulcers because the proximal third is lined by non-glandular stratified squamous epithelium. The majority (80%) of ulcers occur in the proximal third or nonglandular region. In a report of 171 race horses in New Zealand, more gastric ulcers were found in the lesser and greater curvature of the nonglandular region near the Margo plicatus where acids are localized, when compared with the saccus caecus region.[3] Nonglandular squamous mucosa is predisposed to acid injury because it lacks substantial protective mucus and bicarbonate layers.[4,5] Furthermore, the erosive effects of gastric acid are likely the cause of colic signs in horses with gastric ulcers, but generally nonglandular ulcers must be severe to cause abdominal pain.

The distal two thirds of the stomach is lined by glandular mucosa and has extensive protective mucus and bicarbonate layers. The glands in this region secrete hydrochloric acid (HCl) and pepsinogen for digestion.[1,4] This region also contains an extensive capillary network and undergoes rapid restitution of epithelium when injured. Approximately 20% of ulcers occur in this region and may heal rapidly without therapeutic intervention. Moderate to severe ulcers in this region are likely to lead to abdominal pain, especially when they occur at or around the pyloric opening. When abdominal pain is present treatment is indicated.

Horses are continuous gastric HCl secretors,[6] and acid exposure is thought to be the primary cause of EGUS and intermittent abdominal pain associated with gastric ulcers. Gastric HCl secretion is stimulated by the gastrin, histamine and acetylcholine, a neurotransmitter from the Vagus nerve. However, other acids (volatile fatty acids [VFAs], bile acids [BA], and lactic acid [LA]) and enzymes (pepsin), found in the stomach may irritate stomach mucosa. Prolonged exposure of acids to the nonglandular mucosa, in a low pH environment, likely contributes to EGUS and the abdominal pain observed in some horses.

PREVALENCE

The prevalence of gastric ulceration is high in performance horses. Recently, in endoscopic studies performed in Thoroughbred and Standardbred horses actively racing and training, the prevalence of gastric ulcers was 88% (152 of 171).[3] Furthermore, prevalence of gastric ulcers in Swedish Standardbred racehorses in race training was 70% (56 of 80), and ulcers were significantly associated with horses that were in preparatory training and those that had raced in the last month when compared with horses that were fit but did not race in the last month.[7] Also, the prevalence of gastric ulcers was 53% in Danish Pleasure horses and 56% in a study of older horses (mean age 13.1 years).[8,9] Although effective treatments are available for EGUS, these and other studies confirm that the prevalence of gastric ulcers in competition and noncompetition horses remains high.

RISK FACTORS FOR EQUINE GASTRIC ULCER SYNDROME

Although acid injury has been implicated in the cause of EGUS, several risk factors for its development have been identified (**Table 1**).

Table 1	
Clinical signs and risk factors of EGUS	
Clinical Signs Adults	**Risk Factors**
Acute colic	Stress
Recurring colic	Transportation
Excessive recumbency	High-grain diet
Poor body condition	Stall confinement
Partial anorexia	Intermittent feeding
Poor appetite	Intense exercise
Poor performance/training	Racing
Attitude changes	Illness
Stretching often to urinate	NSAID use
Inadequate energy	Management changes
Chronic diarrhea	

Gender, Age, and Temperament

In a previous study there was slightly higher percentage of gastric ulceration in geldings (94%) than in colts (78%) and fillies (82%).[10] Although studies performed in racehorses in active training showed no difference in the prevalence or severity of EGUS between males and females.[3,11]

In a study performed in Standardbred racehorses in training, the severity of gastric ulcers was higher in horses ≥3 years of age than in 2-year-old horses, and the risk of ulcers increased with age in geldings and decreased with age in the mares and stallions. However, this could have been because the older horses had been in race training for a longer period.[7]

Temperament, a nervous disposition, is often discussed as a predisposing factor and has been shown to be associated with gastric ulcers in one study;[12] However, a study of Thoroughbred race horses failed to show the same association.[13]

Exercise Intensity

Horses involved in training and racing are at high risk for EGUS.[13,14] As discussed previously, current prevalence figures show that 70% to 88% of performance horses have EGUS. Recently it was shown that horses running on a high-speed treadmill have increased abdominal pressure and decreased stomach volume.[15] The authors speculated that contraction of the stomach allowed acid from the glandular mucosa to reflux into the nonglandular mucosa leading to injury. Daily exercise may increase the exposure of the nonglandular mucosa to acid explaining the increased prevalence of gastric ulcers in horses in training. Furthermore, an increase in serum gastrin concentration has been shown to occur in exercising horses.[16] This increase in serum gastrin may increase glandular HCl secretion that may lead to acid damage. Continuous acid exposure and ulceration is the primary cause of abdominal pain in horses with EGUS.

Also, the prevalence of gastric ulcers is higher in horses used for racing. In a post mortem study, Thoroughbred race horses in active training had a higher prevalence (80%), when compared with retired horses (52%).[17] These findings support other studies in which horses participating in intense training and racing have a higher prevalence of ulcers compared with horses used for pleasure.[18,19] Also, Swedish race horses in preparatory training and those that had raced during the last month had a significantly higher risk of ulcers that horses that were fit for racing but had not raced during the last month.[7]

Intermittent Versus Continuous Feeding

Horses grazing at pasture have a decreased prevalence of EGUS. During grazing, there is a continuous flow of saliva and ingesta that buffers stomach acid, and stomach pH is ≥4.0 for a large portion of the day. On the other hand, when feed is withheld from horses, before racing or in stabled horses, gastric pH drops rapidly, and the nonglandular mucosa is exposed to an acid environment.[20] However, a recent study found that pastured pregnant and nonpregnant mares had a high prevalence of gastric ulcers.[21] One possible explanation of this high prevalence of gastric ulcers in these pastured mares may be that horses consume less forage during the evening hours compared with daytime hours, which may result in less saliva production and a low pH environment in the proximal stomach. A recent study by Husted and colleagues[22] found that proximal stomach pH was lower in the early morning hours (1:00 to 9:00) regardless of housing (paddock or stable). This may be why pastured and stabled horses are susceptible to EGUS. A low pH environment in the proximal stomach may contribute to ulcer formation in the nonglandular squamous mucosa regardless of housing.

Intermittent feeding has been shown to cause and increase the severity of non-glandular ulcers in horses, and this has been used as a model to consistently produce EGUS.[23] The nonglandular mucosa is the most susceptible to ulceration in horses subjected to intermittent feeding because of its lack of mucosal protective factors. Gastric ulceration was found in 75% of horses fed twice daily and in 57.9% horses fed 3 times a day.[24] Nearly 58% of regularly fed horses had gastric ulcers, whereas 75% of irregularly fed horses had gastric ulcers. Also, a more recent study in Danish pleasure horses found an increased risk of gastric ulceration when forage feeding interval exceeded 6 hours,[25] which suggests that continuous forage feeding may be critical to reducing the risk of gastric ulceration.

Stall Confinement

Stall confinement has been implicated as a risk factor for EGUS.[26] In that study, six of seven horses housed in stalls had gastric ulcers, whereas no horse had gastric ulcers after 7 days turnout to pasture. However, in another study, the prevalence of ulcer severity did not differ significantly between horses stabled full time, horses kept in a stable part time, or horses kept in a pasture full time.[3] One study evaluating housing in horses found that neither proximal stomach nor ventral stomach pH changed signif-icantly in horses housed in stalls alone, housed in stalls with a companion, or housed in a grass paddock.[22] However, pH level in the proximal stomach was lower during the early morning hours regardless of the housing, and feed intake was lowest during these hours. Thus, other factors may play role in stabled horses that increase the risk of EGUS. Stabled horses typically are fed two large meals daily. These meals are traditionally high in grains and consumed rapidly, which lead to a decrease in saliva production and less buffering of stomach contents. Also, high grain diets may be fermented by resident stomach bacteria to VFAs, which in an acid environment may lead to ulceration.[27–29]

High Concentrate Diets

Size and composition of the grain has a profound effect on causing EGUS. Diet has been implicated as a risk factor for EGUS. Serum gastrin concentrations are highest in horses fed high-concentrate diets. Also, high-concentrate diets are high in digestible carbohydrates, which are fermented by resident bacteria, resulting in the production of VFAs. The VFAs in the presence of low stomach pH ($\leq$ 4) cause acid damage to the nonglandular squamous mucosa.[27–29] However, a recent study in horses found that alfalfa hay and a pelleted concentrate diet had lower gastric ulcer scores than horses fed Coastal Bermuda hay.[30] Furthermore, a previous study found that horses fed alfalfa hay and grain had higher stomach pH level and lower ulcer scores when compared with horses fed Brome grass hay without grain.[31] In that later study, the authors speculated that calcium and protein, both high in the alfalfa hay-grain diet, buffered stomach contents resulting in a protective effect on the nonglandular mucosa. Thus, alfalfa hay when fed with or without concentrates may have a protective and antiulcer effect in horses and decrease abdominal pain associated with EGUS.

Nonsteroidal Antiinflammatory Agents

The use of NSAIDs is common in horses presenting with acute abdominal pain. Typically, these horses are given either phenylbutazone or flunixin meglumine intravenously to control pain during a colic episode. These agents, especially flunixin meglumine are very effective in decreasing abdominal pain associated with acute colic, but several side effects have been reported that make their use risky in horses with EGUS. Phenylbutazone and flunixin meglumine have been found to induce gastric ulcers in horses[32] but usually at higher-than-recommended doses. Also, the use of NSAIDs in racehorses has not been shown to be a risk factor for EGUS in other epidemiologic studies.[17–19] Thus, NSAID are thought to cause more severe ulcers in the glandular mucosa because of their effect on prostaglandin inhibition. Prostaglandin inhibition results in decreased mucosal blood flow, decreased mucus production, and increased HCl secretion. Although prostaglandins are also important in the regulation of acid production and sodium transport, it may be their effect on mucosal blood flow that is the most important.[33] Adequate blood flow is necessary to remove hydrogen ions that diffuse through the mucus layer covering the glandular mucosa. Gastric mucosal ischemia may lead to a hypoxia-induced cellular acidosis and release of oxygen-free radicals, phospholipase, and proteases, which may damage the cell membrane leading to necrosis. Although NSAIDs are commonly used, they have the potential to exacerbate EGUS in horses with colic, and one should use them with caution.

Helicobacter spp and other Bacteria

Helicobacter spp (other than Helicobacter pylori) have been isolated from humans and a variety of animals suffering from gastric ulcers and gastritis.[34] Recently, a new enterohepatic Helicobacter species, Helicobacter equorum, was isolated from fecal samples of two clinically healthy horses.[35] Also, Helicobacter equorum DNA was found in the feces of two of seven (28.6%) foals less than 1 month of age and 40 of 59 (67.8%) foals 1 to 6 months of age.[36] Furthermore, Helicobacter-like DNA was detected in the stomach of 10 Thoroughbred horses in Venezuela.[37] In this study, Helicobacter-like DNA was detected in two of seven horses with gastric ulcers, three of five horses with gastritis, five of six horses with both pathologies, and one horse with normal gastric mucosa. Furthermore, 10 of 11 of the horses infected with Helicobacter had either gastric ulcers or gastritis or both pathologies. However, 39% of the horses in that study did not have gastric lesions, so multiple causes are likely.

Once gastric ulcers are present, other bacteria have been implicated in inhibiting ulcer healing. Bacteria, including Escherichia coli, were cultured from the stomach of horses.[38] In rats, which have a compound stomach similar to horses, E Coli administered orally, rapidly colonized acetic acid-induced gastric ulcers and impaired healing.[39] Oral antibiotic treatment with streptomycin or penicillin suppressed bacterial colonization of the ulcer and accelerated ulcer healing. Also, oral administration of lactulose resulted in an increase in *Lactobacillus spp* growth and colonization of the ulcer bed. Accelerated ulcer healing was seen in the rats compared with placebo-treated controls. Thus, bacterial colonization of gastric ulcers in the stomach of horses may delay ulcer healing, and in this case treatment with antibiotics may be indicated.

Clinical Signs of Equine Gastric Ulcer Syndrome

Clinical signs associated with EGUS are numerous and often vague. Acute and recurrent colic, diarrhea, rough hair coat, poor appetite, weight loss, attitude changes, depression, and decreased performance are seen in horses with gastric ulcers.[1,40] Ulcers are more common in horses showing clinical signs of abdominal pain (see **Table 1**).[11] In Thoroughbred horses in race training, gastric ulcers were associated with poor performance, poor hair coat, picky eating or intermittent anorexia, and mild intermittent abdominal pain. Of horses with a client complaint of conditions associated with gastric ulcers or showing subtle signs of poor health, gastric ulcers were identified in 88% to 92% compared with 37% to 52% identified in horses not showing clinical signs. Furthermore, the prevalence of gastric ulceration in the group of horses with poor general appetite was significantly ($P<.0001$) higher (94.8%) compared with horses with good general appetite (48.6%).[42]

In addition to an increased prevalence of ulcers in clinically affected horses, the severity of ulceration may be correlated with the severity of abdominal pain or severity of colic, and 49% of horses presented to a referral hospital for abdominal pain had gastric ulcers.[43] Also, 49% of horses responding to medical treatment had gastric ulcers, whereas a significantly smaller number (32%) that required surgery had gastric ulcers. Furthermore, in that same study, horses with duodenitis proximal jejunitis had a higher prevalence of gastric ulcers compared with horses with other gastrointestinal lesions.

DIAGNOSIS

Diagnosis of EGUS requires a thorough history, physical examination, and a minimum database. Identifying risk factors and clinical signs are also helpful in making a diagnosis. However, gastroscopy is the only definitive diagnosis for gastric ulcers currently available. Standing gastroscopy procedures have been described in detail elsewhere in the literature and require an endoscope of least 2 m to visualize the nonglandular mucosa and margo plicatus and a 2.5 m to 3 m endoscope to visualize the pylorus and proximal duodenum in most adult horses.[1,44,45] Use of a gastric ulcer scoring system allows clinicians to compare gastroscopic findings and monitor healing of ulcers and evaluate efficacy of treatment.[1,46]

Currently, there are no hematologic or biochemical markers to diagnose EGUS. However, a recent report showed that horses with gastric ulcers had lower red blood cell counts (RBC) counts and hemoglobin concentrations than horses that did not have gastric ulcers.[12] Some horses with EGUS may be slightly anemic or have hypoproteinemia, but in the authors' experience, the RBC and hemoglobin concentrations may be low but are rarely outside normal reference ranges.

Other presumptive diagnostic techniques include a sucrose absorption test.[47] Urine sucrose concentrations were significantly higher for horses with gastric ulcer scores greater than 1. Using a urine sucrose concentration cutoff value of 0.7 mg/mL or higher showed an apparent sensitivity of 83% and specificity of 90% to detect ulcers in horses tested using the sucrose permeability test. Thus, this test may provide a simple, noninvasive test to detect and monitor gastric ulcers.

In a recent study, a fecal occult blood test was found to be helpful in the diagnosis of EGUS.[48] The positive predictive value of the fecal occult blood test (FOBT) in horses with EGUS was 90%; however, the negative predictive value was only 17%, which suggests that a horse with a positive FOBT are likely to have a gastric ulcer. In an attempt to improve the negative predictive value of the FOBT, investigators developed another test (SUCCEED Equine Fecal Blood Test, Freedom Health LLC., Aurora, Ohio) that uses specific equine monoclonal antibodies to both albumin and hemoglobin in an easy-to-use kit.[49,50] Recent reports showed an improved predictive value of a negative test (72%), but the predictive value of a positive test was slightly lower (77%). Thus, this new test may be helpful in diagnosing EGUS in horses but should be used as part of a complete workup. A false-positive FOBT result may occur if a recent rectal examination, rectal biopsy, or other rectal trauma has occurred or if the horse has a protein loosing enteropathy.

Unfortunately, laboratory techniques provide only presumptive diagnostic evidence of EGUS, whereas a definitive diagnosis can only be made by endoscopic examination. Therefore, if gastroscopy is not available and ulcers are strongly suspected, it may be worthwhile to start empiric treatment and observe for resolution of clinical signs.[1] If the horse does not respond to treatment, referral to a facility with a gastroscope is indicated.

An effective method the authors have used is to give an antacid (Maalox Suspension, 1 mL/kg body weight [bw]) to which lidocaine (1:1000; 0.5 mL/kg bw) is added and administered via nasogastric tube. If gastric ulcers are the cause of the abdominal pain, then pain should subside within 15 minutes. If abdominal pain continues, then gastric ulcers are less likely, and further diagnostics should be performed.

MANAGEMENT OF EQUINE GASTRIC ULCER SYNDROME

Pain relief, healing, and prevention of secondary complications are the primary goals of antiulcer therapy and management recommendations. The mainstay of pharmacologic treatment of EGUS is to increase stomach pH and suppress HCl acid secretion. Because of the high recurrence rate, effective acid control should be followed by nutritional and dietary management strategies to prevent ulcer recurrence.

Pharmacologic Therapy

Pain management

The management of pain during a colic episode can be difficult, especially if the signs are severe. However, horses with primary or secondary gastric ulceration present with mild bouts of colic that usually respond to therapeutic doses. If EGUS is suspected, then phenylbutazone and flunixin meglumine should be avoided. A single therapeutic dose of phenylbutazone (4.4 mg/kg, intravenous [IV]) or flunixin meglumine (1.1 mg/kg, IV) will probably not result in catastrophic consequences, but repeated doses can further compromise mucosal blood flow, increase stomach acidity, and decrease mucus secretion, which may exacerbate gastric ulcers.

Alternative NSAIDs, like ketoprofen or firocoxib, may be used in horses with colic. Ketoprofen (2.2 mg/kg bw, IV, every 8 hours) was shown to have a less toxic effect on the gastrointestinal tract of horses compared with horses treated with phenylbutazone (4.4 mg/kg bw, IV, every 8 hours).[32] Furthermore, phenylbutazone-treated horses had a significant ($P<.05$) decrease in serum total protein and albumin concentrations and edema of the small intestine and erosions and ulcers of the large colon were observed. Horses in the ketoprofen-treated group did not develop renal papillary necrosis. In horses with dysphagia, gastric reflux or thrombosis of the jugular veins Ketoprofen (1 g) can be administered per rectum and may have some clinical efficacy, but it has low bioavailability.[51]

Recently, firocoxib (Equioxx, Merial Limited; Duluth, Georgia), a new cox-2 inhibitor NSAID, was approved for treatment of lameness in horses. Gastric ulcers were not detected in horses administered firocoxib (0.1 mg/kg, orally, every 24 hours, for 30 days).[52] However, firocoxib is US Food and Drug Administration (FDA) approved for the control of pain and inflammation associated with osteoarthritis in horses, thus, its efficacy in horses with abdominal pain is unknown. Furthermore, currently there is no intravenous formulation of this product, so it cannot be administered orally in horses with abdominal pain and gastric reflux or dysphagia.

The use of tranquilizers such as xylazine, butorphanol, or detomidine are an excellent alternative to NSAIDs in controlling abdominal pain. Xylazine (0.2–0.4 mg/kg) or detomidine (20–40 µg/kg, IV), alpha-2 adrenergic blocking agents, have sedative effects and are potent analgesic agents, with minimal effects on gastric and intestinal motility. Xylazine is short acting (15–20 minutes), whereas detomidine is more potent and is longer acting (30–60 minutes). These drugs allow clinical examination of horses and are indicators of pain severity. If pain is controlled for 2 to 3 hours, then the colic episode is not severe, whereas pain control for less than 15 minutes with either of these agents suggests more severe cause of abdominal pain, for which surgery may be indicated.

Butorphanol tartrate (0.004–0.1 mg/kg, IV), a synthetic narcotic agent, can be administered alone or with xylazine or detomidine. This agent is a potent analgesic agent and can provide temporary relief in horses experiencing abdominal pain. Also, butorphanol can be used pre- or postoperatively to control pain in horses with gastric ulcer. In a recent study, butorphanol (13 µg/kg/h, for 24 hours and a continuous rate infusion [CRI]) administered to horses after abdominal surgery showed significantly lower behavior pain scores when compared with those in saline-treated horses.[53] This could be used in horses with abdominal pain caused by EGUS as a CRI to achieve sustained pain control.

Specific antacid therapy

Once EGUS is diagnosed, therapy should be initiated to achieve the above outlined goals. Some EGUS lesions heal spontaneously, but generally most lesions in performance horses or horses showing clinical signs should be treated with pharmacologic agents. There are many approaches to treating EGUS, but the accepted strategy requires acid-suppressive therapy. Currently, Omeprazole paste (Gastrogard, Merial Limited, Duluth, Georgia) is the only FDA-approved product for treatment and prevention of recurrence of EGUS.[54] The use of proton pump inhibitors offers many advantages over H2 antagonists, which include FDA approval, once-daily administration, and the ability to block gastric acid secretion regardless of stimulus.

Omeprazole

Omeprazole oral paste (4 mg/kg, orally, every 24 hours) inhibits gastric acid secretion for 24 hours in horses.[55] In an acid environment omeprazole is activated to a sulphenamide derivative and binds reversibly to the H+/K+ ATPase in parietal cells and inhibits transport of hydrogen ions into the stomach.[56] Because of its effect on the cell, omeprazole is often called a "proton-pump blocker." The effect on gastric acid secretion is dose and time dependent.[57] Omeprazole is metabolized in the liver and excreted in urine and bile, and significant liver disease may affect the metabolism of the drug. Omeprazole has been found to be an effective treatment for EGUS at a dose of 4 mg/kg orally once daily.[54] A recent study of 565 horses in race training found that 96% of the 147 horses being administered H2 antagonists had gastric ulcers, with 61% considered to be severely affected.[58] Of the horses not receiving H2 antagonists, 88% had gastric ulcers, with 58% considered severe. All of the horses in the study were put on a 28-day course of omeprazole. There was a statistical improvement in performance, weight gain, attitude, appetite, and appearance after treatment. Endoscopically, 65% of the horses with gastric ulcers that were treated were healed, and 94% were improved. The primary reason for the failure of treatment with H2 antagonists was owner compliance and incorrect dosing. A second study found that 99% of spontaneous ulcers in adult horses and foals over 4 weeks of age were improved, with 86.7% healed with omeprazole treatment.[59] Effectiveness of omeprazole was also shown to increase the rate of healing in horses with ulcers and that were removed from race training.[60]

Recently, horses treated with omeprazole (0.5 mg/kg, IV) had an increased mean gastric juice pH level of greater than 4.0, 1 hour after administration.[61] In a study performed to evaluate the efficacy of omeprazole (0.5 mg/kg, IV, every 24 hours) for 5 days, gastric juice pH level was increased significantly from 2.01 ± 0.42 before administration to 4.35 ± 2.31 one hour after administration. Also, pH level increased on day 5 from 5.27 ± 1.74, 24 hours after the fourth dose to 7.00 ± 0.25, one hour after the fifth daily dose. Furthermore, nonglandular gastric ulcer number score significantly decreased after 5 days of treatment; however, none of the ulcers healed. Because of its potent and long duration of action on gastric juice pH, this intravenous formulation of omeprazole may show promise for treatment of EGUS in horses with dysphagia, gastric reflux, or other conditions that restrict oral intake of omeprazole paste. However, because of the variability of acid suppression after the first dose and dose of 1.0 mg/kg, IV, every 24 hours is recommended as a loading dose.

Histamine Type-2 Receptor Antagonists

Histamine stimulates acid secretion from the parietal cells.[62] Histamine type-2 receptor antagonists decrease acid secretion by competitively binding to the histamine receptor, thus blocking histamine attachment and stimulation of gastric acid secretion. Additionally, these agents may inhibit acid secretions stimulated by gastrin and acetylcholine.[63]

Cimetidine

Cimetidine has been used since the early 1980s to treat and prevent ulcers in horses and foals, but there is little scientific evidence in the veterinary literature showing that it has efficacy in the treatment of EGUS. The authors cannot recommend cimetidine for treatment or prevention for EGUS.

Ranitidine

Ranitidine hydrochloride (6.6 mg/kg) is four times more potent than cimetidine.[64] When given orally (6.6 mg/kg, orally, every 8 hours), ranitidine suppresses acid output and maintained a median stomach pH level of 4.6. At a dose of 6.6 mg/kg given orally every 8 hours, ranitidine was able to successfully limit ulcer development in a feed deprivation model.[26] Lower doses (4.4 mg/kg, orally, every 8 hours) given orally were ineffective for treatment of EGUS.[20,65,66] The recent availability of the generic ranitidine has made this drug popular and effective in treating EGUS. Ranitidine (6.6 mg/kg, orally, every 8 hours) has efficacy and in recommended for treatment of EGUS, but owner compliance is difficult.

Although ranitidine has been the most studied, other H2 antagonists have been evaluated experimentally and may allow for less frequent dosing and more effective acid suppression.[67] Bioavailability and pharmacodynamic studies with famotidine (2.8 mg/kg, orally, every 12 hours; 0.3 mg/kg, IV, every 12 hours) in horses[68] suggest that it can be used for treatment of EGUS, but may be cost prohibitive.

Coating or Binding Agents

Sucralfate and bismuth subsalcyclate are two compounds that bind to stomach ulcers and promote healing. Sucralfate is a hydroxyl aluminum salt of sucrose octasulfate and binds to the negatively charged particles in the ulcer bed, buffering HCl by increasing bicarbonate secretion, stimulating prostaglandins production, and adhering to the ulcer bed.[69] In the stomach, sucralfate is converted to a sticky amorphous mass, thought to prevent diffusion of hydrogen into the ulcer. In a clinical trial in horses, sucralfate (22 mg/kg, orally, every 8 hours) did not improve subclinical ulcer healing in 6- and 7-month-old foals. Therefore, sucralfate alone may not be beneficial in treatment of EGUS but can be used in conjunction with acid-suppressive therapy and may be more suited for treatment of right dorsal colitis (colonic ulcers) at a dose of 22 mg/kg, orally, every 6 to 8 hours.

Bismuth-containing compounds may have a coating effect similar to sucralfate. Additionally, it will inhibit the activation of pepsin and increase mucosal secretion.[70] A compound containing 26.25 g of bismuth failed to raise the pH in five horses.[71] Bismuth subsalicylate may be converted to sodium subsalicylate in the gastrointestinal tract, which may cause gastric irritation. Also, salicylates, similar to aspirin, decrease prostaglandin secretion and may further compromise an already damaged mucosa.[72] Thus, compounds containing bismuth are not recommended for treatment of EGUS. However, bismuth is used as part of the therapy in humans with *Helicobacter pylori*–induced gastric ulcers and may be used in horses with chronic recurring gastric ulcers in which *Helicobacter* is suspected.

Synthetic Hormones

Misoprostol, a synthetic PGE 1 analog, is effective in the treatment of gastric and duodenal ulcers in humans. Acid suppression, increased mucosal blood flow, increased bicarbonate secretion, and increased mucosal restitution are mechanisms of misoprostol. In one study, misoprostol (5 μg/kg, orally) increased stomach pH and inhibited gastric acid secretion for 8 hours. Misoprostol is contraindicated in pregnant and nursing horses because of its effect on increasing uterine contraptions. Although no reports of side effects have been reported in horses, side effects reported in other species include diarrhea, cramping, flatulence, and uterine contraction. Side effects are dose dependent.[56]

A somatostatin analog, octreotide acetate, has also been evaluated in horses.[73] Octreotide (0.5 to 5.0 μg/kg) raised the gastric pH level to greater than 4 for approximately 5 hours, with no adverse effects noted. While octreotide use appears to be very safe in human patients, it requires multiple daily dosing and is cost prohibitive in horses. The benefit of using a somatostatin analog is the prevention of hypergastrinemia associated with long-term use of acid suppressive drugs. The hypergastrinemia has a positive tropic effect on gastric cells and may result in proliferation.[74] Because somatostatin inhibits gastrin secretion, this hypertrophy is avoided; however, no case of gastric hypertrophy has been reported in horses after long-term use of acid suppressive drug therapy.

Prokinetic Agents

Prokinetic agents (see the article by Doherty elsewhere in this issue for a review of prokinetic agents) may be valuable as an adjunct therapy in the treatment of EGUS, and when there is adynamic ileus and gastroduodenal reflux. Bethanechol (0.25 mg/kg, IV) and erythromycin lactobionate (0.1 and 1.0 mg/kg, IV) increased solid-phase gastric emptying time in horses.[75] No adverse effects were seen in healthy patients; however, other forms of erythromycin can cause fatal colitis in adult horses at antimicrobial doses. Both prokinetic agents increase gastric emptying versus saline, but bethanechol appeared to be superior. It increased the gastric emptying rate of solid food versus erythromycin and increased gastric emptying rate of liquid versus saline. Bethanechol is a synthetic muscarinic cholinergic agent that is not degraded by acetylcholinesterase. The only side effect of the bethanechol administration was increased salivation. The recommended dose is 0.025 to 0.030 mg/kg subcutaneously every 3 to 4 hours followed by oral maintenance therapy of 0.3 to 0.45 mg/kg 3 to 4 time daily.[75] It is also possible that gastroduodenal reflux may worsen after treatment in patients with a proximal small intestinal obstruction.

Other pharmacologic agents have been used to treat EGUS with mixed success, and their suggested doses are listed in **Table 2**.

Duration of Pharmacologic Treatment

It is difficult to predict how long a nonglandular or glandular gastric ulcer will take to heal, but the initial recommended treatment time for most antiulcer medications is 28 days. However, management changes in addition to pharmacologic therapy can affect healing ulcers. For example, after a feed deprivation model of ulcer induction, ulcers were healed or nearly healed in horses after 9 days of pasture turnout.[26] Omeprazole treatment in Thoroughbred horses kept in training took longer to heal, with 57%, 67%, and 77% healing after 14 days, 21 days, and 28 days of treatment, respectively.[54] In a field trial, horses with spontaneous-occurring ulcers treated with omeprazole showed 86% healing after 28 days of treatment.[59] The authors recommend endoscopic examination after 14 days of omeprazole therapy to determine if the ulcers are healed. If the gastric ulcers are healed, then the dose can be reduced (1–2 mg/kg, PO, q24h) to prevent recurrence of ulcers while the horse remains in race training.[54,76] If the ulcers are still present, then the full 28-day course of

Drug	Dosage	Dosing Interval	Route of Administration
Omeprazole	0.5–1.0 mg/kg	Intravenously	Every 24 hr
Omeprazole (GastroGard)	4 mg/kg (treatment) 1 mg/kg (prevention)	Orally	Every 24 hr
Ranitidine	1.5 mg/kg	Intravenously	Every 6 hr
Ranitidine	6.6 mg/kg	Orally	Every 8 hr
Famotidine	0.3 mg/kg	Intravenously	Every 12 hr
Famotidine	2.8 mg/kg	Orally	Every 12 hr
Misoprostol	5 µg/kg	Orally	Every 8 hr
Sucralfate	20–40 mg/kg	Orally	Every 8 hr
AlOH/MgOH antacids	30g AlOH/15 g MgOH	Orally	Every 2 hr

Table 2
Drug therapy for treatment of EGUS

omeprazole should be followed and the horse further evaluated after that time. When endoscopy is not available, horses should be treated for at least 28 days. It should be noted that clinical signs might resolve before complete healing has taken place. Signs of poor appetite, colic, or diarrhea will usually resolve within a few days after initiating treatment, and the horse is expected to make improvements in body condition and attitude within 2 to 3 weeks. Histamine type 2 antagonist therapy should be continued for at least 28 days, but healing may take longer than 40 days and may not be as effective as treatment with omeprazole paste.[77]

In general it may take longer to treat large ulcers, more severe ulcers, and ulcers in the nonglandular mucosa.[70] In cases in which clinical signs have resolved and the risk factors for ulcer development are low, spontaneous healing of ulcers may occur without further treatment. However, spontaneous healing will not occur in horses that continue intensive training, and ulcers may recur in those successfully treated if therapy is discontinued.[54] If clinical signs attributed to EGUS have not resolved after 48 to 72 hours of treatment, the diagnosis or therapy should be reconsidered.

Environmental, Nutritional, and Dietary Management of Equine Gastric Ulcer Syndrome

Pharmacologic therapy may be necessary to heal both glandular and nonglandular gastric ulcers in horses, but once pharmacologic therapy is discontinued, the ulcer will quickly return if management changes are not instituted. Environmental, nutritional, and dietary management can be initiated during therapy to help facilitate ulcer healing and prevent ulcer recurrence. As mentioned before, intense or long-duration exercise, stall confinement, and diet are risk factors for EGUS. Several management changes can be instituted to decrease severity and prevent ulcer recurrence. A thorough review on the nutritional and dietary management of horses with EGUS is presented elsewhere.[78]

Antibiotics Versus Probiotics

Helicobacter equorum DNA was isolated from the glandular and nonglandular stomach mucosa in horses.[35–37] Also, recently a large population of diverse acid-tolerant bacteria (E coli, Lactobacillus, and Streptococcus spp) were isolated from the gastric contents of horses fed various diets.[38] In rats, which have a compound stomach similar to horses, bacteria (E coli) rapidly colonized acetic acid-induced stomach ulcers and impaired ulcer healing.[38] In this study, oral antibiotic treatment with streptomycin or penicillin suppressed bacterial colonization of the ulcer and markedly accelerated ulcer healing. Also, oral administration of lactulose resulted in an increase Lactobacillus spp growth and colonization of the ulcer bed. This accelerated ulcer healing in these rats compared with placebo-treated controls. In a recent study in horses with spontaneously occurring gastric ulcers, an antibiotic (trimethoprim suphadimidine) or a probiotic preparation containing Lactobacillus sp facilitated healing of gastric ulcers.[79] These data suggest that resident stomach bacteria are important in maintenance and progression of nonglandular gastric ulcers in horses, and treatment with antibiotic or probiotic preparations may facilitate ulcer healing after 2 weeks of treatment, with the full effect occurring after 4 weeks of treatment. Thus, antibiotic treatment may be indicated in horses with chronic nonresponsive gastric ulcers, but more importantly, probiotic preparations containing Lactobacillus and Streptococcus spp may be helpful in prevention of gastric ulcers or may be used as an adjunct to pharmacologic treatment.

Dietary Supplements

A plethora of dietary supplements on the market for horses claim efficacy in treatment and prevention of gastric ulcers. Many of these products have not been tested in the horse, and to date very little scientific evidence exists on their efficacy. Below are several supplements that have some scientific testing or have ingredients that have been shown to be helpful in ulcer treatment and prevention.

Seabuckthorn berry extract

There is an increasing interest in the use of herbs and berries that have therapeutic application in humans and animals. Berries and pulp from the seabuckthorn plant (*Hippophae rhamnoides*) are high in vitamins, trace minerals, amino acids, antioxidants, and other bioactive substances and have been used successfully to treat mucosal injury, including decubital ulcers, burns, and stomach and duodenal ulcers in humans.[80,81] In addition, seabuckthorn berries have been shown to successfully treat and prevent acetic acid–induced gastric ulcers in rats.[82] A recent study was completed to evaluate the efficacy of seabuckthorn berry pulp and extract (3 ounces fed twice daily; SeaBuck Complete, SeaBuck LLC, Midvale, Utah) on the treatment and prevention of gastric ulcers in horses.[83] This preparation of seabuckthorn berry did not significantly decrease nonglandular gastric ulcer scores in eight treated horses when compared with the untreated controls; however, this preparation prevented an increase in gastric ulcer scores after an alternating feed deprivation, ulcer induction model, compared with control horses, which had a significant increase in gastric ulcer scores. Also, gastric ulcer scores in seven of eight seabuckthorn-treated horses either stayed the same or decreased compared with just two of eight of the untreated controls during this period. Although this preparation of seabuckthorn berry did not heal ulcers in these horses, it may be efficacious in the prevention or worsening of nonglandular gastric ulcers in horses during times of stress.

Calcium carbonate supplements

There are many supplements on the market containing calcium carbonate, a primary component of human antacids preparations, namely Tums. These products contain varying concentrations of calcium carbonate and various other herbs and coating agents. The author performed a small study with an antacid preparation containing calcium carbonate (Neigh-Lox, Kentucky Performance Products, LLC, Versailles, Kentucky) to determine efficacy in treatment and prevention of gastric ulcers in horses (Frank M. Andrews, DVM MS, unpublished data, 2001). In that study, four healthy horses were fed hay and a small amount of grain top dressed with 4 ounces of this calcium carbonate supplement twice daily for 3 weeks. There was no significant difference in gastric ulcer scores between control horses and treated horses; however, gastric juice pH remained ≥ 4 for 2 hours after feeding when compared with control horses. Also, in an in vitro study, this supplement, when added to acid damaged stomach tissue, resulted in recovery of sodium transport. Thus, these data suggest that calcium carbonate preparations may have some efficacy in maintaining mucosal integrity, but horses may need to be fed more frequently than twice daily to prevent EGUS.

Oils (corn oil, rice bran oil)

Dietary fats delay gastric emptying time in man and other species.[84] In contrast to most species, a recent study showed that gastric emptying rates were slower in horses fed a high carbohydrate diet compared with horses fed a high fat diet, although these rates were not statistically significant.[85] However, gastric relaxation was significantly greater in horses fed the high carbohydrate diet compared with horses fed the high-fat diet. At this time it seems that supplementation of dietary fat may not have a profound effect on gastric emptying in horses.

In another study, Cargile and colleagues,[86] fed dietary corn oil (45 mL, orally, once daily) by dose syringe to ponies with gastric cannulas. These ponies had a significantly lower gastric acid output and increased prostaglandin concentration in gastric juice when supplemented with corn oil. The authors conclude that corn oil supplementation could be an economical approach to the therapeutic and prophylactic management of glandular ulcers in horses, especially those associated with the use of NSAIDS.

In contrast to the previous study, Frank and colleagues[87] evaluated the antiulcerogenic properties of corn oil, refined rice bran oil, and crude rice bran oil. Horses were fed the oil (8 ounces, once daily, mixed in grain) for 6 weeks. The findings showed no statistical differences in nonglandular ulcer scores among the treatment groups, and glandular ulcers were rare in these horses. In this model, dietary oils did not prevent nonglandular gastric ulcers in these horses, suggesting that dietary oils may not be useful in treatment or prevention of nonglandular ulcers but may be helpful in treatment or prevention of glandular ulcers.

SUMMARY

Equine gastric ulcer syndrome is common in horses and stomach acids, and environmental, nutritional, and dietary factors are likely important causative factors. Upon initial diagnosis of EGUS, treatment should be started with effective pharmacologic agents. Abdominal pain can be a feature of EGUS, and the clinician should avoid NSAIDs to treat the abdominal pain. Prevention of ulcer recurrence primarily depends on environmental and nutritional and dietary management. Finally, the recommendations for horses with EGUS include the following:[78]

1. Keep the horse eating by providing a minimum of 1 to 1.5 kg/100 kg of body weight of long-stem high-quality forage (hay) free-choice throughout the day and night.
2. Feed alfalfa hay or a mixture alfalfa hay to help buffer stomach acid.
3. Feed grain and concentrates sparingly. Give no more than 0.5 kg/100 kg of body weight of grain or grain mixes such as, "sweet feed" and don't feed grain meals less than 6 hours apart.
4. Try corn oil or other dietary supplements, but feed hypertonic electrolyte pastes or supplements after exercise with a grain meal.
5. Consider therapeutic or preventative doses of effective pharmacologic agents in horses that are performing high intensity exercise, traveling or in a high-stress situation. This is especially important in horses with chronic arthritis and one should consider the following:
    Choose NSAIDs that have minimal effects on the gastrointestinal tract. These are firocoxib and ketoprofen.
    Doses of NSAIDs should be titered so that the minimal dose that effectively controls pain should be used.
    If NSAIDs are used, then administering antiulcer medications at preventative or treatment doses should be considered.

REFERENCES

1. Anon. Recommendations for the diagnosis and treatment of equine gastric ulcer syndrome (EGUS). Equine Vet Educ 1999;1(2):122–34.

2. Tobin T, Chay S, Kamerling S, et al. Phenylbutazone in the horse: a review. J Vet Pharmacol Ther 1986;9(1):1–25.
3. Bell RJW, Kingston JK, Mogg TD, et al. The prevalence of gastric ulceration in racehorses in New Zealand. N Z Vet J 2007;55(1):13–8.
4. Murray MJ. Aetiopathogenesis and treatment of peptic ulcer in the horse: a comparative review. Equine Vet J Suppl 1992;13:63–74.
5. Ross IN, Bahari HM, Turneberg LA. The pH gradient across mucus adherent to rat fundic mucosa in vivo and the effect of potential damaging agents. Gastroenterology 1981;81:713–8.
6. Cambell-Thompson ML, Merritt AM. Basal and pentagastrin-stimulated gastric secretion in young horses. Am J Physiol 1990;259:R1259–66.
7. Jonsson H, Egenvall A. Prevalence of gastric ulceration in Swedish Standardbreds in race training. Equine Vet J 2006;38(3):209–13.
8. Andrews FM, Buchanan BR, Smith SH, et al. In vitro effects of hydrochloric acid and various concentrations of acetic, propionic, butyric and valeric acids on bioelectric properties of equine gastric squamous mucosa. Am J Vet Res 2006; 67:1873–82.
9. Luthersson N, Hou Nielsen K, Harris P, et al. Prevalence and anatomical distribution of equine gastric ulceration syndrome (EGUS) in 201 horses in Denmark. Equine Vet J, in press.
10. Sandin A, Skidell J, Haggstorm J, et al. Post mortem findings of gastric ulcers in Swedish race horses older than age one year: a retrospective study of 3715 horses, (1924–1996). Equine Vet J 2000;32:36–42.
11. Rabuffo TS, Orsini JA, Sullivan E, et al. Association between age or sex and prevalence of gastric ulceration in Standardbred racehorses in training. J Am Vet Med 2002;221(8):1156–9.
12. McClure SR, Glickman LT, Glickman NW. Prevalence of gastric ulcers in show horses. J Am Vet Med 1999;215(8):1130–3.
13. Vatistas NJ, Snyder JR, Carlson G, et al. Cross-sectional study of gastric ulcers of the squamous mucosa in thoroughbred racehorses. Equine Vet J Suppl 1999;29: 34–9.
14. Vatistas NJ, Sifferman RL, Holste J, et al. Induction and maintenance of gastric ulceration in horses in simulated race training. Equine Vet J Suppl 1999;29:40–4.
15. Lorenzo-Figueras M, Merritt AM. Effects of exercise on gastric volume and pH in the proximal portion of the stomach of horses. Am J Vet Res 2002;63(11):1481–7.
16. Furr M, Taylor L, Kronfeld D. The effects of exercise training on serum gastrin responses in the horse. Cornell Vet 1994;84:41–5.
17. Hammond CJ, Mason DK, Watkins KL. Gastric ulceration in mature thoroughbred horses. Equine Vet J 1986;18(4):284–7.
18. Murray MJ, Schusser GF, Pipers FS, et al. Factors associated with gastric lesions in thoroughbred racehorses. Equine Vet J 1996;28(5):368–74.
19. Vastista NJ, Snyder JR, Carlson G, et al. Epidemiological study of gastric ulceration in the thoroughbred race horse: 202 horses 1992-1993. Proc Am Assoc Equine Pract 1994;40:125–6.
20. Murray MJ, Schusser GF. Measurement of 24-h gastric pH using an indwelling pH electrode in horses unfed, fed, and treated with ranitidine. Equine Vet J 1993; 25(5):417–21.
21. Le Jeune SS, Neito JE, Dechant JE, et al. Prevalence of gastric ulcers in Thoroughbred broodmares in pasture. Presented at the Proceedings of the 52nd Annual American Association of Equine Practitioners meeting. San Antonio, TX, December 3–6, 2006.

22. Husted L, Sanchez LC, Olsen SN, et al. Effect of paddock vs. stall housing on 24 hour gastric pH with the proximal and ventral equine stomach. Equine Vet J 2008; 40:337–41.

23. Murray MJ. Equine model of inducing ulceration in alimentary squamous epithelial mucosa. Dig Dis Sci 1994;12:2530–5.

24. Feige K, Furst A, Eser MW. Effects of housing, feeding, and use on equine health with emphasis on respiratory and gastrointestinal disease. Schweiz Arch Tierheilkd 2002;144(7):348–55.

25. Luthersson N, Hou Nielsen K, Harris P, et al. Risk factors associated with equine gastric ulcer syndrome (EGUS) in 201 horses in Denmark. Equine Vet J, in press.

26. Murray MJ, Eichorn ES. Effects of intermittent feed deprivation, intermittent feed deprivation with ranitidine administration and stall confinement with ad libitum access to hay on gastric ulceration in horses. Am J Vet Res 1996;57(11): 1599–603.

27. Nadeau JA, Andrews FM, Patton CS, et al. Effects of hydrochloric, acetic, butyric and proprionic acids on pathogenesis of ulcers in the nonglandular portion of the stomach of horses. Am J Vet Res 2003;64(4):404–12.

28. Nadeau JA, Andrews FM, Patton SC, et al. Effects of hydrochloric, valeric and other volatile fatty acids on pathogenesis of ulcers in the nonglandular portion of the stomach of horses. Am J Vet Res 2003;64:413–7.

29. Andrews FM, Buchanan BR, Elliott SB, et al. In vitro effects of hydrochloric acid and lactic acid on bioelectric properties of equine gastric squamous mucosa. Equine vet J 2008;40:301–5.

30. Lybbert T, Gibbs P, Cohen N, et al. Feeding alfalfa hay to exercising horses reduces the severity of gastric squamous mucosal ulceration. Presented at the Proceedings of the 54th Annual meeting of the Am Assoc Equine Pract. Orlando, FL, December 2–5, 2007. p. 525–6.

31. Nadeau JA, Andrews FM, Mathew AG, et al. Evaluation of diet as a cause of gastric ulcers in horses. Am J Vet Res 2000;61(7):784–90.

32. MacAllister CG, Morgan SJ, Borne AT, et al. Comparison of adverse effects of phenylbutazone, flunixin meglumine, and ketoprofen in horses. J Am Vet Med Assoc 1993;202(1):71–7.

33. Navab F, Steingrub J. Stress ulcer: is routine prophylaxis necessary? Am J Gastroenterol 1995;90:708–12.

34. Fox JG. The non-H. pylori helicobacters: their expanding role in gastrointestinal and systemic disease. Gut 2002;50:273–83.

35. Moyaert H, Decostere A, Vandamme P, et al. Helicobacter equorum sp. nov., a urease-negative Helicobacter species isolated from horses faeces. Int J Syst Evol Microbiol 2007;57:213–8.

36. Moyaert H, Haesebrouck F, Dewulf J, et al. Helicobacter equorum is highly prevalent in foals. Vet Microbiol 2009;133(1–2):190–2.

37. Contreras M, Morales A, Garcia-Amado MA, et al. Detection of Helicobacter-like DNA in the gastric mucosa of thoroughbred horses. Lett Appl Microbiol 2007; 45(5):553–7.

38. Al Jassim RAM, Scott PT, Trebbin AL, et al. The genetic diversity of lactic acid producing bacteria in the equine gastrointestinal tract. FEMS Microbiol Lett 2006;248:75–81.

39. Elliott SN, Buret A, McKnight W, et al. Bacteria rapid colonize and modulate healing of gastric ulcer in rats. Am J Physiol Gastrointest Liver Physiol 1998;275: 425–32.

40. Murray MJ. Diagnosing and treating gastric ulcers in foals and horses. Vet Med 1991;8:820–7.
41. Murray MJ, Grodinsky C, Anderson CW, et al. Gastric ulcers in horses: a comparison of endoscopic findings in horses with and without clinical signs. Equine Vet J Suppl 1989;7:68–72.
42. Bezděková B, Jahn P, Vyskočil M, et al. Gastric ulceration, appetite, and feeding practices in standardbred racehorses in the Czech Republic. Acta Vet Brno 2008;77:603–7.
43. Dutkti SA, Perkins S, Murphy J, et al. Prevalence of gastric squamous ulceration in horses with abdominal pain. Equine Vet J 2006;38(4):347–9.
44. Murray MJ, Nout YS, Ward DL. Endoscopic findings of the gastric antrim and pylorus in horses: 162 cases (1996–2000). J Vet Intern Med 2001;15:401–6.
45. Andrews FM, Reinemeyer CR, McCracken MD, et al. Comparison of endoscopic, necropsy and histology scoring of equine gastric ulcers. Equine Vet J 2002; 34(5):475–8.
46. MacAllister CG, Andrews FM, Deegan E, et al. A scoring system for equine gastric ulcers. Equine Vet J 1997;29:430–3.
47. O'connor MS, Steiner JM, Roussel AJ, et al. Evaluation of sucrose concentration for detection of gastric ulcers in horses. Am J Vet Res 2004;65(1):31–9.
48. Pellegrini FL. Results of a large scale necroscopic study of equine colonic ulcers. J Equine Vet Sci 2005;25:113–7.
49. Carter S, Pellegrini FA. The use of novel antibody tools to detect the presence of blood in equine feces. Company Bulletin Freedom Health LLC 2006;1–3.
50. Pellegrini FL, Carter SD. An equine necroscopic study to determine the sensitivity and specificity of a dual antibody test. Company Bulletin Freedom Health LLC 2007;1–2.
51. Corveleyn S, Deprez G, Van Der Weken W, et al. Bioavailability of ketoprofen in horses after rectal administration. J Vet Pharmacol Ther 1996;19(5):359–63.
52. Equioxx, Merial Limited, Duluth, GA. Freedom of Information Summary 2005;13.
53. Sellon DC, Roberts MC, Blikslager AT, et al. Effects of continuous rate intravenous infusion of butorphanol on physiologic and outcome variables in horses after celiotomy. J Vet Intern Med 2004;18(4):555–63.
54. Andrews FM, Sifferman RL, Bernard W, et al. Efficacy of omeprazole paste in the treatment and prevention of gastric ulcers in horses. Equine Vet J Suppl 1999;29:81–6.
55. Daurio CP, Holste JE, Andrews FM, et al. Effect of omeprazole paste on gastric acid secretion in horses. Equine Vet J Suppl 1999;29:59–62.
56. Plumb DC. Veterinary drug handbook. 4th edition. Ames: Iowa State Press; 2002.
57. Andrews FM, MacAllister CM, Jenkins CC, et al. Omeprazole: a promising drug for antiulcer treatment in horses. Proc Am Assoc Equine Pract 1995;41:184–6.
58. MacAllister CG, Sangiah S. Effect of ranitidine on healing of experimentally induced gastric ulcer in ponies. Am J Vet Res 1993;54(7):1103–7.
59. MacAllister CG, Sifferman RL, McClure SR, et al. Effects of omeprazole paste on healing of spontaneous gastric ulcers in horses and foals; a field trial. Equine Vet J Suppl 1999;29:77–80.
60. Murray MJ, Haven ML, Eichorn ES, et al. Effects of omeprazole on healing of naturally-occuring gastric ulcers in Thoroughbred racehorses. Equine Vet J 1997;29(6):425–9.
61. Andrews FM, Frank N, Sommardahl CS, et al. Effects of intravenously administered omeprazole on gastric juice pH and gastric ulcer scores in adult horses. J Vet Intern Med 2006;20:1202–6.
62. Kitchen DL, Merritt AM, Burrow JA. Histamine-induced gastric acid secretion in horses. Am J Vet Res 1998;59(10):1303–6.

63. Brunton LL. Agents for control of gastric acidity and treatment of peptic ulcers. In: Hardman JG, Limbird LE, editors. Goodman and Gilman's the pharmacological basis of therapeutics. Hightstown, NJ: McGraw Hill. p. 901–16.
64. Sangiah S, MacAllister CC, Amouzadeh HR. Effects of cimetidine and ranitidine on basal gastric pH, free and total acid contents in horses. Res Vet Sci 1988; 45:291–5.
65. Holland PS, Ruoff WW, Brumbaugh GW, et al. Plasma pharacokinetics of ranitidine HCl in adult horses. J Vet Pharmacol Ther 1997;20:145–52.
66. Johnson JH, Vatistas N, Castro L, et al. Field survey of the prevalence of gastric ulcers in Thoroughbred racehorses and on response to treatment of affected horses with omeprazole paste. Equine Vet Educ 2001;13(4):221–4.
67. Orsini JA, Dreyfuss DJ, Vecchione J, et al. Effects of a histamine type-2 receptor antagonist (BMY-25368) on gastric secretion in horses. Am J Vet Res 1991;53(1): 108–10.
68. Duran SH. Famotidine. Compendium on Continuing Education for the Practicing Veterinarian 1999;21(5):424–5.
69. Borne AT, MacAllister CG. Effect of sucralfate on healing of subclinical gastric ulcers in foals. J Am Vet Med 1993;202(9):1465–8.
70. MacAllister CG. Medical therapy for equine gastric ulcers. Vet Med 1995;11: 1070–6.
71. Clark CK, Merritt AM, Burrow JA, et al. Effect of aluminum hydroxide/magnesium hydroxide antacid and bismuth subsalicylate on gastric pH in horses. J Am Vet Med 1996;208(10):1687–91.
72. Martindale WH. Metals and some metallic salts. In: Reynolds JEF, editor. The extrapharmacopoeia of Martindale. 28th edition. London: Pharmaceutical Press; 1982. p. 926–46.
73. Sojka JE, Weiss JS, Samuels ML, et al. Effect of the somatostatin analogue octreotide on gastric fluid pH in ponies. Am J Vet Res 1992;53(10):1818–21.
74. Tielemans T, Hakanson R, Sundler F, et al. Proliferation of enterochromaffin-like cells in omeprazole-treated hypergastrinemic rats. Gastroenterology 1989;96: 723–9.
75. Ringger NC, Lester GD, Neuwirth L, et al. Effect of bethanechol or erythromycin on gastric emptying in horses. Am J Vet Res 1996;57(12):1771–5.
76. McClure SR, White GW, Sifferman RL, et al. Efficacy of omeprazole paste for prevention of recurrence of gastric ulcers in horses in race training. J Am Vet Med Assoc 2005;226(10):1681–4.
77. Lester GD, Smith RL, Robertson ID. Effects of treatment with omeprazole or ranitidine on gastric squamous ulceration in racing Thoroughbreds. J Am Vet Med Assoc 2005;227:1636–9.
78. Reese RE, Andrews FM. Nutritional and dietary management of equine gastric ulcer syndrome. Vet Clin North Am Equine Pract 2009;25:79–92.
79. Al Jassim RAM, McGowan T, Andrews FM, et al. Role of bacteria and lactic acid in the pathogenesis of gastric ulceration, Rural Industries Research and Development Corporation (RIRDC), final report, Australia 2008:1–26.
80. Geetha S, Ram MS, Singh V, et al. Anti-oxidant and immunomodulatory properties of seabuckthorn (Hippophae rhamnoides) an invitro study. J Ethnopharmacol 2002;79:373–8.
81. Beveridge T, Li TSC, Oomah BD, et al. Seabuckthorn products: manufacturing and composition. J Agric Food Chem 1999;47:3480–8.

82. Xing J, Yang B, Dong Y, et al. Effects of sea buckthorn (Hippophaë rhamnoides L.) seed and pulp oils on experimental models of gastric ulcer in rats. Fitoterapia 2002;73:644–50.

83. Reese RE, Andrews FM, Elliott SB, et al. The effect of seabuckthorn berry extract (Seabuck Complete) on prevention and treatment of gastric ulcers in horses. Presented at the Proceedings of the 9th International Equine Colic Research Symposium, Liverpool. June 8–11, 2008.

84. Sidery MB, Macdonald IA, Blackshaw PE. Superior mesenteric artery blood flow and gastric emptying in humans and the differential effects of high fat and high carbohydrate meals. Gut 1994;35:186–90.

85. Lorenzo-Figueras M, Preston T, Ott EA, et al. Meal-induce gastric relaxation and emptying in horses after ingestion of high-fat versus high-carbohydrate diets. Am J Vet Res 2005;66:897–906.

86. Cargile JL, Burrow JA, Kim I, et al. Effect of dietary corn oil supplementation on equine gastric fluid acid, sodium, and prostaglandin E_2 content before and during pentagastrin infusion. J Vet Intern Med 2004;18:545–9.

87. Frank N, Andrews FM, Elliott SB, et al. Effects of dietary oils on the development of gastric ulcers in mares. Am J Vet Res 2005;66:2006–11.

Inflammatory Bowel Disease in Horses

Karen A. Kalck, DVM

KEYWORDS
- Inflammatory • Malabsorption • Maldigestion
- Enteritis • Small intestine

TERMINOLOGY

Inflammatory bowel disease (IBD) in the horse is a malabsorptive and maldigestive disorder most commonly affecting the small intestine. Occasionally, in advanced disease, the large intestine is involved also. Malabsorption, defined as defective nutrient uptake or transport by the intestinal mucosa,[1] can affect the absorption of carbohydrates, proteins, fats, vitamins, or minerals, or of any combination of these nutrients. Maldigestion is defined as impaired breakdown of micronutrients.[1] The distinction between maldigestion and malabsorption often is not possible and usually is not clinically relevant.

In adult horses, IBD is recognized as an infiltration of the mucosa and submucosa with abnormal cells.[1] The diagnosis is based on the degree of inflammation and the predominant type of infiltrating leucocyte.[2] The cause of this abnormal cellular infiltrate has been linked to abnormal immune responses to bacterial, viral, parasitic, or dietary antigens.[3] In foals, IBD is associated more commonly with infectious agents causing malabsorption.

TYPES OF INFLAMMATORY BOWEL DISEASE IN THE HORSE
Eosinophilic Enteritis and Multisystemic Eosinophilic Epitheliotrophic Disease

Eosinophilic enteritis is recognized as diffuse inflammatory cell infiltration of the small intestinal mucosa with eosinophils and lymphocytes.[3] A subset of affected horses also suffer from eosinophilic infiltration of other organs and tissues including the skin, liver, pancreas, oral cavity, esophagus, lungs, and mesenteric lymph nodes.[3,4] This more severe form of the disease is known as "multisystemic eosinophilic epitheliotrophic disease" (MEED).

Horses of any sex, age, or breed may be affected with eosinophilic enteritis or MEED, but it seems most common in young (2–4 years of age) Standardbred and Thoroughbred horses.[3,5] Recurrent colic is a common clinical sign with this form of

Department of Large Animal Clinical Sciences, The University of Tennessee College of Veterinary Medicine, 2407 River Drive, Knoxville, TN 37996, USA
E-mail address: kakalck@mail.ag.utk.edu

Vet Clin Equine 25 (2009) 303–315
doi:10.1016/j.cveq.2009.04.008
0749-0739/09/$ – see front matter © 2009 Elsevier Inc. All rights reserved.

IBD, and the disease may be diffuse or focal. Circumferential mural bands can form because eosinophilic enzymes stimulate mural fibrosis that partially obstructs the lumen of the small intestine.[6] This obstruction can lead to low-grade chronic colic or result in an acute episode if significant obstruction and distention occur.[7] Other findings include mucosal ulceration, enlargement of ileal Peyers patches, and mesenteric lymphadenopathy.[1] Horses affected with MEED may have severe dermatitis resembling pemphigus foliaceus with lesions on the face, limbs, ventrum, and coronary bands.[1] The dermatitis may or may not be pruritic and can become secondarily infected if severe.[8] A peripheral eosinophilia is uncommon.[8,9] These horses may have an elevated gamma-glutamyltransferase (GGT) level if the liver is affected.[1]

A specific diagnosis of eosinophilic enteritis can be made via skin biopsy if lesions are present. Biopsy of the rectum or liver also has been useful for diagnosis.[1] Eosinophilic granulomas associated with vasculitis and fibrinoid necrosis of intramural vessels on rectal biopsy are pathognomonic of MEED.[10]

The cause of this form of IBD is thought to be a type I hypersensitivity reaction possibly caused by inhaled, dietary, or parasitic antigens.[11] Therefore elimination of these antigens is a necessary part of the treatment plan. Diet change, anthelmintics, and corticosteroids are all used for treatment of eosinophilic enteritis. Treatment options are discussed in more detail in a later section. Most of the current literature reports that treatment usually is unsuccessful, but occasionally horses do respond favorably.[12]

Granulomatous Enteritis

Granulomatous enteritis is characterized by lymphoid and macrophage infiltration of the mucosal lamina propria with variable numbers of plasma cells and giant cells.[13] There usually is marked villous atrophy, and the ileum typically is the most severely affected portion of the gastrointestinal tract.[14] This condition is similar to Crohn's disease in humans and Johne's disease in cattle. Johne's disease is associated with infection by *Mycobacterium pseudotuberculosis*; although this organism is rarely isolated in horses, *M. avium* has been reported in some cases.[14] In humans who have Crohn's disease, there is excessive activation of mucosal T cells leading to transmural inflammation. This activation is amplified and perpetuated by the release of pro-inflammatory cytokines, and this pathophysiology is assumed to be similar in the horse.[15] Hepatic and pulmonary granulomas also have been reported in horses with granulomatous enteritis.[16]

Horses diagnosed with granulomatous enteritis can be of any age, sex, or breed, but young Standardbred horses are over-represented, and there seems to be a familial predisposition.[1,16] One study showed that more than 80% of the cases of granulomatous enteritis in horses were in Standardbreds, and about 90% of these horses were between 1 and 5 years of age.[14] As with the other forms of IBD, the cause is unknown. Possible causes include an abnormal host inflammatory reaction to intestinal bacteria or dietary components. Aluminum exposure via invading micro-organisms, particularly parasites, also has been linked to granulomatous enteritis in horses.[17]

Lymphocytic/plasmacytic Enteritis

Lymphocytic/plasmacytic enteritis is characterized by excessive infiltration of lymphocytes and plasma cells in the lamina propria of the gastrointestinal tract with the absence of granulomatous change.[18] There is no age, breed, or sex predilection for this form of IBD. It has been suggested that this condition may be an early stage of intestinal lymphosarcoma.[4]

Lymphosarcoma

Intestinal lymphosarcoma can affect horses of any breed, sex, or age and has been reported in a horse with selective IgM deficiency.[19] Some studies have shown alimentary lymphoma primarily to affect young horses, but other reports indicate that older horses are more predisposed.[20] Lesions can be primary or secondary metastases from another site, most commonly mediastinal lymphosarcoma. Horses present with recurrent colic and weight loss, which can be acute despite the progressive nature of the disease process. The presentation of the disease may range from discrete tumors to diffuse infiltrates (**Fig. 1**).[21] Additionally, enlarged mesenteric lymph nodes infiltrated by malignant cells may be detected.[1] Mucosal ulcers may contribute to protein loss in horses with lymphosarcoma. Anemia and thrombocytopenia are common, and lymphocytosis is rare.[5] The prognosis for this form of IBD is poor, because horses usually present in an advanced stage of the disease.

INFECTIOUS CAUSES OF INFLAMMATORY BOWEL DISEASE

Lawsonia intracellularis is an obligate intracellular bacterium found in the cytoplasm of proliferative crypt epithelial cells; infection with this organism also is known as "proliferative enteropathy." Affected horses usually are 3 to 7 months of age and often have been weaned recently.[5] Occasionally infection has been reported in adult horses as well.[21] These foals usually present with hypoproteinemia, ventral edema, and ill-thrift. Concurrent diseases, including respiratory tract infection, dermatitis, parasitism, and gastric ulceration, are common also.[5] Diagnosis is via serology and fecal polymerase chain reaction test. False-negative results are possible because of the intracellular site of infection and intermittent shedding in the feces.[22] Intravenous oxytetracycline (6.6 mg/kg every 12 hours) for 1 week followed by either chloramphenicol (50 mg/kg every 8 hours by mouth [PO]) or erythromycin estolate (15–25 mg/kg every 6–8 hours PO) and rifampin (5–10 mg/kg every 24 hours PO) is the treatment of choice. The oral drug therapy is required for several weeks to months. Treatment often is successful if the disease is not advanced.

Rhodococcus equi infection also has been implicated as a cause of malabsorptive disorder of foals and weanlings. Diarrhea as a result of *R. equi* infection is rare in the

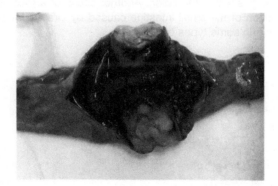

Fig. 1. Small intestinal lymphosarcoma. A discrete nodule within the small intestine of a 5-year-old Warmblood gelding. The horse presented with acute colic necessitating surgical intervention. The affected portion of small intestine was resected. No additional lesions were found during surgery, but biopsy of a mesenteric lymph node revealed metastasis had already occurred.

absence of pulmonary lesions, but pathology caused by the enteric form alone has been reported.[23] Diagnosis is based on clinical signs of concurrent pneumonia in the foal or positive culture from a transtracheal wash or feces. Occasionally culture of the peritoneal fluid also yields a positive diagnosis.[23] Treatment is the same as for *R. equi* pneumonia, although a prolonged course of antibiotic treatment may be necessary. Foals with extrapulmonary *R. equi* infections associated with the pneumonia have a more guarded prognosis than those with pulmonary lesions alone.[23]

DIAGNOSIS
History and Clinical Signs

A thorough history and physical examination of a horse is imperative for the diagnosis of IBD in the horse. The initial examination should include a thorough evaluation of the animal's diet. It is common to encounter horses in poor body condition that results solely from a lack of appropriate and adequate feed intake. Horses with IBD often present with weight loss or failure to gain weight despite adequate nutrition and appetite. Occasionally, depending on the stage of the disease, appetite may be decreased. An oral examination also should be performed to look for dentition problems or signs of tooth root abscessation. These dental abnormalities can lead to reduced feed intake and subsequent weight loss. The physical examination typically is normal with all vital parameters within the reference ranges. The horse may have increased gastrointestinal motility, and signs of hypoproteinemia may be seen as dependent, pitting edema. Occasionally diarrhea may be seen if the large intestine also is affected (**Box 1**).

A history of mild, recurrent colic is common in horses with IBD. An acute, severe colic episode necessitating surgery can occur also. The mild episodes of colic may be attributed to changes in motility caused by the infiltrate within the small intestinal walls. The more severe colic episodes usually are caused by the fermentation of excessive carbohydrate within the large colon. These carbohydrates normally would have been absorbed within the small intestine, but, because of the malabsorptive disease, the carbohydrates are able to reach the colon and undergo fermentation by normal colonic flora, resulting in excessive gas production. This excessive gas production may result in a spasmodic medical colic or progress to a displacement or torsion from the gas within the colon. Another cause of a mild or acute episode of colic is obstruction of the small intestine caused by circumferential mural bands or masses that form in some types of IBD.[7]

Box 1
Differential diagnoses for chronic diarrhea in the horse

Chronic parasitism

Peritonitis

Use of nonsteroidal anti-inflammatory drugs

Inflammatory bowel disease

Salmonellosis

Chronic liver disease

Sand

Minimum Laboratory Database

A minimum database including a complete blood cell count (CBC) and serum biochemistry is indicated. Results of the CBC can be normal or may show a neutrophilia, hyperfibrinogenemia, and anemia that typically is normocytic and normochromic.[21,24] The serum biochemistry often reveals hypoproteinemia characterized by hypoalbuminemia caused by protein-losing enteropathy (**Box 2**). Globulins are variable and can be elevated or decreased depending on the cause of the disease.[21] Other abnormalities may be present, depending on other organ involvement. For example, it is possible to see an elevated GGT with MEED if the liver is affected. A urinalysis also is beneficial, especially if hypoalbuminemia is present, to rule out proteinuria. Fecal flotation for parasites is indicated in any horse with hypoalbuminemia and weight loss. Enteritis with anorexia and weight loss has been described in association with cyathostomiasis in horses.[22]

If the horse presents with diarrhea, additional diagnostics are required for complete evaluation. Fecal cultures for *Salmonella* spp and *Clostridium* spp as well as *Clostridium* toxin assays (*C. difficile* toxin A and *C. perfringens* enterotoxin) are recommended. Additionally, serology and polymerase chain reaction for Potomac horse fever may be warranted, depending on geographic location. Other causes of chronic diarrhea in the horse should be investigated such as the use of nonsteroidal antiinflammatory agents, sand accumulation within the colon, and liver disease.

Rectal Palpation

A thorough rectal examination is indicated in any horse with weight loss and chronic colic. Occasionally, thickened portions of the small intestine can be palpated in horses with IBD. One also should attempt to palpate the sublumbar lymph nodes for enlargement. Any other abnormalities, such as palpably enlarged mesenteric lymph nodes, abdominal masses, or evidence of peritonitis, should be noted.

Abdominal and Thoracic Ultrasound

Transabdominal ultrasound can help confirm small intestinal thickening. Normal duodenal and jejunal wall thickness is 3 mm or less with the bowel being moderately distended.[25] The ileal wall thickness, however, can measure up to 4 to 5 mm in normal horses.[25] It is helpful to obtain an image of several loops of small intestine in one frame. One then can measure from lumen to lumen across two walls and divide the

---

Box 2
Differential diagnoses for weight loss and hypoproteinemia in the horse

Malnutrition

Parasitism

Gastrointestinal ulceration

Inflammatory bowel disease

Neoplasia

Liver disease

Bacterial infection (pneumonia, pleuropneumonia, peritonitis)

Viral infection (infectious anemia)

Chronic renal failure

measurement in half to obtain an individual wall thickness. Occasionally lymphade-nopathy also can be visualized with transabdominal ultrasound. Transrectal ultra-sound also can be used to measure the thickness of the small intestinal wall if specific segments are palpably abnormal. Ultrasound images from horses diagnosed with IBD can be seen in **Fig. 2**.

All other portions of the gastrointestinal tract should be evaluated ultrasonograph-ically. Special attention should be given to the right dorsal colon, looking for any thick-ening or evidence of ulceration that could be associated with right dorsal colitis. The liver, kidneys, and spleen should be evaluated for any abnormalities, and the entire abdomen should be scanned for evidence of a mass. An abbreviated thoracic ultra-sound examination should be performed to rule out pleural fluid accumulation as a differential diagnosis for hypoalbuminemia.

Abdominocentesis

An abdominocentesis should be performed in any horse with hypoproteinemia. Results are helpful in ruling out peritonitis as a cause of the low protein. In most cases of IBD the peritoneal fluid is normal, although neoplastic cells may be seen on the cytologic examination in lymphosarcoma cases.[26] The absence of neoplastic cells does not rule out a diagnosis of lymphosarcoma, however. An increased number of neutrophils or eosinophils in the peritoneal fluid may be found in horses with eosino-philic infiltrative disease.[1] Fluid should be collected into ethylenediaminetetraacetic acid and a culture tube and sent immediately to a laboratory for total protein

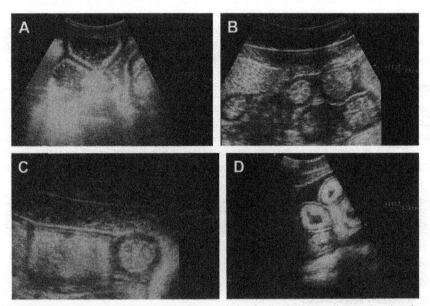

Fig. 2. Ultrasound. In A and B the thickness of the wall of the small intestine has been measured across two adjacent walls. The resulting measurement is the value of two wall thicknesses. Note the hypoechoic ring around each bowel segment, indicating thickening within that segment. (C) Image taken before treatment of a horse diagnosed with eosino-philic enteritis. The measurement is taken across only one wall of the small intestine wall. (D) A second horse with an advanced case of eosinophilic enteritis that initially responded to treatment but then relapsed. The horse was euthanized soon after this image was obtained.

concentration, total nucleated cell count, and cytologic evaluation. The plain sample can be submitted for bacterial culture and sensitivity if deemed necessary by macroscopic or cytologic evaluation.

Gastroscopy with Duodenal Biopsy

Gastroscopy can confirm or rule out gastric ulceration as a cause of the hypoproteinemia. The procedure also can be diagnostic of a gastric carcinoma.[27] All portions of the gastric mucosa should be evaluated, and the duodenum can be entered with skillful manipulation of the endoscope. A biopsy can be diagnostic of IBD if the duodenum is involved. In early or segmental disease (especially focal eosinophilic strictures), however, the lesions may be missed.[28] Other disadvantages of this type of biopsy are the small sample size and the lack of a full-thickness biopsy. Only a mucosal and possibly a submucosal sample is obtained with this procedure.

Once the duodenum has been entered with the endoscope, a standard biopsy instrument is passed through the biopsy channel of the endoscope. At least three biopsy samples should be taken, and mucosal bleeding at biopsy site is indicative of adequate sample size.[1] Care should be taken to avoid the opening of the common bile duct in the proximal duodenum.

Rectal Biopsy

Rectal biopsy can be of benefit in suspected cases of IBD. The procedure is simple, and requires little specialized equipment. An accurate diagnosis can be made in approximately one third of horses with IBD.[21] The most common diagnosis from a rectal biopsy is inflammatory disease of a rather nonspecific nature (**Box 3**).[10]

This finding, however, can be beneficial in narrowing the differential diagnoses in the case. The question that often arises is what variations can be considered normal in a rectal biopsy. Neutrophils are not found within the surface epithelium or crypts in control specimens, so when seen they always are considered pathologic.[10] Neutrophils normally can be found within the lamina propria in normal rectal biopsies, however. Lymphocytes and plasma cells also can normally be found in the lamina propria of the rectum, but a hypercellularity in this area is considered abnormal.[10] When lymphocytes and plasma cells are observed within the epithelium, differential diagnoses of cyathostominosis, granulomatous disease, alimentary lymphoma, or lymphocytic/plasmacytic IBD should be considered.[1] Eosinophilic infiltration of the lamina propria and submucosal layers of the rectum also can be considered normal.[10] False-negative results also are possible when evaluating rectal biopsy specimens, especially if disease is restricted to the small intestine. In one study, a diagnosis of malignant lymphoma was confirmed solely by rectal biopsy in only one of seven affected horses.[10]

A rectal biopsy can be obtained from a standing horse with minimal restraint, although sedation may be required for safety reasons. A sharp uterine biopsy instrument is used to obtain the biopsies. The clinician obtaining the biopsy should first evacuate the rectum

---

Box 3
Differential diagnosis for increased cells in an intestinal biopsy

Inflammatory bowel disease

Diarrhea

Cyathostominosis

manually. Then, using a gloved hand and well-lubricated arm, the clinician inserts the uterine biopsy instrument into the rectum, carefully guarded by the hand of the clinician. It is recommended that the sample be obtained from the dorsolateral position (11 o'clock and 1 o'clock locations) of the rectum, approximately 30 cm proximal to the anal sphincter.[10] A mucosal fold is isolated with the gloved hand, the instrument is advanced, the jaws are opened to capture the fold, and the biopsy is placed in 10% formalin for histopathology.[10] A second biopsy may be obtained for culture of *Salmonella* spp. Complications are unusual, but excessive bleeding can occur.

Exploratory Surgery

The best diagnostic sample for IBD is a full-thickness biopsy from the affected portion of the small intestine. This sample can be obtained via exploratory surgery by either flank laparotomy or ventral midline incision. Unfortunately, these biopsies are invasive and usually are not performed for the diagnosis of IBD. Affected horses are not always good candidates for major exploratory surgery because complications caused by hypoproteinemia and the catabolic state of the patient are common.[21] If performed, biopsies should be taken from grossly abnormal intestine or, if all is grossly normal, from three different sections of intestine.[1] Care should be taken in obtaining full-thickness biopsies from abnormal intestine, because dehiscence is a rare but fatal complication. The samples should be placed in formalin. Additional samples, such as biopsies of the cecum, colon, and mesenteric lymph nodes, may be warranted.

Absorption Tests

The oral glucose absorption test (OGAT) is relatively simple to perform and does not required specialized equipment. The test also is inexpensive and can be completed stall-side. The horse should be in a relatively quiet environment free of unusual noises or activity, which could influence blood glucose values. Following a 12- to 18-hour fast, the unsedated horse is administered glucose at 1 g/kg body weight as a 20% solution via nasogastric tube.[29] Blood samples then are collected every 30 minutes for 2 hours (including the baseline sample) and every 60 minutes for another 4 hours.[27] In a normal horse, the plasma glucose level should rise to higher than 185% of baseline by 120 minutes[29] and should return to normal by 6 hours.[27] In a modified version of this test, only one sample is taken at 120 minutes following glucose administration.[30] Horses typically fall into one of three groups based on the results of the OGAT.[31] Horses showing normal absorption are considered to have normal small intestine. Partial absorption (an increase of 115%–185%) indicates the presence of inflammatory infiltrate, villous atrophy, or intestinal wall edema, possibly with normal histopathology. Partial absorption also can occur with enhanced use of glucose or delayed gastric emptying. When the curve indicates total malabsorption (< 115% increase), the horse is suspected of having diffuse small intestinal disease.

Although the OGAT is a straightforward diagnostic test, several factors can influence the results, including dietary history, gastric emptying rate, intestinal transit, age, hormonal effects, and the metabolic state of horse.[32] For example, if a horse is in a catabolic state for other reasons but has normal absorption, the curve may show false-positive results (a flat line) because of the rapid use of the administered glucose. Alternatively, in a horse with abnormal absorption that is overly stressed, the plasma glucose may be artificially elevated resulting in a false-negative result. Other reasons for false-positive results that have been reported include gastric impactions (delayed gastric emptying) and colonic cyathostominosis.[30]

A second, more specialized, absorption test is the administration of D-xylose rather than glucose. The benefits of this test over the OGAT are that the D-xylose concentration in the blood is not affected by hormonal influences or metabolism.[33] Gastric emptying, intestinal motility, intraluminal bacterial overgrowth, and renal clearance still can affect the results, however.[1] The procedure is similar to the OGAT. Following a 12- to 18-hour fast, the unsedated horse is administered D-xylose at 1 g/kg body weight as a 10% solution via nasogastric tube. Blood samples are taken at baseline and every 30 minutes for 3 hours. In a normal horse, xylose levels should peak at more than 20 mg/dL 60 to 90 minutes following administration. Results are interpreted in much the same way as with the OGAT. A flat curve has been recorded in cases of bacterial overgrowth, parasitism, and idiopathic villous atrophy.[34,35] The curve also can be abnormal in the absence of histopathologic changes to the small intestine if the disease is not diffuse.[1] Examples of possible resulting curves are shown in **Fig. 3**. Complications from either absorption test are extremely rare, but the oral dose of carbohydrate could cause a horse predisposed to laminitis to develop an acute episode.

Nuclear Scintigraphy

Nuclear scintigraphy with technetium-99m–labeled hexamethylpropyleneamine oxime–labeled leucocytes has been used in an attempt to detect small intestinal pathology.[36] This procedure is noninvasive but requires specialized facilities equipped for handling radioactive materials. The outcome of the study performed using this technique showed that it could detect nonspecific intestinal pathology. Some horses with pathology, however, were normal when tested, resulting in false-negative results.[36]

TREATMENT AND PROGNOSIS

In general, long-term treatment of IBD in horses is reported to be unsuccessful.[21] When treated appropriately, however, horses can improve and even recover. Treatment is aimed at decreasing the horse's exposure to possible dietary, parasitic, or environmental inciting antigens.

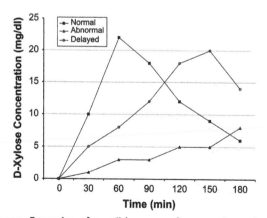

Fig. 3. D-xylose curves. Examples of possible curves from D-xylose absorption tests. The squares represent a curve of a normal horse, with peak D-xylose concentration greater than 20 mg/dL by 60 minutes. The triangles represent a flat line resulting from a horse with complete malabsorption. The open circles represent a delayed response that may occur with partial absorption in the small intestine.

Dietary recommendations include providing the horse with a highly digestible, well-balanced feed. Feeding smaller amounts more frequently also may help by increasing digestion and absorption. Corn oil can be added to the ration for extra fat and calories.[21] The composition of the feedstuffs also may be important. Feeds with a high fiber content such as grass hay and pasture grasses are converted from cellulose to volatile free fatty acids in the cecum.[1] This diet decreases the requirement of the small intestine to participate in digestion. Also, placing the horse on a diet with one ingredient, a monodiet, may help eliminate possible inciting antigens. A type of diet often recommended is oats supplemented with corn oil and grass hay as the roughage source.

Special recommendations for parasite control may be indicated for horses diagnosed with IBD. Even low levels of parasites that normally accumulate between deworming episodes can be a trigger for inflammation in affected horses. It is recommended that horses with IBD be treated with a daily dewormer such as pyrantel tartrate (Strongid C). It also is important to remember that horses maintained on a daily deworming product must be treated with an ivermectin and praziquantel product in the spring and fall to eliminate bots and tapeworms, because those parasites are not prevented by the daily deworming. The use of the daily deworming product removes parasites from contact with the horse's immune system, thereby eliminating a natural hyposensitization process.

Corticosteroids are the treatment of choice in horses confirmed to have IBD. These drugs are used to decrease the intestinal inflammation associated with the disease.[21] A prolonged, tapering course is required, and administration is parenteral initially because of the malabsorption process. The initial dose is 0.05 to 0.1 mg/kg intramuscularly (IM) for 2 to 4 weeks and then tapered depending on the response of the patient.[9] It is important to re-evaluate the horse's progress before switching to orally administered dexamethasone. A sample dosing schedule is given in **Box 4**. Prednisolone also may be considered as an alternative or successive treatment to dexamethasone but is more expensive.

An additional treatment option that can be considered is metronidazole for its antimicrobial and anti-inflammatory effects.[21] This treatment is used with varying success in humans who have Crohn's disease.[1] Hydroxyurea, an antineoplastic drug, has been shown to improve some horses with MEED and is used to treat humans who have hypereosinophilia syndrome.[1] Last, in horses diagnosed with lymphosarcoma, chemotherapy can prolong survival up to 6 to12 months.[1]

Box 4
Sample dosing schedule for horse with inflammatory bowel disease

This schedule is intended only to serve as a starting point, because all horses respond differently, and the dosing schedule should be adjusted to meet each individual horse's needs.

Medication: dexamethasone 2 mg/mL

  0.05 mg/kg IM daily for 3 weeks

  0.03 mg/kg IM daily for 3 weeks

Re-evaluate horse clinically

  0.03 mg/kg PO daily for 3 weeks

  0.03 mg/kg PO every other day for 6 weeks

Abbreviations: IM, intramuscularly; PO, orally.

Response to treatment is variable and reportedly is better with eosinophilic and lymphocytic/plasmacytic types than with granulomatous enteritis.[1] The overall prognosis for this disease is reported to be guarded to poor,[21] often because the disease is in an advanced stage at the time of diagnosis. If the disease is focal, surgical resection of the affected bowel can be curative, but this situation is unusual.[20,37] Some horses do respond favorably to corticosteroids, however.[9] In the author's experience, if the horse is treated properly and for the appropriate length of time, the prognosis is better than reported in other published reports. Approximately 50% of horses seem to show significant improvement or resolution of clinical signs, excluding horses diagnosed with lymphosarcoma, a diagnosis that always carries a poor prognosis. Occasionally horses with IBD may require lifelong, low-dose treatment with corticosteroids to remain symptom free.[1] There are complications associated with the prolonged used of corticosteroids in horses. Treated animals have an increased susceptibility to infections and may develop symptoms similar to those in animals affected with hyperadrenocorticism (Cushing's disease), such as muscle wasting and a dull haircoat.[21] These side effects do seem to resolve if the corticosteroid treatment is discontinued. The possible development of laminitis as a complication following administration of corticosteroids also should be discussed with the owner.

SUMMARY

IBD historically has been regarded as a rare clinical syndrome of horses but probably is underdiagnosed. Simple diagnostic tests are available to support a clinical diagnosis of IBD and can be accomplished even in a nonhospital setting. Although most current literature indicates IBD in horses is a grave diagnosis, it is possible to treat these patients successfully.

REFERENCES

1. Mair T, Pearson GR, Divers TJ. Malabsorption syndromes in the horse. Equine Vet Educ 2006;18(6):383–92.
2. Divers T, Pelligrini-Masini A, McDonough S. Diagnosis of inflammatory bowel disease in a Hackney pony by gastroduodenal endoscopy and biopsy and successful treatment with corticosteroids. Equine Vet Educ 2006;18(6):368–71.
3. Schumacher J, Edwards JF, Cohen ND. Chronic idiopathic inflammatory bowel diseases of the horse. J Vet Intern Med 2000;14:258–65.
4. Barton M. Diagnosis and treatment of enteritis and inflammatory bowel disease. Paper presented at the AAEP Focus Meeting. Quebec, Canada, July 31–August 2, 2005.
5. Roberts M. Proliferative and inflammatory intestinal diseases associated with malabsorption and maldigestion. In: Reed S, Bayly WM, Sellon DC, editors. Equine internal medicine. 2nd edition. St. Louis (MO): Saunders; 2004. p. 878–84.
6. Scott E, Heidel JR, Snyder SP, et al. Inflammatory bowel disease in horses: 11 cases (1988–1998). J Am Vet Med Assoc 1999;214(10):1527–30.
7. Southwood L, Kawcak CE, Trotter GW, et al. Idiopathic focal eosinophilic enteritis associated with small intestinal obstruction in 6 horses. Vet Surg 2000;29:415–9.
8. Nimmo Wilkie J, Yager JA, Nation PN, et al. Chronic eosinophilic dermatitis: a manifestation of a multisystemic eosinophilic, epitheliotropic disease in five horses. Vet Pathol 1985;22:297–305.
9. McCue M, Davis EG, Rush BR, et al. Dexamethasone for treatment of multisystemic eosinophilic epitheliotropic disease in a horse. J Am Vet Med Assoc 2003; 223(9):1320–3.

10. Lindberg R, Nygren A, Persson SGB. Rectal biopsy diagnosis in horses with clinical signs of intestinal disorders: a retrospective study of 116 cases. Equine Vet J 1996;28(4):275–84.

11. Hillyer M, Mair TS. Multisystemic eosinophilic epitheliotrophic diseases in a horse: attempted treatment with hydroxyurea and dexamethasone. Vet Rec 1992;130: 392–5.

12. Carmalt J. Multisystemic eosinophilic disease in a Quarter Horse. Equine Vet Educ 2004;16:231–4.

13. Meuten D, Butler DG, Thomson GW, et al. Chronic enteritis associated with the malabsorption and protein-losing enteropathy in the horse. J Am Vet Med Assoc 1978;172:326–33.

14. Lindberg R. Pathology of equine granulomatous enteritis. J Comp Pathol 1984; 94:233–47.

15. Fiocchi C. Inflammatory bowel disease: aetiology and pathogenesis. Gastroenterology 1998;115:182–205.

16. Sweeney R, Sweeney CR, Saik J, et al. Chronic granulomatous bowel disease in three sibling horses. J Am Vet Med Assoc 1986;188(10):1192–4.

17. Fogarty U, Perl D, Ensley S, et al. A cluster of equine granulomatous enteritis cases: the link with aluminium. Vet Hum Toxicol 1998;40(5):297–305.

18. Kemper D, Perkins GA, Schumacher J, et al. Equine lymphocytic-plasmacytic enterocolitis: a retrospective study of 14 cases. Equine Vet J Suppl 2000;32: 108–12.

19. Perryman LE, Wyatt CR, Magnuson NS. Biochemical and functional characterization of lymphocytes from a horse with lymphosarcoma and IgM deficiency. Comp Immunol Microbiol Infect Dis 1984;7(1):53–62.

20. Taylor S, Pusterla N, Vaughan B, et al. Intestinal neoplasia in horses. J Vet Intern Med 2006;20:1429–36.

21. Barr B. Infiltrative intestinal disease. Vet Clin North Am Equine Pract 2006;22:e1–7.

22. Stampfli H, Oliver OE. Chronic diarrhea and weight loss in three horses. Vet Clin North Am Equine Pract 2006;22:e27–35.

23. Davis J. Medical disorders of the small intestine. In: Smith B, editor. Large animal internal medicine. 4th edition. St. Louis (MO): Mosby; 2009. p. 723–31.

24. Sweeney R. Laboratory evaluation of malassimilation in horses. Vet Clin North Am Equine Pract 1987;3:507–14.

25. Desrochers A. Abdominal ultrasonography of normal and colicky adult horses. Paper presented at the AAEP Focus Meeting. Quebec, Canada, July 31–August 2, 2005.

26. Mair T, Hillyer MH. Clinical features of lymphosarcoma in the horse: 77 cases. Equine Vet Educ 1992;18:149–56.

27. Tamzali Y. Chronic weight loss syndrome in the horse: a 60 case retrospective study. Equine Vet Educ 2006;18(6):372–80.

28. Evens S, Bonczynski JJ, Broussard JD, et al. Comparison of endoscopic and full-thickness biopsy specimens for diagnosis of inflammatory bowel disease and alimentary tract lymphoma in cats. J Am Vet Med Assoc 2006;229(9):1447–50.

29. Roberts M, Hill FWG. The oral glucose tolerance test in the horse. Equine Vet J 1973;5:171–3.

30. Murphy D, Reid SWJ, Love S. Modified oral glucose tolerance test as an indicator of small intestinal pathology in horses. Vet Rec 1997;140:342–3.

31. Mair T, Hillyer MH, Taylor FGR, et al. Small intestinal malabsorption in the horse: an assessment of the specificity of the oral glucose tolerance test. Equine Vet J 1991;23(5):344–6.

32. Jacobs K, Bolton JR. Effect of diet on the oral glucose tolerance test in the horse. J Am Vet Med Assoc 1982;180(8):884–6.
33. Bolton J, Merritt AM, Cimprich RE, et al. Normal and abnormal xylose absorption in the horse. Cornell Vet 1976;66:183–97.
34. Brown C. The diagnostic value of the d-xylose absorption test in horses with unexplained chronic weight loss. British Veterinary Journal 1992;148:41–4.
35. Roberts M. Malabsorption syndromes in the horse. Compendium on Continuing Education for the Practicing Veterinarian 1985;7:S637–46.
36. Menzies-Gow N, Weller R, Bowen M, et al. Use of nuclear scintigraphy with ^{99m}Tc-HMPAO-labelled leucocytes to assess small intestinal malabsorption in 17 horses. Vet Rec 2003;153:457–62.
37. Schumacher J, Moll HD, Spano JS, et al. Effect of intestinal resection on two juvenile horses with granulomatous enteritis. J Vet Intern Med 1990;4(3):153–6.

Impactions of the Small and Large Intestines

Amy E. Plummer, DVM

KEYWORDS

- Colic • Impaction • Ileal impaction • Cecal impaction
- Large colon impaction • Small colon impaction

Impactions of the small and large intestines are frequently determined to be the cause of colic in horses. An impaction is an accumulation of dehydrated ingesta in a portion of the digestive tract. Most commonly, the term "impaction" is used when discussing this condition in the ascending (large) colon; however, impactions can also occur in other segments of the intestine. Impactions cause simple obstructions of the intestinal tract and do not generally cause ischemia or necrosis of the bowel unless they become severe.

Impactions are typically located at sites where the intestinal diameter deceases. These sites include the pelvic flexure (the transition from the left ventral colon to the left dorsal colon) and the transition from the right dorsal colon to the transverse colon. Additionally, impactions can occur at sites that contain sphincters, such as the ileal–cecal–colical orifice. The specific pathogenesis for impactions is not fully understood, although risk factors have been identified for several types of impactions. The clinical onset for most impactions is slower than what is seen with strangulating lesions, and horse owners may notice mild clinical signs over an extended period of time.

The treatment of specific types of impactions will be discussed later in this article, but in general it includes withholding feed until the impaction passes, rehydrating the ingesta, and, if necessary, administering analgesic agents. In severe cases, surgery may be necessary to relieve the impaction. Initially, as with any type of colic, feed should be withheld as soon as the condition is recognized. Because the abdominal pain associated with these conditions is often mild, horses will continue to eat. Furthermore, before reintroducing feed to a horse with an impaction, the impaction should be resolved and this should be confirmed, most commonly by performing a repeated rectal examination (with pelvic flexure impactions) or by observing that an adequate volume of feces has passed.

The use of analgesics is necessary to reduce pain and intestinal spasms that occur at the impaction sites. Pain control for horses with impactions is relatively easy compared with that for horses with more severe colic, and often requires smaller

---

Large Animal Clinical Sciences, The University of Tennessee, College of Veterinary Medicine, 2407 River Drive, Knoxville, TN 37996, USA
E-mail address: aeplummer@gmail.com

Vet Clin Equine 25 (2009) 317–327
doi:10.1016/j.cveq.2009.04.002
0749-0739/09/$ – see front matter © 2009 Elsevier Inc. All rights reserved.

vetequine.theclinics.com

amounts and less frequent administration of medications to attain pain control. Flunixin meglumine (0.5–1.1 mg/kg/12 hours, IV) is a nonsteroidal anti-inflammatory drug considered to be one of the best analgesics for colic (visceral) pain; however, phenylbutazone (4.4 mg/kg, IV) can be just as effective in some horses. Agents such as flunixin meglumine and phenylbutazone inhibit cyclooxygenase production, which in turn prevents the formation of prostaglandin, which is active in causing increased blood flow, irritation, and inflammation. If flunixin meglumine alone is not sufficient to control pain, especially in horses in which gastrointestinal distention is a feature, xylazine is the drug of choice. Xylazine is a nervous system depressant and an alpha-2 adrenergic agonist. It has effects on the presynaptic and postsynaptic receptors of the central and peripheral nervous systems, and these actions reduce intestinal spasms. It provides analgesia and sedation to horses with impactions. Generally, xylazine (0.1–0.2 mg/kg, IV; 0.2–0.3 mg/kg, IM) can be used to provide analgesia and sedation; however, smaller or larger doses could be used for horses with variable pain. It provides short periods (15–120 minutes) of pain relief.

Detomidine (2.5–5.0 µg/kg, IV or IM), a more potent alpha-2 agonist than xylazine, can be used judiciously to provide analgesia; however, this potent analgesic may mask severe pain. Whenever detomidine is used, the horse should be monitored frequently, including taking notice of mucus membrane color, capillary refill time, or other serious degradations in clinical parameters.

Opioids (eg, butorphanol, 0.01–0.02 mg/kg, IV or IM) can be used in combination with alpha-2 agonists to provide neuroleptanalgesia. Opiods are known to stop colon motility and thereby provide temporary pain relief.

Spasmolytics have been used to provide analgesia by decreasing spasms in numerous species, including horses that are having colic episodes. N-butylscopolammonium bromide (Buscopan, Boehringer Ingelheim, GmbH, Germany; 0.3 mg/kg, IV, slowly) has recently been approved for use in horses in the United States. This agent is an antimuscarinic and anticholinergic agent that is used specifically as an antispasmotic. When used, it is important to not administer an overdose or use the drug for a prolonged period of time because it can cause prolonged ileus. Additionally, this drug is known to increase the heart rate for approximately 30 minutes after administration, so the heart rate can not be used as an accurate indicator of increased pain during this time.

Fluid therapy (enteral or parenteral) should be administered with the goal of systemic rehydration and hydration of the ingesta to allow resolution of the impaction. Enteral administration of fluids will be discussed in more detail in the section of this article that covers large colon impactions. The goal of balanced intravenous fluid therapy is to decrease the plasma protein concentration (ie, overhydration) and produce increased intestinal secretion in the areas of the impaction. To accomplish this, fluid rates of approximately 120 to 240 mL/kg/day (2–4 times the maintenance fluid rates) must be used. When administering intravenous fluids at these rates, it is important to monitor concentrations of electrolytes (sodium, potassium, and chloride).

Laxatives are used to resolve impaction, and those commonly used include mineral oil, magnesium sulfate, dioctyl sodium sulfosuccinate, and psyllium. Mineral oil (5–10 mL/kg, by way of a nasogastric tube) may not penetrate the mass of firm ingesta as well as some of the other laxatives. Mineral oil is useful as a marker for intestinal transit time and should be evident as staining on the perineal area for 12 to 18 hours after administration.

Magnesium sulfate (1 gm/kg, in 2 liters of water, by way of a nasogastric tube, every 12–24 hours), an osmotic cathartic and promotes water moving into the intestinal lumen, thereby softening the impaction. It is important the horse is systemically hydrated when using magnesium sulfate, as toxicity has been reported in dehydrated horses.[1]

Dioctyl sodium sulfosuccinate (DSS; 16.5 to 66 mg/kg, mixed in 1 liter of water, by way of a nasogastric tube) has historically been advocated by some to be useful in the treatment of impactions. As an anionic surfactant, it facilitates water penetration into the firm ingesta by decreasing surface tension. There have been reports of overdosing, and there is a low margin of safety with this medication. A maximum dose of 0.2 g/kg has been reported, but one report suggested that toxic signs were seen in a normal horse that was administered 50 mg/kg by way of a nasogastric tube.[2,3] There are no recent studies evaluating the efficacy or clinical use of DSS, so it should be used with caution in horses that have impaction colic.

Although the majority of impactions can be managed medically, in more severe impactions, surgical treatment is necessary. Generally, surgery is required in horses that have uncontrolled pain or for those that do not respond to medical therapy. Surgical treatments will be discussed individually in the following sections of this article that cover each type of impaction.

DUODENAL AND JEJUNAL IMPACTIONS

Impactions of the duodenum and jejunum are rare, and reports in the literature are limited to case reports and case series. There have been reports of duodenal impactions caused by the ingestion of cracked corn, a corncob, wood, a phytobezoar, a trichophytobezoar, and persimmon fruit.[4–9] Clinical signs of duodenal impactions are similar to those of other small intestinal obstructions, and horses often have significant nasogastric reflux. Diagnosis of duodenal impactions is usually made at surgery or necropsy, and treatment is on a case-by-case basis, depending on the nature of the impaction.

Primary jejunal impactions with feed are rare. Jenjunal impactions are typically secondary to intestinal adhesions, ischemia, or a diverticulum. Diagnosis is based on clinical signs of colic and evidence of a small intestinal obstruction (ie, excessive nasogastric reflux). Surgery is often required to treat the primary inciting cause.

ILEAL IMPACTIONS

Ileal impaction is a leading cause of nonstrangulating small intestinal obstruction in horses. These impactions are more commonly diagnosed in the southeastern United States. Feeding coastal Bermuda grass hay has been identified as a risk factor for ileal impactions in horses.[10] Also, changes in the feeding of hay (eg, introduction of a round bale to a pasture) have been identified as risk factors for the development of ileal impaction. Additionally, infection with the intestinal tapeworm *Anaplocephala perfoliata* has been shown to have a strong association with ileal impactions in horses in the United Kingdom.[11] One report found a significantly higher rate of ileal impactions in the fall (September–November), whereas other reports have not identified a seasonal distribution.[12]

Horses with ileal impactions show signs consistent with small intestinal obstruction with copious nasogastric reflux. Differentiating an ileal impaction from a strangulating small intestinal lesion or anterior enteritis can be difficult. Abdominal pain varies from mild to severe, depending on the duration of the impaction and the degree of small intestinal and gastric distention.[10,12,13] Most horses have decreased gastrointestinal borborygmi and an increased heart rate.[10,12,13] Nasogastric reflux is commonly obtained, but may be absent if the impaction has been present for a short period of time.[10,12,13] A rectal examination performed early in the course of the impaction may allow the examiner to palpate a dough-like mass on the right side of the abdomen just medial to the cecum.[14] More commonly, there is such severe small intestinal distention that it is not possible to palpate the impaction.[10,12,13] Examination of peritoneal fluid can be helpful in determining whether the small intestine is ischemic and compromised (either associated with the impaction or in cases in which a strangulating lesion is present). Peritoneal fluid samples in horses with ileal impactions are typically clear yellow and have normal WBC count (<10,000 cells/μl) and normal to slightly elevated total protein concentration (< 3 gm/dL).[10,12]

Historically, surgical treatment for ileal impactions was advocated based on a study that reported higher survival rates for horses that underwent surgery sooner after the onset of clinical signs.[13] More recently, there were reports of successful medical treatment for horses with ileal impactions that had a stable cardiovascular status and were responsive to pain medication.[14] As discussed earlier in this article, differentiating between an ileal impaction and a strangulating obstruction can be difficult. If the diagnosis is unclear, early surgical intervention may increase the survival rate for horses that have a prolonged course of disease.

Medical therapy for ileal impactions involves intravenous rehydration using balanced polyionic fluids at two to three times the maintenance rates (120–180mL/kg/day), the use of pain control methods, and serial examinations of the severity of small intestinal distention and peritoneal fluid samples. Unlike other, more distal impactions, decompression of the stomach by collecting nasogastric reflux is critical in the treatment of ileal impactions, and the use of oral fluids or other medications should be avoided. It is important to evaluate the response to pain relief methods in horses with continuous nasogastric reflux. Continued pain after stomach decompression may indicate a more serious small intestinal disease.

Surgical treatment should be pursued when horses are unresponsive to medical therapy and pain medications or to changes in the peritoneal fluid WBC and total protein concentration, which may suggest that the bowels are compromised. By softening the impaction through extraluminal massage with fluid in the bowel orad to impaction, the impaction can be manually reduced at surgery.[12,13] Some authors advocate the injection of a saline and DSS solution (dioctynate oral solution; 1.5 L saline with 60 mL DSS) into the impaction using an 18-gauge needle to minimize the trauma to the bowel if the impaction is not easily reduced.[12] Historically, bypass procedures including jejunocecal bypass with or without ileal resection were advocated as part of the surgical correction.[13] Because of numerous complications and the high success rates of extramural massage without a bypass procedure, such procedures are no longer performed unless the bowel is compromised or there is ileal hypertrophy.[12]

Horses with ileal impactions have a good prognosis as long as they are treated early. Parks and colleagues,[13] in a retrospective study of 75 horses, found that survival decreased with the increasing duration of clinical signs. Most of the horses in this study had surgery with an enterotomy or a bypass procedure. Horses can successfully be treated medically, provided they have a stable cardiovascular status, controllable pain, the resolution of small intestinal distention on rectal examination, and no evidence of significant changes in the peritoneal fluid.

CECAL IMPACTIONS

Impaction of the cecum is the most common pathologic condition affecting the cecum, accounting for 5% of horses seen with intestinal impaction and up to 4.1% of horses seen at referral hospitals for colic.[15,16] The incidence of cecal rupture in horses with cecal impactions has been reported to be as high as 57%.[17] Cecal impactions have previously been classified into two types: cecal impactions with the cecum filled with dehydrated ingesta and cecal dysfunction with the cecum filled with fluid and ingesta.[18]

This article focuses on the first type of cecal impactions. The pathogenesis of cecal impaction is likely multifactorial, and the specific cause for any individual case is usually unknown. There are anecdotal reports of cecal impactions being associated with poor dentition, decreased water intake, feeding of coarse roughage, administration of nonsteroidal anti-inflammatory drugs, and infestation with *A perfoliata*.[17,19,20] Horses hospitalized for diseases unrelated to the gastrointestinal tract, predominantly those that are musculoskeletal in origin, have been identified to have cecal impactions.[17] Today, most such horses are placed under general anesthesia and receive nonsteroidal anti-inflammatory drugs. Abnormalities in cecal motility, as opposed to mechanical obstruction caused by firm ingesta, are believed to be the main cause of impaction in such cases. One report found that Arabian, Appaloosa, and Morgan horses are at increased risk for cecal impaction, whereas other reports have not found specific breeds at increased risk.[15,17,20,21] Several reports have found that older horses (>15 years old) are at increased risk for developing cecal impactions.[15,20,21]

Typically, horses with cecal impactions show mild to moderate signs of colic, and the signs of pain may continue for several days.[15,17,21–23] Alternatively, the condition in some horses will progress rapidly and the cecum will rupture before proper treatment can be initiated.[15,17,21] In a recent respective of 114 horses that were treated for cecal impactions, the median heart rate was 46 beats per minute and the median capillary refill time was 2 seconds. The majority of the clinical laboratory findings were not significantly different from normal values, and evidence of systemic dehydration was the most consistent abnormality. Most horses with cecal impactions did not have any net nasogastric reflux. Peritoneal fluid parameters are usually within normal limits, unless the impaction had become so severe that the bowel wall was compromised, which was likely to be the result of pressure necrosis.[15] Thus, findings of these and other studies highlight evidence that cecal impactions cause mild changes as seen by way of physical examination and laboratory tests and that careful rectal palpation is critical in the diagnosis of cecal impactions. The earliest abnormality felt during a rectal examination is reportedly increased tension on the ventral cecal band.[20] It can be difficult to differentiate horses with cecal distention from horses with large colon distention. To aid in the diagnosis of cecal impaction, it is important to remember that the cecum is attached to the dorsal body wall and therefore it is not possible to pass a hand dorsally over a distended cecum.

Treatment for cecal impactions is controversial, with some veterinarians advocating medical therapy and others surgical intervention.[15,17,20,21,24] Some authors recommend surgical intervention only in cases that are refractory to medical therapy or in cases with severe cecal distention, whereas others recommend early surgical intervention.[15,17,20,25,26] If surgical intervention is performed, the decision must be made whether a typhlotomy is performed or a typhlotomy with a cecal bypass procedure. Regardless of the therapy selected, it is important to recognize that there are numerous reports of horses diagnosed with cecal rupture that had histories of only mild colic and that all owners should be informed of the risk for cecal rupture when treating cecal impactions.

Medical therapy for cecal impactions includes using pain control methods, withholding feed and fluids to soften the mass, and using prokinetic agents to improve cecal emptying. Because pain is known to decrease gastrointestinal motility, the judicious use of analgesics is important in the treatment of cecal impactions. Flunixin meglumine (0.5–1.1 mg/kg, IV, every 12 hours) is used as well as xylazine (0.1–0.2 mg/kg, IV). Because pain with cecal impactions is often mild, it is imperative to monitor the impaction using repeated rectal examinations and not rely on response to pain medications alone. In the author's opinion, detomidine should not be used in cecal impactions unless surgery is not a treatment option for the horse. There are currently no reports specifically addressing the usefulness of *N*-butylscopolammonium bromide in cecal impactions.

Feed should be withheld from horses during treatment. Because colic signs are often mild in horses with cecal impactions, the horses will often continue to eat if given the opportunity. Owners often do not recognize that this can lead to more severe impaction. Oral laxatives (eg, mineral oil and magnesium sulfate) are often administered once a day to aid in rehydrating the impaction. It is important to remember that horses with cecal impactions can pass mineral oil around the impaction and that this can not be used as a marker of resolution of the impaction.

Fluid therapy should be administered with the goal of systemic rehydration and hydration of the ingesta to allow resolution of the impaction. This can be accomplished by an enteral or parenteral route. There are several studies looking at enteral fluid therapy for treatment of colon impactions; however, none specifically address the use of this route for horses with cecal impactions. It is the author's experience that using this route can make cecal impactions in horses more painful and does not aid in the treatment of cecal impactions as well as it does in ascending (large) colon impactions. Typically, balanced polyionic fluids at rates of approximately 120 to 240 mL/kg/day (2–4 times the maintenance fluid rates) must be used.

Prokinetic agents may be used in horses with cecal impaction. Commonly, yohimbine (0.15 mg/kg, mixed in 1 liter of fluid and administered over 30 minutes, IV, every 12 hours) has been advocated for the treatment of cecal impaction (F.M. Andrews, personal communication, 2009). Yohimbine, an alpha-2 adrenergic antagonist, has been reported to improve gastric emptying in horses after exposure to endotoxins.[27]

During medical treatment for cecal impactions, it is imperative that the horses be carefully monitored and that frequent rectal examinations are performed because cecal rupture may occur in these horses. In a recent retrospective study, the decision for surgical intervention was based on the severity of pain at the time of admission, the persistence of pain or an increase in the severity of pain while hospitalized, the severity of cecal distention on rectal examination, or failure to respond to medical treatment.[15] Some authors have advocated surgical intervention in horses with cecal impactions that are refractory to medical therapy or in horses with severe cecal distention, and other authors advocate early surgical intervention in most cases.[17,20] Results of the previously mentioned study[15] found that although medical treatment can be successful in some horses with cecal impactions, early surgical intervention is critical in horses that are not responding to this medical therapy (which consisted of IV fluids, analgesics, and oral mineral oil).

Surgical treatment of cecal impactions involves evacuation of the cecal contents and, in some cases, cecal bypass.[15,17,25–29] Bypass procedures were originally developed in an effort to decrease the recurrence of the cecal impaction.[22,25,28–30] Typhlotomy is most commonly used to evacuate the cecal contents. Cecocolic anastomosis (which is not currently recommended because of problems with cecal tympany) and ileocolic and jejunocolic anastomosis have been reported to be used as bypass procedures.[25,28,29] In the author's retrospective study, only 2 of the 37 horses that were treated surgically had bypass procedures performed. Postoperative care is the same as with other abdominal surgery procedures.

The prognosis for discharge from the hospital is good.[15] In a recent report of 114 horses with cecal impaction, 44 of 54 (81%) horses treated medically were discharged, whereas 34 of 37 (91.8%) horses treated surgically and allowed to recover were discharged from the hospital. Eleven of 114 (9.6%) horses were euthanized after initial examination, and 12 of 37 (32%) horses treated surgically were euthanized at surgery because of existing cecal rupture. Follow-up information was reported for 47 of the horses, and the long-term survival rate (alive after >1 year) was 91%. The recurrence rate for cecal impaction was 13% (6/47 horses).

ASCENDING (LARGE) COLON IMPACTIONS

Large colon impaction is common in horses, and it was seen in 13.4% of the cases of colic treated at one referral center.[31] The same study reported that 53.7% (79/147) of the horses that had a change in their routine within 2 weeks of their colic episode were at risk.[31] However, decreased exercise because of stall confinement, increased time spent in a stable, recent change in an exercise program, cribbing behavior, a history of travel within 24 hours of a colic episode, and not having ivermectin or moxidectin anthelmintic administered were identified as risk factors for the development of large colon impactions in a different study.[32] Decreased water consumption is often believed to be a factor in the development of impactions, possibly because of cold weather, a lack of available water, or broken automatic watering systems in stalls. Poor dentition is also a common risk factor for developing large colon impactions. Mares and middle-aged horses are more commonly diagnosed with large colon impactions.[31]

The majority of large colon impactions occur at the sites where bowel luminal diameter decreases. The pelvic flexure is the most common site, and such impactions occurred in 103 of 147 (70.1%) horses in one study.[31] Additional impaction sites include the left ventral colon in 30 of 147 (20.4%) horses and the right ventral and dorsal colons in 14 of 147 (9.5%) horses.

Clinical signs vary depending on the severity of the impaction. Pain is generally mild to moderate, with few horses showing severe colic signs. Interestingly, 70 of 147 (47.6%) horses in one retrospective study did not show any signs of abdominal pain on admission to the referral center.[31] In the same study, 50 of 147 (34%) horses had mild signs of abdominal pain, 16 of 147 (10.9%) had moderate pain, and the remaining 11 of 147 (7%) showed severe pain. Most horses have decreased or absent gastrointestinal borborygmi. Diagnosis is generally made using rectal palpation. Impactions of the pelvic flexure and the ventral colons are generally palpable; however, impactions of the right dorsal colon can be difficult to palpate and distinguish from cecal impactions. It is important to differentiate impactions, which consist of increased amounts of feedstuff and are often firm, from a dehydrated colon, which can also be firm but is generally secondary to some other type of colic. The use of peritoneal fluid analysis can be helpful in determining whether the bowel is compromised, and peritoneal fluid WBC and total solids are usually within normal limits in most horses with large colon impactions.

Medical treatment for large colon impactions is generally successful. Horses will often respond to oral medications given by way of nasogastric tubes and analgesics alone. The horses should be kept off feed until the impaction resolves. Mineral oil (1 gallon by way of a nasogastric tube once a day) can be given, but it is important to remember that the oil can pass around the impaction. Magnesium sulfate (1 g/kg once a day for 2–3 days in 2 liters of water, by way of a nasogastric tube) is believed to cause rehydration of the feces and can be used in horses that are not systemically dehydrated. Flunixin meglumine (0.5–1.1mg/kg/12 hrs, IV) is usually the analgesic of choice.

When the previous treatments are not successful in resolving the impaction or the impaction is believed to be severe, more aggressive therapies may be necessary. Although most studies describe the use of intravenous fluids, there have been recent discussions of using high volumes of oral fluids to resolve impactions without systemically "overhydrating" the horse.[33,34] A study found that the use of enteral and intravenous fluids with enteral magnesium sulfate increases colonic and fecal hydration and causes plasma expansion in horses with colonic impaction.[34] That study also found that the use of enteral fluids (10 L/hr for 6 hours by way of an 18-F equine enteral feeding tube) produced more changes in the hydration of the ingesta and feces than did the use of intravenous fluids (10 L/hr for 6 hours) with 1 g/kg magnesium sulfate in 1 liter of water, which were administered at the beginning of the study. Additionally, there was a trend towards more defecation with the use of enteral fluids, supporting the hypothesis of the gastrocolic reflex stimulation with enteral fluid therapy. Some horses in that study did show abdominal discomfort resulting from the high volume of enteral fluids. Current recommendations include the use of enteral fluids with a balanced electrolyte solution given by way of a nasogastric tube at 5 to 10 L/hr. There are "homemade" recipes described in other texts for making balanced enteral fluids using tap water, salt, potassium chloride, and sodium bicarbonate.

In addition to enteral fluids, intravenous fluids are often administered and are necessary if the horse has cardiovascular compromise or electrolyte abnormalities. These fluids are often administered at two to three times the maintenance rates. In addition to flunixin meglumine, xylazine (0.3–0.8 mg/kg, IV or IM, every 2–4 hrs) can be used without clinically apparent detrimental effects on motility.[31] Some clinicians also use butorphenol (0.02 mg/kg, IV or IM, every 6–8 hrs), detomidine (0.1 mg/kg, IV, every 6–8 hrs), or a combination of any two of these to control pain. Regardless of the analgesics administered, it is important to clinically assess the horse's response to the pain medication and its cardiovascular status throughout medical treatment.

Surgery is indicated if abdominal pain is not controllable, there are significant changes in the peritoneal fluid, or there is deterioration of the cardiovascular status. Twenty four of 147 horses (16%) in one retrospective study required surgery.[31] Rupture of the bowel is a risk when these horses are taken to surgery because of the weight of the colon. The risk for rupture should be discussed with the client before surgery. A ventral midline celiotomy and pelvic flexure enterotomy is performed to allow evacuation of the ingesta from the colon. Often, the colon must be evacuated before it is completely exteriorized from the abdomen to prevent tearing.

The prognosis for horses with large colon impactions is excellent, and the prognosis is better for horses treated medically than for those treated surgically. In the retrospective study by Dabareiner and White,[31] the long-term survival rate was 95.1% for medically treated horses and 57.8% for surgically treated horses. The most common complications cited with large colon impaction therapy were thrombophlebitis of the jugular vein and diarrhea. The study found that 32% (33/100) of the horses that were available for follow-up examinations had one or more episodes of colic after discharge from the hospital, which was higher than expected. The authors speculated that this could be the result of those horses having colonic dysfunction that led to the first impaction or that the impaction caused permanent damage that predisposed the horse to subsequent colic episodes.

DESCENDING (SMALL) COLON IMPACTIONS

Impactions are reportedly one of the most common conditions of the small colon (affecting 34% of horses with small colon disease), yet one study has found that only 2.5% of the horses presented for acute abdominal pain have small colon impactions.[35,36] Similar to other types of impactions, poor-quality roughage, poor dentition, a lack of water, and motility disorders have been suggested to be risk factors for small colon impactions.[36] Some studies have found a seasonal distribution of small colon impactions, with most cases being seen in the fall and winter; however, other studies have not identified seasonal distribution.[36–38] Horses older than 15 years of age, American miniature horses, and ponies were identified in one study to have increased risk for development of small colon impactions, whereas other studies have not found age and breed to be risk factors.[35–38] Horses diagnosed with small colon impactions are also commonly diagnosed with colitis; however, it remains undetermined whether the impactions occur primarily followed by colitis or the impactions are a result of colitis. One recent retrospective study identified horses with small colon impactions to be 10.8 times more likely to have diarrhea at the time of admission than horses admitted with large colon impactions.[38] The authors were unable to determine whether diarrhea was present before the impactions or vise versa. Two studies have determined that horses treated surgically for small colon impaction may be at increased risk for developing salmonellosis, with one of the studies stating that 43% of the surgically treated cases included fecal cultures that were positive for *Salmonella*.[36,37] It remains unknown if there is a causal association between small colon impactions and salmonellosis.

Clinical signs for horses with small colon impactions are similar to signs seen with other types of impactions. The most commonly reported clinical signs are abdominal pain (with the majority of cases described as mild to moderate), increased heart rates, and decreased manure production.[36,37] Lack of borborygmi and abdominal distention were the next most consistently reported clinical signs reported in one study, whereas another study found diarrhea and decreased appetite to be the next most commonly reported clinical signs.[36,37] Additional signs include fever, straining to defecate, depression, and nasogastric reflux.[36,37] Clinical pathology values are usually within normal values in the majority of horses with small colon impactions; however, some horses show leukopenia with a left shift.[36,37]

A definitive diagnosis of small colon impaction is usually made by rectal palpation (21/28 of the cases in one study, and 70/84 of the cases in another study).[36,37] Most of the remaining cases are diagnosed at surgery.[36,37] In addition to the impaction being felt on rectal exam, gas distention of the cecum or large colon and edematous or roughened rectal mucosa were reported in several cases.[36,37]

Similar to other impactions, treatment for small colon impactions can be either medical or surgical. A recent retrospective study reported that 23 of 44 (52%) cases were treated medically and 21 of 44 (48%) cases were treated surgically.[38] Previous reports had 47 of 84 (56%) cases treated medically with the remainder treated surgically in one, and 10 of 28 (36%) cases treated medically and 18 of 28 (64%) cases treated surgically in the other.[36,37]

Medical therapy includes the use of balanced polyionic intravenous fluids at two to three times the maintenance rate as well as oral fluids given by way of a nasogastric tube. Osmotic laxatives are also commonly used and given as described previously in this article. Flunixin meglumine and sedatives are used to manage pain. Although the use of standing enemas has been described, the risk associated with rectal tears is high and this procedure is not commonly performed in adult horses. Additional treatments more specific to small colon impactions include the use of antibiotics (penicillin and gentocin) if the horse is leukopenic or *Salmonella typhimurium* antiserum.[36]

Surgery is most commonly done if the horse is not responding to medical therapy, there is severe abdominal distention, or the horse is not responding to analgesia. If peritoneal fluid is abnormal (eg, increases in proteins, white blood count, red blood cell count, or bacteria) surgery should be strongly considered because some impactions can cause pressure necrosis of the small colon bowel wall. Most commonly, a ventral midline celiotomy and high enema are performed with the surgeon using gentle transmural massage from within the abdomen while an assistant passes a tube and delivers water by way of the rectum. Some surgeons also advocate performing a large colon enterotomy to evacuate the large colon to reduce the risk for reimpaction in the immediate postoperative period.

The reported prognosis for small colon impactions ranges from fair to good. In a recent report, 21 of 23 (91%) horses treated medically and 20 of 21 (95%) horses treated surgically survived to discharge.[38] Fever and diarrhea are the most commonly reported posttreatment (medical or surgical) complications.[38]

REFERENCES

1. Henninger R, Horst J. Magnesium toxicosis in two horses. J Am Vet Med Assoc 1997;211:82–5.
2. Freeman D, Ferrente PL, Palmer JE. Comparison of the effects of intragastric infusions of equal volumes of water, dioctyl sodium sulfosuccinate, and magnesium sulphate on fecal composition and output in clinically normal horses. Am J Vet Res 1992;53:1347–53.
3. Moffat R, Kramer L, Lerner D, et al. Studies on dioctyl sodium sulfosuccinate toxicity: clinical, gross and microscopic pathology in the horse and guinea pig. Can J Comp Med 1975;39:434–41.
4. Bohanon T. Duodenal impaction in a horse. J Am Vet Med Assoc 1988;192:365–6.
5. Bridges E, Jamison KC, Lowder MQ. Duodenal phytobezoar with secondary perforating gastric ulcer in an adult equine horse. Vet Clin North Am Equine Pract 1993;15:34.
6. Dixon R. Intestinal obstruction in a gelding. Aust Vet J 1965;41:20–2.
7. Green P, Tong JMJ. Small intestinal obstruction associated with wood chewing in two horses. Vet Rec 1988;123:196–8.
8. Turner T. Trichophytobezoar causing duodenal obstruction in a horse. Comp Contin Educ Pract Vet 1986;8:977–8.
9. Wilson R, Scruggs DW. Duodenal obstruction associated with persimmon fruit digestion by two horses. Equine Vet Sci 1992;12:26–8.
10. Little D, Blikslager AT. Factors associated with the development of ileal impaction in horses with surgical colic: 78 cases (1986–2000). Equine Vet J 2002;34(5): 464–8.
11. Proudman C, French NP, Trees AJ. Tapeworm infection is a significant risk factor for spasmotic colic and ileal impaction colic in the horse. Equine Vet J 1998;30: 194–9.
12. Hanson R, Wright JC, Schumacher J, et al. Surgical reduction of ileal impactions in the horse: 28 cases. Vet Surg 1998;27:555–60.
13. Parks A, Doran RE, White NA, et al. Ileal impaction in the horse: 75 cases. Cornell Vet 1989;79:83–91.
14. Hanson R, Schumacher J, Humburg J, et al. Medical treatment of horses with ileal impactions: 10 cases (1990–1994). J Am Vet Med Assoc 1996;208(6):898–900.
15. Plummer A, Rakestraw PC, Hardy J, et al. Outcome of medical and surgical treatment of cecal impaction in horses: 114 cases (1994–2004). J Am Vet Med Assoc 2007;231(9):1378–85.
16. White N. Epidemiology and etiology of colic. In: NA W, editor. The equine acute abdomen. Philadelphia: Lea & Febiger; 1990. p. 49–64.
17. Campbell M, Colahan PC, Brown MP, et al. Cecal impaction in the horse. J Am Vet Med Assoc 1984;184(8):950–2.

18. Dabareiner R, White NA. Diseases and surgery of the cecum. Vet Clin North Am Equine Pract 1997;13:303–15.
19. White N. Diseases of the cecum. In: NA W, editor. The equine acute abdomen. Philadelphia: Lea & Febiger; 1990. p. 369–74.
20. Collatos C, Romano S. Cecal impaction in horses: causes, diagnosis and medical treatment. Comped Contin Educ Pract Vet 1993;15(7):976–81.
21. Dart A, Hodgson DR, Snyder JR. Ceacal disease in equids. Aust Vet J 1997;75: 552–7.
22. Ross M, Martin BB, Donawick WJ. Cecal perforation in the horse. J Am Vet Med Assoc 1985;187:249–53.
23. White N, Lessard P. Risk factors and clinical signs associated with cases of equine colic. Presented at the 32nd Annual Meeting of American Association of Equine Practitioners, 1986.
24. Roberts C, Sloan DE. Cecal impactions managed surgically by typhlotomy in 10 cases (1988–1998). Equine Vet J Suppl 2000;32:74–6.
25. Ross M, Tate LP, Donawick WJ, et al. Cecocolic anastomosis for the surgical management of cecal impaction in horses. Vet Surg 1986;15:85–92.
26. Craig D, Pankowski R, Car B, et al. Ileocolostomy–a technique for surgical management of equine cecal impaction in horses. Vet Surg 1987;16:451–5.
27. Meisler SD, Doherty TJ, Andrews FM, et al. Yohimbine ameliorates the effects of endotoxin on gastric emptying of the liquid marker acetaminophen in horses. Canadian Journal of Veterinary Research 2000;64:208–11.
28. Ross M, Orsini JA, Ehnen SJ. Jejunocolic anastomosis for the surgical management of recurrent cecal impaction in a horse. Vet Surg 1987;16:265–8.
29. Gerard M, Bowman KF, Blickslager AT, et al. Jejunocolostomy or ileocolostomy for treatment of cecal impaction in horses: nine cases (1985–1995). J Am Vet Med Assoc 1996;209:1287–90.
30. Symm W, Nieto JE, VanHoogmoed L, et al. Initial evaluation of a technique for complete cecal bypass in the horse. Vet Surg 2006;35:674–7.
31. Dabareiner R, White NA. Large colon impaction in horses: 147 cases (1985–1991). J Am Vet Med Assoc 1995;206(5):679–85.
32. Hillayer M, Taylor FG, Proudman CJ, et al. Case control study to identify risk factors for simple colonic obstruction and distension colic in horses. Equine Vet J 2002;34:455–63.
33. Hallowell G. Short communication: retrospective study assessing efficacy of treatment of large colonic impactions. Equine Vet J 2008;40(4):411–3.
34. Lopes M, Walker BL, White NA, et al. Treatments to promote colonic hydration: enteral fluid therapy versus intravenous fluid therapy and magnesium sulphate. Equine Vet J 2002;34(5):505–9.
35. Dart A, Snyder JR, Pascoe JR, et al. Abnormal conditions of the equine descending (small) colon: 102 cases (1979–1989). J Am Vet Med Assoc 1992;200(7): 971–8.
36. Rhoads W, Barton MH, Parks AH. Comparison of medical and surgical treatment for impaction of the small colon in horses: 84 cases (1986–1996). J Am Vet Med Assoc 1999;214(7):1042–7.
37. Ruggles A, Ross MW. Medical and surgical management of small-colon impaction in horses: 28 cases (1984–1989). J Am Vet Med Assoc 1991;199(12):1762–6.
38. Frederico L, Jones SL, Blickslager AT. Predisposing factors for small colon impaction in horses and outcome of medical and surgical treatment: 44 cases (1999–2004). J Am Vet Med Assoc 2006;229(10):1612–6.

Enteroliths and Other Foreign Bodies

Rebecca L. Pierce, BVetMed, MRCVS

KEYWORDS

• Colic • Enterolith • Fecalith • Bezoar • Foreign body

ENTEROLITHIASIS

Enteroliths are formed in the ampulla coli of the right dorsal colon from mineral deposition arranged in concentric layers around a central nidus.[1–3] Enteroliths can cause either a partial or complete obstruction of the right dorsal or transverse or small colon. Although many horses have been affected by enterolithiasis and it is not a new problem, the specific pathogenesis of enterolith formation is still not understood completely.[4]

Enteroliths have been reported as a cause of colic since the 1800s. Horses owned by millers were noted to be more affected than the rest of the population.[3,5] Reports of enteroliths decreased in frequency until an increase in the frequency of cases was observed in the 1980s.[3,5,6] California and areas of the southwest have a higher prevalence of enterolithiasis than other regions of North America.[3,7,8] In two previous reports, enterolithiasis has been identified in 1.7% and 15.1% of horses presenting for colic.[8,9] One of these reports also stated that enterolithiasis was diagnosed in 27.5% of horses that underwent an exploratory celiotomy because of colic.[8] Other authors have reported that 45%, 57%, and 71% of horses with enterolithiasis had a primary enterolith obstruction occurring in the small colon.[1,8,9] Obstruction caused by an enterolith was diagnosed in 35% of horses presenting for small colon disorders.[10] The reported numbers reflect various regions in which enteroliths are common and horses are predisposed.

Several different shapes of enteroliths have been described, but spherical or tetrahedral are commonly described (**Fig. 1**).[11] Tetrahedral stones are most commonly observed when more than one enterolith is present.[1,2,4,5,7] Horses may develop more than one enterolith, and multiple enteroliths have been reported in 28%, 39%, 45%, or 52% of horses diagnosed with enterolithiasis (Pierce RL, unpublished observations, 2008).[1,8,12]

The weight of removed stones can vary, but reported weights range from 200 g up to 9 kg. A median of 0.2 kg and an average of 200 g to 1.5 kg has also been reported.[5,9] Size is also variable, but reported diameters range from 1 to 15 cm.[3,4]

Department of Large Animal Clinical Sciences, The University of Tennessee College of Veterinary Medicine, 2407 River Drive, Knoxville, TN 37996, USA
E-mail address: rpierc10@utk.edu

Vet Clin Equine 25 (2009) 329–340
doi:10.1016/j.cveq.2009.04.010
0749-0739/09/$ – see front matter © 2009 Elsevier Inc. All rights reserved.

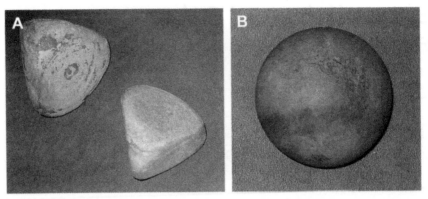

Fig. 1. (*A*) Tetrahedral-shaped enterolith. (*B*) Round enterolith removed from the small colon.

Etiology

The nidus at the center of the enterolith is most commonly sand or a small stone; however, hair or a piece of metal such as a wire or nail have also been identified.[1–3,5] When the mineral is deposited around cloth, rope, or hay net, an irregular-shaped concretion is formed (**Fig. 2**).[1,13] The rate of formation seems to be variable and may be affected by pH, mineral availability, and colonic motility.[12] Because of certain breed predilections and a familial trends[8] for developing enterolithiasis, a genetic component affecting colonic motility, colonic pH, colonic mineral content, or digestive enzymes has been hypothesized.[3,7,8,12,14] As more research is done regarding the physiologic mechanisms affecting enterolith formation, it may be possible to target specific genes involved in their regulation.[15]

Enterolith composition in horses is magnesium ammonium phosphate (struvite).[2,4] This differs from that in other species in which intestinal concretions are commonly calcium salts.[1,4] Sodium, sulfur, potassium, and calcium have also been identified in varying quantities.[4] The formation of struvite crystals has been linked to Mg^{2+} supersaturation, the presence of NH^{4+}, and PO_4^{3-} in an alkaline (pH $\geq$7.0) enviroment.[4,6,12,16] In experimental ponies fed magnesium oxide, an increase in

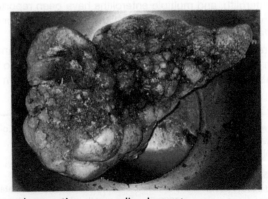

Fig. 2. Irregular-shaped concretion surrounding hay net.

colonic pH was observed.[6] So besides providing substrate for formation, dietary magnesium may also affect colonic pH to favor enterolith formation.

Furthermore, feeding alfalfa hay has been reported to be a risk factor for enterolith formation.[3,8,9,16,17] Alfalfa hay has a higher protein concentration when compared with grass hay. The metabolism of proteins by colonic bacteria results in ammonia formation and leads to an alkaline pH within the colon.[12]

Because of the struvite component, excess dietary levels of dietary magnesium, phosphorus, and nitrogen have been hypothesized to contribute to enterolith formation.[1,12] Alfalfa hay, especially in California, has excess magnesium,[5] protein, and phosphorus, and[15] increased colonic mineral content was reported in horses fed a high alfalfa diet.[15,16]

Mineral content of the water has also been examined as a potential contributor to enterolith formation[5] as a result of increased magnesium concentrations. However, the contribution of dietary magnesium, from alfalfa hay, may contribute more to enterolith formation, but the combination of diet and water sources may have an additive effect.[5]

Wheat bran has also been hypothesized as a risk factor for enterolith formation. Wheat bran contains high concentrations of phosphorus, magnesium, and protein.[3,5] However, in recent studies, this association was not observed.[16,17]

Other risk factors for enterolith formation include confinement housing of at least 50% of the day, limited access to pasture grazing, and decreased colonic motility.[4,8,9] There may be a positive effect on colonic motility and exercise, and this positive effect may be negated in stall-confined horses.

Colonic hypomotility has also been reported as a risk factor in horses with enterolithiasis.[12,16] Decreased exercise has been linked to increased retention time for particulate matter within the intestinal tract. Because horses without access to pasture were found to have higher colonic mineral concentrations, there may be a potential dilutional effect of grass on ingested alfalfa.[16]

Signalment

Enteroliths have been recognized in certain breeds. Arabians are at higher risk for enteroliths when compared with other breeds.[3,6–8] In several reports, 19% to 56% of enterolith cases were reported in Arabian or Arabian crosses (Pierce RL, unpublished observations, 2008).[7–11] Morgan horses (Pierce RL, unpublished observations, 2008),[6,8] and American Miniature Horses.[9] Furthermore, Saddlebreds[8] have also been identified as high-risk groups compared with other breeds for developing enterolithiasis. Also, in several reports Quarter horses contributed to 24% to 27% of all enterolith cases, but did not appear to be overrepresented when compared with overall hospital population (Pierce RL, unpublished observations, 2008).[8,11] When compared with overall hospital populations, some breeds have been considered to be underrepresented, including Thoroughbreds and Warmbloods (Pierce RL, unpublished observations, 2008).[8,11] In a study comparing the location of the enterolith within each breed, enteroliths in Arabians and thoroughbreds were found more frequently in the large colon (67%, 73%) than in the small colon (33%, 27%) (Pierce RL, unpublished observations, 2008).

Gender predilection for enterolith formation has not been observed (Pierce RL, unpublished observations, 2008).[1,6,9,11] Several investigators have reported that stallions were underrepresented within study groups (Pierce RL, unpublished observations, 2008).[8] The exact cause of this underrepresentation is not known but may be explained by the effects of male hormones (testosterone) on colonic motility.

Also, thoroughbreds may be underrepresented because they represent a younger group (<5-year-old Thoroughbred horses) and may have skewed these results.

The mean age of horses identified with enteroliths ranged from 9 to 14.5 years (Pierce RL, unpublished observations, 2008).[1,7–9,11] Other studies identified older aged horses were more likely to have enterolith at surgery; however, this may reflect owners' willingness to pursue surgery or referral in older horses. Also, implementation of preventative measures in susceptible populations may slow the rate of enterolith formation, thus, a diagnosis may be made in older horses. In one study, the mean age for horses with large colon enterolithiasis was 15.3 years and that of the small colon was 13.3 years ($P < .005$) (Pierce RL, unpublished observations, 2008). This observation may reflect the difference in time required for enterolith formation in the large colon. Horses with a true enterolith (lamellar deposition of crystal) are not commonly reported in horses younger than 2 to 4 years of age (Pierce RL, unpublished observations, 2008).[7,11] Concretions that form around objects such as bits of baling twine, lead rope, hay net, cloth, or rubber tend to be removed from younger horses.[18]

History and Presentation

The obstruction usually occurs where the diameter of the transverse colon narrows or within the small colon. Because the diameter of the right dorsal colon is generally larger than the diameter of the enterolith, affected horses generally suffer from a partial intestinal blockage.[3] The enterolith may transiently occlude the opening of the smaller transverse colon resulting in signs of colic.[7,8] Once the enterolith shifts, the right dorsal and transverse colons are not obstructed, and signs of colic pass. Affected horses may suffer from several minor bouts of colic before a diagnosis of enterolithiasis.[2,8] Signs of abdominal pain of affected horses tend to be mild and respond to basic medical therapies consisting of analgesics, mineral oil, or water given via nasogastric tube.[1,3] Owners of affected horses have noticed weight loss, reduced performance, behavioral changes, anorexia, decreased defecation, and passage of enteroliths in feces (Pierce RL, unpublished observations, 2008).[2,3,7,8] Horses in high-risk areas showing signs of intermittent colic signs, poor performance, or anorexia should be evaluated for enterolithiasis.

Clinical signs of a horse with enterolithiasis are consistent with a partial or complete intestinal blockage.[3,8] Initially, cardiovascular parameters are within normal limits[2,3,7,8] but changes in clinical signs, increased heart rate, and respiratory rate are frequently observed as the condition progresses.[1,9] Clinical parameters seem to worsen as the enterolith moves into the small colon.[8] A recent study found that heart rate was ≥60 beats per minute in 56% of small colon enterolith obstructions compared with 10% in horses with large colon enteroliths (Pierce RL, unpublished observations, 2008). The average heart rate for a small colon enterolith obstruction (65 beats per minute) was higher when compared with heart rate in large colon obstructions (56 beats per minute).[8]

Clinical signs of abdominal discomfort vary according to the degree of intestinal distention. The time from onset of clinical signs to presentation to the veterinarian was greater than 12 hours[1] and averaged 24 or 36 hours in horses with enterolithiasis (Pierce RL, unpublished observations, 2008).[9]

Generally, horses presenting with a small colon enterolith obstruction do not seem to be as affected by prior episodes of colic as horses with a large colon enterolith obstruction (Pierce RL, unpublished observations, 2008).[8] This observation can be explained that the smaller-sized enterolith does not act like an intermittent hinge-ball valve as in the partial large colon obstructions. In contrast, the diameter of the small colon and the enterolith is similar, so an obstruction in this region is generally complete and is accompanied by gas distention of the colon and cecum. Horses with enteroliths lodged in the small colon present with more severe signs of pain, including tachycardia and gas distention, secondary to a complete obstruction.[3,7] Obstruction in this portion of the intestinal tract are more likely to present with or develop changes on hematology and abdominocentesis if treatment is delayed.[1,3,7-9] As pressure necrosis of the intestine occurs, peritoneal fluid analysis shows an increase in protein and white blood cell count.[3,9]

Diagnosis

A presumptive diagnosis of enterolithiasis is based on signalment and a thorough history in regions in which this condition occurs frequently. A definitive diagnosis of enterolithiasis can be made using abdominal radiography, performing exploratory celiotomy or necropsy, or occasionally on rectal palpation. Rectal palpation findings are generally inconclusive as the enterolith is rarely palpable.[2,7,8] Often, a history of chronic colic and presenting clinical signs of intermittent or continuous abdominal pain, large intestinal gas distention,[1,8,19] and scant, dry feces within the rectum are highly suggestive of enterolithiasis.[1,3]

Radiographic examination can be used to detect enteroliths in the colon. Generally, four overlapping views are performed.[10] An enterolith can be identified on radiographs by their shape, a smooth rounded border that is often silhouetted against gas, a uniform increased density, and occasionally a radiodense nidus (**Fig. 3**).[12] Radiography as a diagnostic test, has an overall sensitivity of 73% and positive and negative predictive value of 96.4% and 67.5%, respectively.[10] A concurrent feed impaction in the colon may hide the enterolith from view on radiographs, producing a false–negative result. When possible, having horses fast for 24 to 36 hours before radiographic examination can decrease gut fill and improve the diagnostic quality of the films. Large colon enteroliths were positively identified radiographically in 74% and 84% of radiographed horses (Pierce RL, unpublished observations, 2008).[10] To a lesser extent, small colon enteroliths were identified on radiographs in 42% and 54% of radiographed horses (Pierce RL, unpublished observations, 2008).[10] The high degree of false–negative findings for diagnosing small colon enterolithiasis on radiography has been described by others.[3,10] The reason for this may be the smaller size of the small colon enterolith compared with the larger colonic enteroliths. The presence of multiple enteroliths may improve the likelihood of positively identifying an enterolith on radiographic examination.[10] In a study, radiographic examination positively identified 54% of horses with a small colon enterolith; 83% of those had multiple stones (Pierce RL, unpublished observations, 2008).

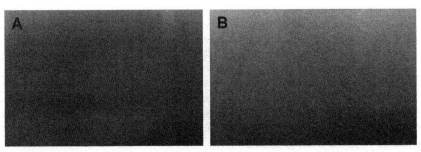

Fig. 3. Radiographs of (*A*) solitary enterolith and (*B*) multiple enteroliths.

Surgical Removal

As mentioned before, a positive diagnosis of enterolithiasis can be made during an exploratory celiotomy. During exploratory celiotomy, an enterolith can be identified by palpating the dorsal, transverse, or small colon. If an enterolith is found, it is important to fully evaluate the rest of the colon for any remaining enteroliths. Also, enteroliths can be an incidental finding, so evaluation for the presence enteroliths should be a part of any exploratory celiotomy.

Large colon

Although a flank approach has been described for removing enteroliths,[1,9] a ventral midline approach with the patient in dorsal recumbency is most commonly performed. Preoperative antibiotics (penicillin 20,000 IU/kg, intravenously [IV], every 6 hours and gentamicin 6.6 mg/kg, IV, every 24 hours) and analgesics (flunixin meglumin 1.1 mg/kg, IV, every 12 hours or every 24 hours) are administered before and continued after surgical induction. The enterolith is generally palpable at the junction between the right dorsal and transverse colon. The large colon is exteriorized, and a pelvic flexure enterotomy is performed to evacuate colon contents. It is important to clear the dorsal and transverse colon of any feed material to facilitate exteriorization of the enterolith and minimize contamination at the enterotomy site. Once the colon is emptied, the enterolith is balloted gently up into the exteriorized dorsal colon. Allowing fluid distention of the colon around the enterolith can ease its movement from the transverse colon. Smaller enteroliths can be removed via the pelvic flexure enterotomy. Extending the abdominal incision cranially may facilitate exteriorization of larger enteroliths.[12] The enterolith is moved to a location that is accessible for its removal, and any excess fluid within the intestinal lumen is evacuated via the pelvic flexure enterotomy. Stay sutures are placed at either end of the enterolith. A barrier drape and saline-soaked lap sponges are placed around the colon containing the enterolith. An enterotomy, centered over the enterolith, is performed in the right dorsal colon. If there are multiple enteroliths to be removed, the dorsal colon enterotomy should be centered so the largest enterolith is removed first.[12] The enterotomy can be closed in two layers (continuous appositional oversewn by an inverting pattern) using synthetic absorbable suture material. The intestine is cleaned with sterile saline-soaked sponges before closure between suture layers and then lavaged with saline before replacing the colon within the abdomen.

Small colon

The majority of small colon obstructions caused by an enterolith occur in the most proximal aspect of the small colon, making adequate surgical exposure difficult or impossible. Short mesenteric attachments prevent the proximal and distal aspects of the small colon from being exteriorized, making an enterotomy or a resection and anastomosis in these areas challenging. Enteroliths in these areas lead to a high risk for peritoneal contamination, especially during manipulation. Difficulties encountered during surgery of the small colon have been described previously and include inflammation, enterotomy dehiscence, peritonitis, rupture, adhesion formation, and vascular compromise.[12,20,21]

Before removal of the enterolith from the small colon, a pelvic flexure enterotomy is performed, and a thorough evacuation of the entire large colon should be performed. This will reduce the amount of fibrous feed material passing through the colon postoperatively and ensure removal of all enteroliths. If the obstruction is in the most proximal aspect of the small colon and cannot be exteriorized, it can be moved by retropulsion of the enterolith through the transverse colon and then into the ascending colon using retrograde flushing and external massage.[22,23] A partial thickness teniotomy consisting of a neuromuscular incision has also been described to increase luminal diameter and facilitate movement of proximally located enteroliths.[24] If the enterolith is located in an accessible portion of the small colon, the obstructed portion of colon is exteriorized and isolated using sponges and drapes. An assistant's hand can be placed proximal to the enterolith aid in keeping the bowel exteriorized.[12] Stay sutures are placed adjacent to the enterolith, and an enterotomy is made through the antimesenteric taenia. Closure of a small colon enterotomy is performed in two layers (simple appositional oversewn with an inverting pattern) using absorbable suture material. Minimal inversion should be applied to preserve the luminal diameter.

Bowel ischemia is likely with small colon obstructions secondary to increased intraluminal pressure (**Fig. 4**).[25] Focal areas of pressure necrosis are commonly encountered, and either a partial or wedge resection can be performed or the weakened area can be reinforced by suture.[3] Resection and anastomosis can be performed if the ischemic portion of colon is accessible. In one study, six horses with small colon enterolithiasis were euthanized intraoperatively because of poor prognosis and another seven ruptured during surgical manipulation.[8]

Postoperative Complications and Survival

Postoperative care includes monitoring of physical parameters and supportive treatment. Feces are generally passed within 24 hours after surgery but may be delayed if the large colon was thoroughly emptied at surgery. Antibiotics and analgesics are administered to most horses 3 to 5 days postoperatively. Other supportive treatments such as IV fluid therapy with electrolyte supplementation or therapies to treat endotoxemia (see chapter on endotoxemia treatment) are administered based on the pre- and postoperative status and clinical and laboratory findings of the patient. In recent studies, peritonitis occurred at a low frequency, so insertion of abdominal drains or abdominal lavage is generally not necessary unless extensive peritoneal contamination occurred at surgery. Use of intraoperative suction, barrier draping, thorough evacuation of the colon content before performing the enterotomy, and lavage after enterotomy closure will decrease the potential for peritonitis.

Most horses can be fed small amounts 12 to18 hours after surgery. If the small colon was affected, feeding a complete pelleted diet in the initial postoperative period is

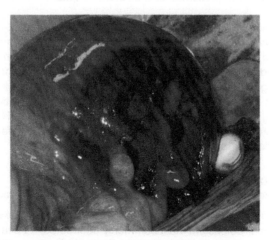

Fig. 4. Rupture of the small colon secondary to enterolith obstruction.

preferable to reduce the bulk of fecal material passing through the enterotomy site and inflamed and edematous small colon. Grass, if available, is also preferable to feeding hay in the initial postoperative period. Administration of fecal softeners such as mineral oil, flax seed oil, or magnesium sulfate may also be used to decrease irritation of the enterotomy site.

Postoperative complications have been reported in horses with enterolithiasis. Diarrhea after surgery is a common sequela in horses with enterolithiasis, especially when a pelvic flexure enterotomy in performed.[26] This diarrhea is probably caused by irritation secondary to surgical manipulation. Also, the postobstruction hypermotility and increased fluid loss may also play a role. Diarrhea was reported in 40.9% and 11.7% cases of postoperative enterolithiasis.[8,9]

Incisional complications have been reported in 8.1% and 44.1% of horses with enterolithiasis.[7,8] Contributing factors to incisional problems include difficulty exteriorizing the affected portion of intestine (primarily the proximal small colon), which may necessitate performing an enterotomy. Incisional trauma to the bowel associated with emptying the large colon may be the reason for complications.[27,28]

Septic peritonitis was found in 2.8%, 17.6%, 18.2%, and 33% horses with enterolithiasis.[1,7-9] Contamination of the abdominal cavity may occur from traumatized, ischemic bowel or necrosis at the incision site from the presence of the enterolith. Also, dehiscence at the incision site is potential source leakage. Other reported complications of enterolith cases were adhesions in 1.8%[8] and laminitis in 9.1% and 3.4%.[8,9]

Survival after surgical removal of enteroliths has improved over time as techniques and aftercare have advanced. Early reported survival rates range from 47% to 70%.[1,7] More recent reports show short-term survival rates of 92% to 96%, whereas long-term survival was reported to be similar, 93%.[8,9]

Recurrence and Prevention

Although the actual rate of recurrence is difficult to determine, horses with a history of enterolithiasis may be predisposed to further formation. One study reported the recurrence rate to be 7.7%.[8] This rate may actually be higher because horses can remain asymptomatic as another enterolith forms in the large intestine. Also, in previous studies, recurrence rates may have been underestimated because horses may have been lost to follow-up or presented to a different hospital the next time an enterolith was diagnosed.

Recommendations to reduce recurrence or formation in "at risk" horses can be made. The majority of the horses' diets should come from pasture or grass hay, and alfalfa-based products should be avoided.[17] Feeding psyllium to prevent nidus accumulation and enhance intestinal motility has also been recommended. Feeding apple cider vinegar (112–205 mL, orally, every 12 hours) to ponies was shown to decrease colonic pH, but its efficacy at reducing enterolith formation is unknown.[29] Also, maintaining enteroliths in a colonic environment with a pH ≤6.6 has been reported to decrease their weight.[6] As we learn more about factors influencing enterolith formation, further recommendations can be made.

OTHER FOREIGN BODIES
Fecaliths, Phytobezoar, Trichobezoar, Phytotrichobezoar, and Phytoconglobates

Other foreign bodies occur anywhere within the intestinal tract; however, the terminal transverse and small colons are most commonly obstructed.[19] Fecaliths are made up of discrete concretions of inspissated fecal material.[13,30] Although they are primarily made up of feed material, fecaliths are more concrete with a distinct shape when compared with a general feed impaction. Their formation generally is associated with poor-quality diet, poor mastication, or reduced water intake.[13] In average-sized adult horses they have been described to be 8 to 12 cm wide and 15 to 20 cm long[20] and 4 to 6 cm in diameter in Miniature foals.[30] Fecaliths have been reported in 7% of horses presenting with small colon disease, but this number may be higher in regions with a lower prevalence of eneroltihiasis.[11]

Small colon fecaliths are most commonly identified in young (<1 year) or older (>15 years) horses.[11] Ponies and American Miniature Horses have been shown to having a higher risk for forming fecaliths.[11,13]

Phytoconglobates are matted concretions of plant material.[13] When the concretions involve the deposition of struvite minerals, they are referred to as "bezoars."[19] Phytobezoars are primarily composed of plant material, trichobezoars of hair, and phytotrichobezoars a combination of the two.[13,20] The small intestine and cecum have been identified as areas of obstruction in case reports (**Fig. 5**).[31,32] Chewing hair or tails is performed by younger horses and weanlings and can result in the formation of trichobezoars.

Foreign Bodies

Reports of obstructive colic secondary to ingested foreign material seem to primarily affect young horses (<3 years). They have been reported as a cause of colic in 2% of horses presenting for small colon disease.[11] Causes of foreign body impaction have been identified as rubberized fencing, tires, baling twine, feed sacks, lead ropes, cloth material, and plastic bags.[18,33–35] Presentation and clinical signs reflect the location of the obstruction. The transverse and small colon are most commonly affected,[18] but obstruction has also been reported of the stomach and small intestine.[33]

Presentation

Similar to the other obstructive conditions discussed in this chapter, horses may remain asymptomatic after ingesting the foreign material. One study recorded that at least 2 years had passed since the horse had exposure to the identified foreign material, and another horse presented within 2 months of exposure.[18] A careful history to include asking the client if there is a missing leg wrap or other foreign material can be helpful in identifying foreign body impaction.

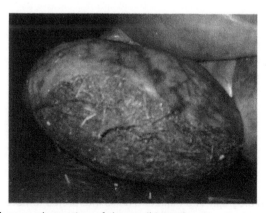

Fig. 5. Phytotrichobezoar obstruction of the small intestine.

Presentation reflects the portion of intestinal tract that is occluded and whether the obstruction is partial or complete. Similar to an enterolith, an obstruction of the small colon is complete, so these animals present with abdominal distention, tachycardia, and moderate to severe signs of abdominal pain.[34] Diagnosis can be suspicious based on signalment and clinical signs. Abdominal radiography can be performed on miniatures, foals, and some weanlings with better detail compared with an adult. Generally, the main findings are signs of gas distention of the large colon and cecum,[36] but occasionally the obstruction may be identified (**Fig. 6**).

Treatment

Based on clinical signs and abdominal pain, an exploratory celiotomy is generally recommended. Medical therapy consisting of intravenous fluids, enemas, and trocarization[30,36] can be initiated but rarely is curative. At surgery, the obstruction is identified, and the large colon content is evacuated via a pelvic flexure enterotomy. If the obstruction is located within the proximal small colon or transverse colon, it can be manipulated using fluid distention to move it up into the dorsal colon (similar to an enterolith) and removed at the pelvic flexure or dorsal colon enterotomy. An obstruction of the small colon can be removed by an antimesenteric enterotomy as described for enteroliths. A high enema and external massage of the intestine can also be performed under general anesthesia to break up a fecalith, and it can then be expressed through the rectum. Care needs to be exercised during manipulation of the small colon because the same concerns for mural pressure exist as for enterolithiasis (**Fig. 7**).

In several cases involving a large, fibrous foreign body obstruction, an enterotomy was made in the large colon through which the surgeon's hand was introduced into the lumen of the intestine to remove obstruction.[18,23] Whichever approach is performed, a thorough evacuation of the large colon content is necessary to prevent recurrence of an obstruction in the immediate postoperative period. A younger horse or American Miniature has a smaller intestinal lumen compared with a full-sized horse, so if a small colon enterotomy is performed, close attention needs to be paid to ensure the lumen is not overly narrowed during closure.

Postoperative care is similar to that described in the section on enterolithiasis. Because of the inflammation present in the colon, these horses need a judicious return to feeding, and avoidance of fibrous feedstuff is important to decrease the likelihood of a postoperative feed impaction. A complete, easily digestible pelleted ration in a dry or

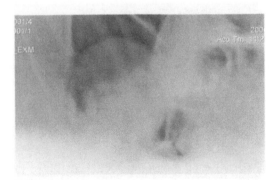

Fig. 6. Abdominal radiograph of a miniature horse interpreted to have gas distention and defined opacity consistent with a fecalith.

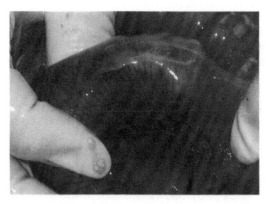

Fig. 7. Mural compression secondary to fecalith impaction in a miniature foal.

mash form is preferred over hay in the initial postoperative period. Administration of fecal softeners can also be initiated to prevent the passage of hard or dry feces.

REFERENCES

1. Blue M. Enteroliths in horses-a retrospective study of 30 horses. Equine Vet J 1979;11(2):76–84.
2. Blue M, Wittkopp RW. Clinical and structural features of equine enteroliths. J Am Vet Med Assoc 1981;179(1):79–82.
3. Murray R, Green EM, Constantinescu GM. Equine enterolithiasis. Compendium on Continuing Education 1992;14(8):1104–11.
4. Hassel D, Schiffman PS, Snyder JR. Petrographic and geochemic evaluation of equine enteroliths. Am J Vet Res 2001;62(3):350–8.
5. Lloyd K, Hintz HF, Wheat JD, et al. Enteroliths in horses. Cornell Vet 1987;77: 172–86.
6. Hintz H, Lowe JE, Livesay-Wilkins P, et al. Studies on equine enterolithiasis. Proc Am Assoc Equine Pract 1988;24:53–9.
7. Evans D, Trunk DA, Hibser NK, et al. Diagnosis and treatment of enterolithiasis in equidae. Compendium on Continuing Education 1981;3(10):383–90.
8. Hassel D, Langer DL, Snyder JR, et al. Evaluation of enterolithiasis in equids: 900 cases (1973–1996). J Am Vet Med Assoc 1999;214(2):233–7.
9. Cohen N, Vontur CA, Rakestraw PC. Risk factors for enterolithiasis among horses in Texas. J Am Vet Med Assoc 2000;216(11):1787–94.
10. Dart A, Snyder JR, Pascoe JR, et al. Abnormal conditions of the equine descending (small) colon: 102 cases (1979–1989). J Am Vet Med Assoc 1992;200(7): 971–8.
11. Hassel D. Enterolithiasis. Clin Tech Equine Pract 2002;1(3):143–7.
12. Yarbrough T, Langer DL, Snyder JR, et al. Abdominal radiography for diagnosis of enterolithiasis in horses: 141 cases (1990–1992). J Am Vet Med Assoc 1994; 205(4):592–5.
13. Schumacher J, Mair TS. Small colon obstructions in the mature horse. Equine Vet Ed 2002;14(1):19–28.
14. Beard W, Robertson JT, Getzy DM. Enterotomy technique in the descending colon of the horse. Effect of location and suture pattern. Vet Surg 1989;18(2): 135–40.

15. Hassel D, Spier SJ, Aldridge BM, et al. Influence of diet and water supply on mineral content and pH within the large intestine of horses with enterolithiasis. Vet J. In press.
16. Hassel D, Rakestraw PC, Gardner IA, et al. Dietary risk factors and colonic pH and mineral concentrations in horses with enterolithiasis. J Vet Intern Med 2004;18:346–9.
17. Hassel D, Aldridge BM, Drake CM, et al. Evaluation of dietary and management risk factors for enterolithiasis among horses in California. Res Vet Sci 2008;85: 476–80.
18. Boles C, Kohn CW. Fibrous foreign body impaction colic in young horses. J Am Vet Med Assoc 1977;171(2):193–5.
19. Rakestraw P, Hardy J. Large intestine. In: Auer S, editor. Equine surgery. 3rd edition. St. Louis (MO): Saunders; 2006. p. 468–9.
20. Keller S, Horney FD. Disease of the equine small colon. Compendium on Continuing Education for the Practicing Veterinarian 1985;7(2):113–20.
21. Ruggles A, Ross MW. Medical and surgical management of small-colon impaction in horses: 28 cases (1984–1989). J Am Vet Med Assoc 1992;199(12):1762–6.
22. Taylor T, Valdez H, Norwood GW, et al. Retrograde flushing for relief of obstructions of the tranverse colon in the horse. Eq Pract 1979;1(5):22–8.
23. Foerner J. Diseases of the large intestine. Vet Clin North Am Equine Pract 1982; 4(1):129–46.
24. Hassel D, Yarbrough TB. A modified teniotomy technique for facilitated removal of descending colon enteroliths in horses. Vet Surg 1998;27(1):1–4.
25. Faleiros R, Macoris DG, Alessi AC, et al. Effect of intraluminal distention on microvascular perfusion in the small colon. Am J Vet Res 2002;63:1292–7.
26. Cohen N, Honnas CM. Risk factors associated with development of diarrhea in horses after celiotomy for colic: 190 cases (1990–1994). J Am Vet Med Assoc 1996;209(4):810–3.
27. Phillips T, Walmsley JP. Retrospective analysis of the results of 151 exploratory laparotomies in horses with gastrointestinal disease. Equine Vet J 1993;25(5): 427–31.
28. Honnas C, Cohen ND. Risk factors for wound infection following celiotomy in horses. J Am Vet Med Assoc 1997;210(1):78–81.
29. Hintz H, Hernandez T, Soderholm V, et al. Effect of vinegar supplementation on pH of colonic fluid. Equine Nutrition Symposium 1989;116–8.
30. McClure J, Kobluk C, Voller K, et al. Fecalith impaction in four miniature foals. J Am Vet Med Assoc 1992;200(2):205–7.
31. Turner T. Trichophytobezoar causing duodenal obstruction in a horse. Compendium on Continuing Education 1986;8:977–8.
32. Maconochie J, Newman IM, Newton-Tabrett D. Phyto-trichobezoars in the cecum of horses in the Northern Territory. Aust Vet J 1968;44(2):81–2.
33. Getty S, Ellis DJ, Krehbiel JD, et al. Rubberized fencing as a gastrointestinal obstruction in a young horse. Vet Med 1976;71:221–3.
34. Gay C, Speirs VC, Christie BA, et al. Foreign body obstruction of the small colon in six horses. Equine Vet J 1979;11(1):60–3.
35. van Wuijckhuise-Sjouke L. Three cases of obstruction of the small colon by a foreign body. Vet Q 1984;6(1):31–6.
36. Yvorchuk-St. Jean K, Debowes RM, Gift LJ, et al. Trichophytobezoar as a cause of transverse colon obstruction in a foal. Cornell Vet 1993;83(2):169–75.

New Perspectives in Postoperative Complications After Abdominal Surgery

Andreas Klohnen, DVM

KEYWORDS

- Colic surgery • Postoperative incisional complications
- Postoperative ileus • Postoperative signs of colic

Abdominal exploratory surgeries are one of the most commonly performed surgeries in equine practice. Although most cases of equine abdominal pain resolve either spontaneously or with medical treatment, some cases would be fatal if surgical intervention was not pursued.[1] As a result of our better understanding of the causes of colic, improved diagnostic modalities to pinpoint the cause of colic, improved anesthesia techniques, improved surgeons skills, and much improved postoperative care and detection of complications earlier, survival rates have been improving vastly over the last 15–20 years.[1] Despite the increase in surgical case survival rates and vast improvements in postoperative care, equine abdominal surgery for gastrointestinal (GI) diseases carries a high mortality rate and complication rate.

This article focuses on postoperative complications after equine abdominal surgery, new ways to prevent complications, and treatment methods. A more general review of postoperative complications was completed by Mair and colleagues,[1] Dukti and White,[2] and Hackett and Hassel.[3] The most common postoperative complications after equine colic surgery are listed in **Box 1**.

CATHETER-RELATED THROMBOPHLEBITIS

Thrombophlebitis is an unpopular secondary complication to intravenous catheterization. Thrombophlebitis is defined as thrombosis of a vein with inflammation of the vessel wall. Septic thrombophlebitis is defined as an infected thrombus. Clinical signs related to vein thrombophlebitis include soft tissue swelling around the catheter entry site, pain upon soft tissue palpation around the catheter site, secondary entry wound catheter site discharge, firm swelling of the catheterized vein, fever spikes, head swelling, and lower limb swelling as a result of the complete vein occlusion.

Chino Valley Equine Hospital, 2945 English Place, Chino Hills, CA 91709, USA
E-mail address: topgun96@att.net

Vet Clin Equine 25 (2009) 341–350
doi:10.1016/j.cveq.2009.05.003   **vetequine.theclinics.com**

Box 1

Postoperative complications in horses undergoing abdominal surgery

Jugular vein thrombophlebitis

Incisional infection during the hospitalization stay, acute hernia formation during the initial hospitalization versus hernia formation after an incisional infection has healed and the body wall formed a hernia, and acute dehiscence of the abdominal wall during the recovery period or the initial hospitalization

Postoperative pneumonia

Postoperative signs of intestinal ileus

Repeated signs of colic during the initial hospitalization or after discharge from the hospital

Signs of colitis or diarrhea[3]

Peritonitis (secondary to intestinal necrosis or leakage of an enterotomy site and leakage of an anastomosis)[2]

Intra-abdominal hemorrhage[2]

Ultrasonographic evaluation of the surrounding soft tissue and the catheterized vein can be used to confirm thrombophlebitis and monitor the extend of the thrombophlebitis.[4] Lateral thoracic veins and cephalic veins appear to thrombose at a higher and faster rate compared to jugular veins. Lateral thoracic veins and cephalic veins catheters and their skin entry sites need to be protected by bandages. It is believed that the bandages increase the risk of venus stasis, which increases the risk of a potential thrombus formation. In a recent private practice review of cases that had multiple different vein catheterizations (jugular vein, cephalic vein, and lateral thoracic vein), it was determined that 65% of the cephalic veins and 85% of the lateral thoracic veins thrombosed.[5]

In a recent review of short term complications in horses undergoing colic surgery, 21 of 252 had evidence of jugular vein thrombosis.[6] In this case series, horses with signs of postoperative abdominal pain and horses that developed signs of postoperative shock had a significantly higher rate of jugular vein thrombosis.[6]

In another review of short term complications after colic surgery, 15 of 747 horses had evidence of varying degrees of jugular vein thrombosis.[7] Horses with signs of postoperative ileus appeared to have a higher rate of jugular vein thrombosis. In a separate review of each of the years in the 3-year study, horses in the third year appeared to have a higher rate of jugular vein thrombosis. In this case series, the single most effective way to prevent jugular vein thrombosis or to decrease the incidence of jugular vein thrombosis appeared to be that all horse handlers started to wear surgical gloves.

POSTOPERATIVE INCISIONAL COMPLICATIONS

In equine GI surgery, the abdominal closure is one of the most important components of the surgical procedure and can contribute to possible postoperative complications that could influence the overall outcome. Several different types of suture material and suture patterns for closure of the linea alba or sheath of the rectus muscle have been investigated.[8] One study suggested that closure of the linea alba with a simple continuous suture pattern is superior in bursting strength when compared to an inverted cruciate suture pattern.[9] Another study investigated biomechanical properties of the equine adult linea alba in regards to tissue bite size and type of suture material.[10]

The study concluded that the optimal tissue bite size in adult horses is 15 mm from the edge of the linea alba.[10]

Postoperative incisional complications include incisional swelling, local infection, suture sinus formation, hematoma formation, incisional drainage, incisional dehiscence, and hernia formation. Overall, incisional complications can develop in 40% of horses that have intestinal surgery,[11] with incisional drainage reported in 32% to 36% of horses, dehiscence in 3% to 5%, and hernia formation in 6% to 17%.[11-13] Another recently published study demonstrated that horses with incisional infections are 62.5 times more likely to develop an incisional hernia compared to horses without incisional problems.[14]

Many different factors associated with incisional complications have been identified and include the age of the horse, size (weight) of the horse, type of incision, type of suture material, method of closure, degree of surgical trauma, length of surgery, and possible difficulties associated with anesthetic recovery.[15-18] A more recent study by Mair and Smith found significant differences in rates of incisional complications in relation to total plasma protein concentration and gut sounds at admission, administration of intraperitoneal heparin, dissection of the linea alba prior to closure, and application of wound coverage (stent bandage or incise drape).[6]

Surgical site infections can be a substantial cause of morbidity in the post-surgical period in horses that have undergone an exploratory celiotomy. The financial implications associated with an extended period of hospitalization for treatment of ventral midline incisional problems and the use of a newly designed abdominal bandage[19] can significantly contribute to hospital charges.

The possible role of surgical sutures in the cause of surgical site infection has been researched extensively, because bacterial contamination of suture material within a surgical wound may increase the virulence of a surgical site infection.[20] The prevention and treatment of surgical site infections is one of the main surgical challenges, and antibacterial-coated suture material may play a role in the prevention of post-surgical infection. Zone of inhibition assays showed that antibacterial (triclosan) coated 2-0 polyglactin 910 sutures provide an antimicrobial effect sufficient to prevent in vitro colonization by *Staphylococcus aureus* and *Staphylococcus epidermis*.[21] Several other in vitro and in vivo studies have evaluated the efficacy of antibacterial coated suture material.[22]

A recently completed study in horses evaluated the clinical effect of antibacterial (triclosan) coated 2-0 polyglactin 910 suture material on the likelihood of incisional complications following ventral midline exploratory celiotomies in 100 horses with abdominal pain.[22] In this study, it was hypothesized that the antibacterial effect of triclosan may decrease the likelihood of incisional complications following ventral midline exploratory celiotomy.[22] The results of this study revealed that antibacterial (triclosan) coated 2-0 polyglactin 910 did not decrease the likelihood of incisional complications in this horse population.[22] Furthermore, there was a slight increased incidence of incisional edema when triclosan coated 2-0 polyglactin 910 was used.[22] Peri-incisional edema may affect local tissue oxygen tension at the incisional site and may result in delayed wound healing, suppression of local immune function and provide an optimal environment for bacterial growth.[22] Thus the clinical relevance and benefits of antibacterial suture material in equine ventral midline closure remains questionable and there may potentially be adverse effects when using triclosan coated suture material.[22]

Only one previously completed study evaluated the potential problem associated with intraoperative culturing of abdominal incisions during colic surgeries and postoperative incisional infections, and it did not find a significant association.[14] Another recently completed study[23] tried to evaluate the exact time frame when these abdominal incision infections are contracted and what type of bacteria (whether acquired from the horse or being nosocomial in origin) is responsible for postoperative incisional infections.[23] In this study, the surgical procedures had been classified as clean if no enterotomy was performed or clean-contaminated if an intestinal lumen was exposed. The results of this study indicate that pre-surgical and intra-surgical cultures rarely yielded any significant growth, indicating appropriate abdominal preparation and maintenance of aseptic technique during surgery.[23] However, infections tended to occur in horses that had significant bacterial growth after recovery and 24 hours after surgery.[23] The results of the study suggest that the period of time for acquiring infections occurs after abdominal closure.[23] This study indicates the need for the continuation of appropriate asepsis and protection of the surgical site in the immediate post-surgical period.[23] However, the duration of postoperative protection needed to significantly reduce surgical site infections is uncertain, but it seems prudent to maintain sterility in the area for the 24-hour period immediately after surgery. It appears that routine application of an antimicrobial incise drape is not sufficient in preventing contamination of the surgical site during recovery. A second study is currently underway, evaluating the use of a more aseptic incisional support during the recovery room period and postoperative period.[24] A previous study evaluated the use of a postoperative abdominal bandage and showed a decrease in incisional problems in the postoperative period.[25]

Once a horse has an incisional infection, treatment options for ventral midline and paramedian skin incision complications have been documented previously in literature.[8] As previously reported, horses with incisional drainage are much more likely to develop incisional hernias or to acutely disrupt all layers of the abdominal wall. In one study, the single most important risk factor for herniation was an incisional infection. An incisional infection increased the risk for future herniation by 17.8 times.[13] In another study, the risk of future incisional hernia formation increased by 62.5 times after having an incisional infection.[14]

If a postoperative incisional infection can not be prevented, it is imperative to avoid a future suture line hernia. A recently completed study evaluated the use of a newly designed postoperative hernia belt/abdominal bandage in horses with postoperative incisional complications (**Fig. 1**).[26] The results of this study compare favorably to the reported literature numbers. In this study, only 85 of 993 (8%) horses had evidence

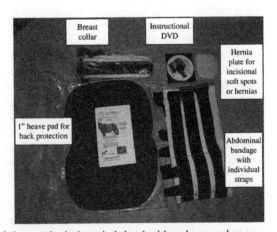

Fig. 1. Contents of the newly designed abdominal bandage package.

of incisional complications.[26] The hernia formation rate in this study was 6% of horses with incisional complications and 0.5% of all horses undergoing an exploratory celiotomy in the study period.[26] All horses were individually measured for a custom newly designed abdominal bandage, and three measurements are required for the newly designed abdominal bandage (**Fig. 2**).

The first measurement is around the girth, just caudal (5–10 cm caudal) to the withers. The second measurement is taken around the largest or widest part of the abdomen (it is recommended to add 2 inches to the measured length for a pad, and the pad should be at least 1 inch thick). The third measurement involves measuring the length of the abdominal incision.

The newly designed abdominal bandage allows for daily wound care and daily inspection of the abdominal incisions.[26] As a result of the edema reduction and the firm and even pressure on the healing ventral midline skin incision or healing paramedian skin incision, abdominal hernias can be prevented.[26] Overall, this study demonstrated that the use of the newly designed abdominal bandage reduced the length of time each horse with incisional drainage needed to be treated and that the incidence of incisional hernia formation, despite incisional drainage, is reduced to very low numbers compared to published literature reports.[1,2,26]

Dehiscence of the body wall, with or without exposure of the abdominal content, is the most serious wound complication after an exploratory celiotomy. Many different causes and factors have been described in the literature that lead to possible body wall failures. Once a body wall fails or any other secondary closure of the body wall is necessary, an abdominal wire repair is needed.[27] A horse with secondary abdominal wire repair should be wearing the newly designed abdominal bandage for daily wound care. In a previous study, one horse that acutely disrupted the body wall layers healed with small dimples along the ventral midline skin incision and very small dimples in the paramedian stab incisions for the wire placement.[26]

POSTOPERATIVE PNEUMONIA

Abdominal exploratory surgeries are performed as a potential life saving procedure. One of the most serious postoperative complications can be the development of postoperative pneumonia. There are several reports on horses with pleuropneumonia after shipping or exercise.[28] Only one case report describes the outcome of a thoroughbred

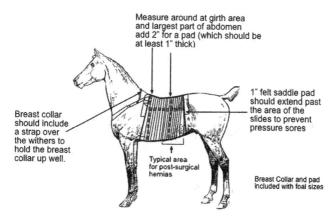

Fig. 2. How to measure for the newly designed abdominal bandage. (*Courtesy of* CM Equine Products, Norco, CA; with permission.)

racehorse who developed postoperative hematogenic pleuropneumonia and died.[29] In a recent short-term complication review of 300 horses undergoing colic surgery, none of the horses undergoing one celiotomy developed signs of postoperative pneumonia.[6] A second study evaluated short-term complications in a group of 747 horses undergoing exploratory celiotomies for signs of abdominal pain.[7] In this group, 4 of 747 horses developed postoperative hemorrhagic pneumonia.[7] Two of the horses had enteroliths removed during surgery, and the other two horses had small intestinal strangulation obstructions as their primary surgical lesions. All four horses had varying degrees of intra-operative naso-gastric reflux. Two of the horses developed postoperative signs of thrombophlebitis, and all four horses developed high fevers (103.5°–106°F) between 5–8 days postoperatively. In all four horses, a trans-tracheal wash was performed, and several resistant bacteria were identified. All four horses were treated with antimicrobials, and the two horses with enteroliths as the primary diagnosis survived to discharge from the hospital and are doing well. The two horses with small intestinal strangulation obstructions as their primary diagnosis were euthanized as a result of complications caused by the hemorrhagic pneumonia.

POSTOPERATIVE SIGNS OF ABDOMINAL PAIN

Abdominal exploratory surgeries for signs of colic are one of the most frequently performed emergency surgeries. The decision to performed surgery is based mainly on physical examination, abdominal ultrasonography findings, abdominal radiography findings, and ultimately response to pain medication. Most horses undergoing an emergency exploratory celiotomy do not show any further signs of abdominal pain after surgery. Signs of abdominal pain after surgery (lying down for an excessive time period, restlessness, flank watching, stretching out, kicking at the abdomen, pawing, and rolling) are all considered abnormal and not desirable. The origin of postoperative pain in horses can be multi factorial, and every effort should be made to determine the cause of postoperative abdominal pain. In a recent review by Mair and Smith,[6] 64 of 227 horses (28.2%) showed signs of abdominal pain after a single laparotomy. In another large case study by Klohnen,[7] 209 of 747 horses showed signs of postoperative abdominal pain. Most of the horses with signs of postoperative abdominal pain respond to medical therapy, especially if the cause of abdominal pain was attributed to postoperative ileus. One hundred ninety of the seven hundred forty seven horses were diagnosed with signs of postoperative ileus[7,35] and treated with intravenous lidocaine. A small percentage of horses will not respond to medical therapy and will require a second exploratory celiotomy.[1–3]

Mair and colleagues[1] summarized many different published studies on evidence based medicine in regards to the decision making process on when to pursue a second laparatomy. In one report, the decision to pursue a second laparatomy was made within 24 hours after the first surgery.[30] The primary reason for the repeat laparotomy was an initial surgical error. Typically, in a private practice setting, horses are taken back to surgery if medical therapy is unsuccessful.[7] Forty six of seven hundred forty seven horses required a second laparotomy, and none of the horses were taken back to surgery within the first 24 hours after the first surgery. There are many other reasons (besides signs of postoperative ileus) that may contribute to postoperative signs of colic.[3]

POSTOPERATIVE ILEUS

Postoperative ileus is an important cause of morbidity and mortality in the postsurgical period for horses with colic. The diagnosis has classically been made on the basis of postoperative reflux obtained through nasogastric intubation and possible postoperative signs of abdominal pain in conjunction with reflux. According to veterinary literature, postoperative ileus mainly has been defined by the volume of reflux that is recovered from a horse during a 24 hour period.[6,30–32] This is neither a definitive nor accurate method of diagnosing postoperative ileus.

Although the exact causes of postoperative ileus are not fully understood, it has been postulated that an imbalance of sympathetic and parasympathetic inputs to the GI tract results in a reduction in propulsive motility, contributing to or causing signs of ileus.[8] Abdominal ultrasonography is a proven diagnostic modality in the preoperative diagnosis of small intestinal lesions and is potentially a useful diagnostic imaging technique to assess distention, contractility, wall edema, and motility of small intestine postoperatively.[33,34]

In a recently completed study, postoperative intestinal ileus was defined by the presence of multiple (n >3) distended loops of small intestine with decreased intestinal contractility and motility.[35] It was the study hypothesis that routine ultrasonographic examination of the postsurgical abdomen would allow for a more definitive and accurate detection of decreased small intestinal motility, indicating a diagnosis of postoperative ileus. Furthermore, a comparison was made between signs of postoperative ileus observed with abdominal ultrasound and naso-gastric reflux.[35]

The results of the study demonstrate that abdominal ultrasound is a reliable method for the diagnosis and monitoring of postoperative signs of intestinal ileus and is potentially a more useful technique than the current analysis of gastric reflux volume.[35] In addition, the study demonstrated that both small intestinal and large intestinal lesions can contribute to postoperative ileus of the small intestine. Interestingly, 88% of the small intestinal ileus cases were associated with a strangulating obstruction,[35] supporting the view that ischemia and intestinal stress at surgery may contribute to intestinal ileus.[30] However, it is also interesting to note that 41% of postoperative ileus cases were diagnosed as having a primary large intestinal lesion.[35] The study further concluded that abdominal ultrasonography appeared to be more accurate in the detection and diagnosis of postoperative intestinal ileus compared to reflux obtained by way of a naso-gastric tube.[35]

POSTOPERATIVE ADHESIONS

Abdominal exploratory celiotomies for signs of acute or chronic colic episodes are one of the most common surgeries performed in equine practice. Postoperative adhesions are one of the possible postoperative complications that can be encountered. Most adhesions are formed in the early postoperative period (30 days after surgery).[36] The extent and exact location of the adhesions will determine if they are a clinical problem or will remain "silent."[36] Adhesions become a clinical problem when they form constrictive bands or when they either compress or anatomically distort the intestines.

Despite numerous research and clinical investigations, postoperative adhesions after exploratory celiotomies continue to present clinical complications and challenges to equine surgeons. In human abdominal surgery, the most common method used for adhesion prevention is the use of high molecular weight polymers and application of physical barriers to focal lesions to prevent adhesion formation between serosal surfaces.

The use of a high molecular weight hydrophilic polymer solution (sodium carboxymethylcellulose [SCMC]) has been shown to reduce the adhesion formation rate and severity of experimentally induced adhesions in ponies[37] and horses.[38] In a more recent clinical study, it was advocated that the use of SCMC improved survival in colic patients.[39]

It was the author's hypothesis in a recently completed study[36] that horses in which 1% SCMC was used intraoperatively would have a lower incidence of adhesion compared to horses without the use of SCMC. Once the initial SCMC results became available, two other groups of horses were evaluated (before and after the use of SCMC).[36] The results of this study[36] did not support the findings that had been previously outlined during the research studies.[37,38] Overall, 644 horses had an exploratory celiotomy over a 4-year period with an adhesion rate of 7.3%.[36]

To the best of the author's knowledge, the Chino Valley Equine Hospital postoperative adhesion rate prior to and after the use of SCMC was 3.6% and 3.8%, respectively.[36] These numbers are in contrast to a confirmed adhesion rate during the use of SCMC that had increased to 24.6%.[36] After careful evaluation of all three study groups, it was determined that no other variables had changed besides the use of the SCMC.[36] The overall results of this study[36] were surprising, and further investigations are underway to determine why the horses in the SCMC group had a higher adhesion rate compared to the non SCMC group of horses. Currently, the use of 1% SCMC is not recommended in clinical cases.[36]

SUMMARY

This article summarizes several new aspects of postoperative complications in horses after abdominal surgery. A more extensive review may be found in the articles by Mair and colleagues,[1] Dutki and White,[2] and Hackett and Hassel.[3]

REFERENCES

1. Mair TS, Smith LJ, Sherlock CE. Evidence-based gastrointestinal surgery in horses. Vet Clin North Am Equine Pract 2007;23:267–92.
2. Dukti S, White N. Surgical complications of colic surgery. Vet Clin North Am Vet Equine Pract 2008;24:513–34.
3. Hackett ES, Hassel DM. Colic: nonsurgical complications. Vet Clin North Am Equine Pract 2008;24:535–55.
4. Gardner SY, Reef VB, Spender PA. Ultrasonographic evaluation of horses with thrombophlebitis of the jugular vein: 46 cases (1985–1988). Jam Vet Med Assoc 1991;199(3):370–3.
5. Klohnen A. Private practice case review of vein thrombosis. J Am Vet Med Assoc, submitted for publication.
6. Mair TS, Smith LJ. Survival and complication rates in 300 horses undergoing surgical treatment of colic: short-term complications. EVJ 2005;37(4):303–9.
7. Klohnen A. A 3 year review of horses undergoing exploratory celiotomies for acute and chronic signs of abdominal pain: short term survival rates and short term complication rates in 747 horses. Vet Surg, submitted for publication.
8. Hardy J, Rakestraw PC. Postoperative care and complications associated with abdominal surgery. In: Auer JA, Stick JA, editors. Equine surgery. 3rd edition. St. Louis (MO): Saunders Elsevier; 2006. p. 506–9.
9. Magee AA, Galupo LD. Comparison of incisional bursting strength of simple continuous and inverted cruciate patterns in the equine linea alba. Vet Surg 1999;28:442–7.
10. Trostle SS, Wilson DG, Stone WC, et al. A study of the biomechanical properties of the adult equine linea alba: relationship of tissue bite size and suture material to breaking strength. Vet Surg 1994;23:435–41.

11. Wilson DA, Baker GJ, Boero MJ. Complications of celiotomy incisions in horses. Vet Surg 1995;24:506–14.
12. Kobluk CN, Ducharme NG, Lumsden JH, et al. Factors affecting incisional complications rates associated with colic surgery in horses: 78 cases (1983–1985). J Am Vet Med Assoc 1989;195:639–42.
13. Gibson KT, Curtis CR, Turner AS, et al. Incisional hernias in the horse. Incidence and predisposing factors. Vet Surg 1989;18:360–6.
14. Ingle-Fehr JE, Baxter GM, Howard RD, et al. Bacterial culturing of ventral median celiotomies for prediction of postoperative incisional complications in horses. Vet Surg 1997;26:7–13.
15. Honnas CM, Cohen ND. Risk factors for wound infection following celiotomies in horses. J Am Vet Med Asoc 1997;210:78–81.
16. Galuppo LD, Pasco JR, Jang SS, et al. Evaluation of iodophor skin preparation techniques and factors influencing drainage from ventral midline incisions in horses. J Am Vet Med Asoc 1999;215:963–9.
17. Stone WC, Lindsay WA, Mason DA, et al. Factors associated with acute wound dehiscence following equine abdominal surgery. Proceedings of the Fourth Equine Colic Research Symposium 1991(52).
18. French NP, Smith J, Edwards GB, et al. Equine surgical colic: risk factors for postoperative complications. Equine Vet J 2002;34:444–9.
19. Klohnen A, Lores M. Management of post-operative abdominal incisional complications with a hernia belt: 85 horses (2001–2005). American College of Veterinary Surgeons Symposium. Chicago (IL), 2007.
20. Edmiston CE, Seabrook GR, Goheen MP, et al. Bacterial adherence to surgical sutures: can antibacterial-coated sutures reduce the risk of microbial contamination? J Am Coll Surg 2006;203:481–9.
21. Rothenburger S, Spangler D, Bhende S, et al. In vitro antimicrobial evaluation of Coated VICRYL* Plus Antibacterial Suture (coated polyglactin 910 with triclosan) using zone of inhibition assays. Surg Infect (Larchmt) 2002;3(Suppl 1):S79–87.
22. Klohnen A, Brauer T, Bischofberger A, et al. Incisional complications following exploratory celiotomies: does antimicrobial (triclosan) coated suture material decrease the likelihood of incisional infection? Presented at the 17th Annual Scientific Meeting, European College of Veterinary Surgeons. Basel, 2008.
23. Klohnen A, Biedrzycki A. A new approach to the detection of incisional site infections after colic surgeries. Vet Surg, submitted for publication.
24. Klohnen A. Comparison of post-operative incisional infection rate in horses undergoing exploratory celiotomies being protected by either an loban bandage or an extensive abdominal bandage in the recovery room. Vet Surg, submitted for publication.
25. Smith LJ, Mellor DJ, Marr CM, et al. Incisional complications following exploratory celiotomy: does an abdominal bandage reduce the risk? Equine Vet J 2007;39:277–83.
26. Klohnen A, Lores M. Management of post-operative abdominal incisional complications with a newly designed abdominal hernia belt: 85 horses (2001–2005). Presented at the 17th Annual Scientific Meeting, European College of Veterinary Surgeons. Basel, 2008.
27. Tulleners EP, Donawick WJ. Secondary closure of infected abdominal incisions in cattle and horses. J Am Vet Med Assoc 1983;182:1377–9.
28. Mair TS, Lane JG. Pneumonia, lung abscesses and pleuritis in adult horses: a review of 51 cases. Equine Vet J 1989;21:175–80.

29. Seung-ho R, Joon-gyu K, Ung-bok B. A hematogenic pleuropneumonia caused by postoperative septic thrombophlebitis in a thoroughbred gelding. J Vet Sci 2004;5:75–7.

30. Freeman DE, Hammock P, Baker P, et al. Short- and long-term survival and prevalence of postoperative ileus after small intestinal surgery in the horse. Equine Vet Suppl 2000;32:42–51.

31. Merritt AM, Blickslager AT. Post-operative ileus: to be or not to be? Equine Vet J 2008;40:295–6.

32. Freeman DE. Postoperative ileus (POI): another perspective. Equine Vet J 2008; 40:297–8.

33. Klohnen A, Vachon A, Fischer AT. Use of diagnostic ultrasound in horses with signs of acute abdominal pain. J Am Vet Med Assoc 1996;209:1597–601.

34. Klohnen A. Abdominal ultrasonography in the equine colic patient: a validation of the technique. Presented at the 17th Annual Scientific Meeting, European College of Veterinary Surgeons. Basel, 2008.

35. Klohnen A, Biedrzycki A. Detection of postoperative ileus with the help of abdominal ultrasound in horses after colic surgery. Equine Vet J, submitted for publication.

36. Klohnen A, Rafetto J. Bischofberger A, et al. Adhesion formation rate after exploratory celiotomies in horses with and without intra-abdominal use sodium carboxymethylcellulose: a 4 year study. Presented at the American College of Veterinary Surgeons Symposium. San Diego, CA, 2008.

37. Moll H, Schumacher J, Wright J, et al. Evaluation of sodium carboxymethylcellulose for prevention of experimentally induced abdominal adhesions in ponies. Am J Vet Res 1991;52:88–91.

38. Hay WP, Mueller PO, Harmon BG, et al. Once percent carboxymethylcellulose prevents experimentally induced adhesions in horses. Vet Surg 2001;30:223–7.

39. Fogle CA, Mathew PG, Yvonne AE, et al. Analysis of sodium carboxymethylcellulose administration and related factors associated with postoperative colic and survival in horses with small intestinal disease. Vet Surg 2008;37:558–63.

Postoperative Ileus: Pathogenesis and Treatment

Thomas J. Doherty, MVB, MSc

KEYWORDS

• Ileus • Horse • Endotoxemia • Macrophages • Prokinetics

Ileus, a disruption of normal gastrointestinal motor activity, is a common complication after abdominal surgery. Gastrointestinal recovery is faster after laparoscopic procedures in human beings, and this is primarily because of the decreased intestinal manipulation.[1] The stomach and colon are the portions of the gastrointestinal tract most severely affected by postoperative ileus (POI) in horses.[2] The incidence of POI in horses may be as high as 20%, and the mortality rate may reach 40%.[3–5] A disruption in coordination of gastrointestinal myoelectrical activity has been seen in the early postoperative period in the horse.[2,6] Postoperative ileus in horses is often complicated by endotoxemia.[7]

CAUSES OF ILEUS

A number of causes of POI have been proposed and include anesthesia, activation of inhibitory spinal and sympathetic reflexes, humoral agents, and inflammation.[8] Anesthesia, per se, has minimal effects on transit of ingesta in rats[9] and on myoelectrical activity in horses;[10] however, opioids contribute to POI in human patients.[11]

A 5-cm skin incision, whether over the abdomen or back, had no effect on intestinal transit in rats; in contrast, a 5-cm incision into the abdominal fascia and muscle or into the abdominal cavity delayed transit.[12] A 5-cm laparotomy caused a significantly greater delay in transit than did a 1-cm laparotomy, regardless of whether the intestines were handled.[12] This inhibitory effect of the abdominal incision on intestinal motility appears to be mediated by a sympathetic reflex and alpha$_2$ receptors, because it was blocked by either guanethidine or yohimbine.[12] Laparotomy alone, under general anesthesia, had minimal effects on intestinal motility in mice, and eventration and light manipulation of intestine, using cotton-tipped applicators, did not significantly increase transit time.[12] In contrast, laparotomy combined with standard intestinal manipulation significantly delayed transit.[13] Postoperative ileus has an early or acute phase and a late phase.

Department of Large Animal Clinical Sciences, The University of Tennessee College of Veterinary Medicine, 2407 River Drive, Knoxville, TN 37996, USA
E-mail address: tdoherty@utk.edu

Vet Clin Equine 25 (2009) 351–362
doi:10.1016/j.cveq.2009.04.011
0749-0739/09/$ – see front matter © 2009 Elsevier Inc. All rights reserved.

Acute Phase

Activation of mechanoreceptors or nociceptors, stimulates afferent nerve fibers, which in turn activate spinal and supraspinal reflexes that inhibit motility.[14] This response can be inhibited by removing the coeliaco-mesenteric plexus, indicating the involvement of a peripheral reflex.[15] The role of a neural mechanism is verified by the fact that the effect of intestinal manipulation on transit in the rat was significantly blocked by the nonspecific adrenergic blocker, guanethidine, and the alpha$_2$ adrenergic antagonist yohimbine, administered 3 hours after surgery.[16]

Late Phase

Researchers have sought a peripheral mechanism to explain the late phase of POI because the acute phase should not be expected to persist after cessation of stimulation. Much research has been directed at characterizing a population of resident macrophages in the intestinal muscularis. These macrophages are inactive under normal conditions;[17] however, the use of lymphocyte function-associated antigen-1 (LFA-1), which is expressed on the surface of leukocytes and mediates cell adhesion as a cellular activation marker, has shown that resident macrophages become activated by surgical manipulation.[18]

Intestinal manipulation releases lipid mediators and degradation products of the extracellular matrix that activate macrophages in the muscularis, and initiate an inflammatory response.[19] This results in the induction of a variety of cytokines, nitric oxide (NÖ), and prostaglandins (PGs). Up-regulation occurs in the expression of adhesion molecules (ICAM-1), tumor necrosis factor-alpha (TNFα) and interleukins 1 (IL-1) and 6 (IL-6) in the vascular epithelium of the muscularis, causing infiltration of circulating leukocytes.[20] Infiltrating leukocytes release additional mediators such as NÖ and prostanoids, and together these events lead to intestinal inflammation, which inhibits intestinal smooth muscle contractility, leading to POI.[16,20] The inflammatory component can be reduced significantly by cyclooxygenase-2 (COX-2) inhibitors.[21] Changes indicative of macrophage activation occur by 3 hours after intestinal manipulation in human patients, as evidenced by increased mRNA encoding for IL-6, COX-2, and inducible nitric oxide synthase (iNOS).[22]

By the first postoperative day, polymorphonuclear neutrophils (PMN), monocytes, mast cells, and T cells have extravasated into the intestinal muscularis in rodents.[18] Cell numbers increase significantly by 24 hours postoperatively, and, although the cell count decreases by day 7, it is still significantly increased over baseline values.[18] There is a strong correlation between the intensity of intestinal manipulation and the magnitude of intestinal infiltration, and the degree of inhibition of circular muscle contractility is strongly correlated with the magnitude of intestinal infiltration.[23]

It is reasonable to suspect that POI results from a similar mechanism in the horse, and NÖ appears to mediate an inhibitory role in the circular muscle of the equine ventral colon and jejunum.[24,25] Postoperative intestinal leukocyte count increased in horses after intestinal ischemia;[26] however, there appears to be no information on the effects of intestinal manipulation on leukocyte infiltration in nonischemic intestines.

POSTOPERATIVE PANENTERIC INFLAMMATORY EFFECT

The development of motor dysfunction in parts of the gastrointestinal tract not directly involved in surgical manipulation has been described in rats.[27] This panenteric response is associated with up-regulation of pro-inflammatory mediators.[27]

A significant impairment of small intestine transit has been shown in a rat model of colonic manipulation;[28] and transit impairment even occurred when the small intestinal was surgically isolated, by means of an ileal loop ileostomy, to eliminate the possibility of a downstream barrier to flow.[29] Colonic manipulation induces an inflammatory response in the muscularis of the small intestine that is initiated and maintained by the release of lipopolysaccharide (LPS) from the colon.[29] The role of LPS in the inflammatory response is verified by the fact that when the intestinal flora is eliminated by pretreatment with oral polymyxin and neomycin, small intestinal dysfunction is prevented. Also, intestinal function is largely unaffected after colonic manipulation in Toll-like receptor 4–deficient mice, which do not respond to LPS.[29] Small intestinal dysfunction is significantly blocked by the administration of COX-2 and iNOS inhibitors, indicating that prostaglandins and NÖ have a role in panenteric dysfunction of smooth muscle.[29]

NEURAL MECHANISMS OF ILEUS

Neural mechanisms of particular importance in ileus are the inhibitory adrenergic and somatosensory pathways and sensitization of primary afferent neurons.[30]

Adrenoreceptors

Alpha$_2$ adrenoreceptors in the intestine modulate the release of acetylcholine and have an important role in POI and LPS-induced ileus.[30,31] Guanethidine and yohimbine ameliorated delayed gastric emptying and colonic transit induced by small intestinal manipulation, indicating an inhibitory role for the sympathetic system on manipulated intestine.[30] Alpha$_2$ receptor stimulation of the inflamed postoperative intestinal muscularis has a significant role in aggravating POI.[32] Stimulation of alpha$_2$ receptors on intestinal macrophages increases expression of iNOS mRNA, which potentiates release of NÖ.[32] Yohimbine decreases expression of iNOS in LPS-treated mice.[33]

Inflammatory-Mediated Neuronal Modulation

Inflammation or distention of the gastrointestinal tract sensitizes polymodal sensory fibers,[34] and intestinal activation results in a prolonged activation of primary afferent neurons.[31] COX-2 expression causes an increase in the nuclear phosphorylation product Fos, which is used to map functional excitatory pathways in the central nervous system.[21] An increase in expression of Fos has been demonstrated within the spinal cord of rats 24 hours after intestinal manipulation, indicating ongoing neuronal activation, as spinal expression of Fos peaks 2 hours after stimulation.[35]

Prostaglandins (PGs) play a major role in POI in rodents, with PGE$_2$ having an inhibitory effect on intestinal motility and a sensitizing effect on intestinal primary afferent nerves.[36] Thus, PGs appear to be a critical link between inflammation and neuronal activation. Intravenous infusion of PGE$_1$ suppressed myoelectrical activity in the stomach and small and large colon and contractile force of the left dorsal colon and small intestinal in horses.[37]

PATHOGENESIS OF LIPOPOLYSACCHARIDE-INDUCED ILEUS

Endotoxemia and bacteremia occur in human patients after manual decompression of the intestine,[38] and endotoxemia occurs commonly in horses with colic.[7] In one study, LPS inhibited gastric and colonic activity in ponies.[39] In horses, LPS reduced cecal blood flow and the frequency of colonic and cecal contractions, and these changes were ameliorated by yohimbine.[40] Yohimbine blocked the inhibitory effect of LPS on liquid-phase gastric emptying in horses.[41]

A systemic LPS challenge induces iNOS mRNA and COX-2 synthase within the intestinal muscularis in rats.[42] It is suggested that LPS-induced activation of macrophages is caused by lipid mediators and degradation products of the extracellular matrix in a manner similar to manipulation-induced activation. Activation of Toll-like receptors, which are expressed on macrophages, is responsible for initiating the inflammatory cascade.[43] This activation is verified by the inability of LPS to affect smooth muscle contractility in TLR4 knockout mice.[44] In rats, intraperitoneal administration of LPS induced a 21-fold increase in staining for LFA-1 in the intestinal muscularis 1 hour after administration, and this is accompanied by a significant infiltration of neutrophils, mast cells, and monocytes.[45]

OPIOIDS AND ILEUS

Data on the effects of morphine on intestinal motility in horses are conflicting. In a study of horses undergoing nonabdominal surgeries, 3 of 51 horses had postoperative colic after a single dose of morphine, yet this incidence did not differ significantly from the group not receiving morphine, in which 2 of 33 horses had colic.[46] Horses undergoing orthopedic procedures had a fourfold risk of the development of postoperative colic if given morphine;[47] however, no association was found between morphine administration and the incidence of colic in horses undergoing magnetic resonance imaging or nonabdominal surgery.[48] Prolonged administration of morphine to awake, healthy horses delayed gastric emptying and prolonged intestinal transit, but these effects were ameliorated by the peripheral opioid antagonist, N-methyl naltrexone (NMN).[49] Conversely, NMN failed to influence POI in a surgical model of intestinal manipulation in rodents.[13]

HYPOCALCEMIA AND ILEUS

Many horses undergoing emergency abdominal surgery have either a low ionized blood calcium concentration at presentation, or hypocalcemia develops over time.[50,51] Moreover, low serum ionized calcium has been reported in horses with ileus.[52] The tendency to develop hypocalcemia is greater with a small intestinal lesion, gastroduodenitis, or endotoxemia, and the probability of ileus developing is high for horses with low plasma ionized calcium.[50] The severity of the illness is the most important prognosticator of the ionized calcium status.[50]

EFFECTS OF PERIOPERATIVE FLUID AND SALT ADMINISTRATION ON ILEUS

Gastric emptying was delayed when hypoalbuminemia was induced experimentally in dogs, and the delay in transit was attributed to edema of the gastric wall.[53] In rats, experimental induction of intestinal edema delayed intestinal transit.[54] The increase in transit time was caused by increased expression of iNOS in the intestine, because pretreatment with a selective iNOS inhibitor decreased iNOS expression without affecting the degree of edema.[54] In human subjects, traditional fluid therapy caused a greater delay in recovery of gastrointestinal function than did a restricted intake of fluid and salt.[55]

Effects of Hypertonic Saline

Hypertonic saline (HTS) exerts beneficial immunomodulatory effects by modulating pro- and anti-inflammatory molecules. In an intestinal ischemia model in rats, a decrease in activation of TNFα and nuclear factor kappa B (NF-κB) after HTS occurred independently of an increase in the anti-inflammatory cytokine IL-10.[56] Also, HTS decreased ICAM-1 expression in a hepatic ischemic–reperfusion model in rats[57] and decreased the expression of iNOS in an intestinal ischemic model.[58]

The use of HTS to treat POI in human patients was described in 1926.[59] In three patients with POI, 60 to 70 mL of 20% or 30% NaCl administered intravenously over 2 minutes was followed quickly by the passage of flatus and ultimate resolution of ileus.

Effects of Hetastarch

Hetastarch down-regulates proinflammatory mediators in endotoxemic rats.[60] Hetastarch decreased expression of adhesion molecule and neutrophil adhesion in endothelial cells from human subjects by direct inhibition of integrin-mediated interactions.[61]

DECREASING SEVERITY OF ILEUS

Dysfunction of intestinal smooth muscle in POI is multifactorial. Prostaglandin production via COX-2 has an important role, as has cytokine production. The adrenergic proinflammatory pathway, consisting of alpha$_2$ up-regulation of NÖ production in recruited monocytes and intestinal resident macrophages, intensifies the inflammatory response. There are a number of strategies that should be considered to reduce the severity of POI.

Pretreat with Nonsteroidal Anti-Inflammatory Drugs

The inflammatory component of POI can be significantly reduced by COX-2 inhibitors.[21] Pretreating rats with ketorolac prevented a decrease in intestinal transit after intestinal manipulation.[62] Phenylbutazone prevented an LPS-induced delay in gastric emptying of liquids in horses,[63] and phenylbutazone or flunixin meglumine improved intestinal myoelectrical activity in LPS-treated horses.[64]

Minimize Size of Abdominal Incision

The laparotomy incision should be as small as possible because long incisions adversely affect intestinal transit.[12]

Minimize Intestinal Manipulation

Because the degree of inhibition of circular muscle contractility is related directly to the magnitude of leukocyte infiltration, which in turn depends on the intensity of intestinal manipulation, every effort should be made to reduce intestinal trauma.[23]

Minimize Intestinal Edema

Edema inhibits transit by increasing the expression of iNOS and subsequent formation of the inhibitory neurotransmitter NÖ.[54] Formation of intestinal edema can be decreased by judicious use of crystalloid solutions and by maintaining plasma oncotic values close to normal. Treatment with HTS should be considered for its anti-inflammatory effects, as should hetastarch because of its oncotic and anti-inflammatory effects.

Intraoperative Use of Intravenous Lidocaine

The antinociceptive,[65] antihyperalgesic,[66] and anti-inflammatory[67] effects of lidocaine justify its use intraoperatively. Intraoperative lidocaine decreased the duration of POI in human patients.[65,68] Administration of lidocaine (0.025 mg/kg/min) intraoperatively to horses undergoing abdominal surgery, followed by an infusion (0.05 mg/kg/min) for 24 hours after surgery, caused a decrease in jejunal diameter and cross-sectional area compared with the control group, and the investigators interpreted this decrease to be caused by an increase in jejunal contractility.[69]

Decrease the Effects of Endotoxemia

Pretreatment with an NSAID will reduce LPS-induced PG formation. Polymyxin B ameliorates the effects of LPS administration to horses.[70] Yohimbine reduces the expression of iNOS in LPS-treated rats and improves intestinal transit.[31]

Treat for Hypocalcemia

Treatment of horses for hypocalcemia was associated with a higher probability of survival.[52]

Prophylactic Use of Alpha₂ Antagonists

Because of the efficacy of alpha₂ antagonists in modulating iNOS expression, prophylactic use of drugs, such as yohimbine, might be considered after the horse recovers from anesthesia.[31] In addition, yohimbine was partially effective in preventing POI in a surgical model in ponies.[2]

PROKINETIC DRUGS

Lidocaine and erythromycin are the most commonly used prokinetics,[71] but the evidence to support the use of either drug for treating POI is lacking. It is also important to realize that most studies of prokinetics have been performed on normal horses, and the results may not apply to horses with POI. This statement is supported by the fact that the contractile response of intestinal smooth muscle to bethanechol is significantly impaired in POI.[45]

Lidocaine

The evidence of a prokinetic effect for lidocaine in the postoperative period is weak, but the evidence supports the use of intraoperative lidocaine to prevent POI. Lidocaine administration to horses after laparotomy failed to restore myoelectrical activity of the jejunum.[72] Nevertheless, lidocaine treatment resulted in shorter hospitalization time in horses with POI or enteritis.[73] Horses should benefit from a lidocaine infusion in the postoperative period because of its anti-inflammatory and antinociceptive actions.

Alpha₂ Antagonists

Alpha₂ antagonists improved POI in rats,[30,31] human beings,[74] and horses,[2] and LPS-induced ileus in mice,[33] rats,[9] and horses.[41] Yohimbine down-regulated the production of iNOS and attenuated the effect of intestinal manipulation and LPS on transit and intestinal smooth muscle contraction.[31,33] Atipamezole, administered postoperatively, improved transit after laparotomy in rats.[75]

In ponies, yohimbine (150 μg/kg intravenous [IV]), when administered before induction of anesthesia and at 3-hour intervals postoperatively, was partially effective in ameliorating POI in a surgical model.[2] Co-administration of metoclopramide improved its effect; however, that study used only three ponies per treatment group.[2] In horses, yohimbine (75 μg/kg IV over 30 minutes) ameliorated the effects of LPS on contractility of the cecum and colon and improved cecal blood flow.[40] Yohimbine (250 μg/kg over 30 minutes) blocked the LPS-induced delay in gastric emptying in horses.[41]

Administration of yohimbine (150–250 μg/kg) as a slow infusion in the early postoperative period is warranted based on the experimental evidence. Alpha₂ antagonists should be administered as a slow infusion to avoid adverse effects, such as excitement and tachycardia.

Drugs Acting as 5-Hydroxytryptamine Receptors

Prokinetics in this class include metoclopramide, cisapride, and tegaserod. Cisapride is no longer available in North America.

Metoclopramide

Metoclopramide is considered to be ineffective in promoting peristalsis in the colon.[76] Nevertheless, metoclopramide decreased transit time of plastic spheres in an intestinal manipulation model of equine POI[2]; however, the study involved only three ponies and used relatively high doses of metoclopramide, which resulted in behavioral effects.[2] In horses, a continuous infusion of metoclopramide (0.04/mg/kg/h) decreased the duration of ileus after small intestinal resection compared with intermittent treatment or no treatment.[77] Pretreatment with metoclopramide (0.15 mg/kg over 30 minutes) was partially effective in resolving LPS-induced gastric stasis in horses.[78] The clinical use of metoclopramide is limited by its ability to induce behavioral effects and its apparent lack of effect on large intestine.

Tegaserod

Tegaserod, a selective agonist at 5-HT$_4$ receptors, decreased transit time in normal horses, but there is no information concerning its effects in horses with POI.[79]

Erythromycin

Erythromycin lactobionate, a macrolide antibiotic with activity at motilin receptors, is most commonly used as a prokinetic for prevention and treatment of cecal impactions.[71] In healthy horses, erythromycin significantly increased myoelectrical activity in the cecum and right ventral colon and increased the rate of cecal[80] and gastric emptying.[81] Erythromycin induced significant increases in myoelectrical activity in the ileum and pelvic flexure, but not in the cecum, during the immediate postoperative period.[6] Overall, these findings do not support the use of erythromycin as a prokinetic in horses with POI.

Parasympathomimetic Drugs

Neostigmine and bethanechol increase availability of acetylcholine at muscarinic receptors. Bethanecol is no longer available for clinical use in North America. Neostigmine increased myoelectrical activity in the ileum, cecum, and right ventral colon and increased the rate of cecal emptying in healthy horses;[82] however, it delayed gastric emptying in another study.[83] Neostigmine does not appear to have been evaluated in horses with POI.

SUMMARY

Drugs used in the postoperative period appear to be ineffective as prokinetics in horses with POI; therefore, efforts should be directed at ameliorating POI by using the least traumatic surgical techniques, administration of NSAIDs, administration of polymyxin B to horses with endotoxemia, and judicious selection and use of intravenous fluids. Administering lidocaine intraoperatively seems warranted based on evidence from human studies. There is strong evidence for the efficacy of alpha$_2$ antagonists, such as yohimbine, to prevent NÖ release. Concurrent administration of metoclopramide may improve the efficacy of yohimbine.

REFERENCES

1. Piskun G, Kozik D, Rajpal S, et al. Comparison of laparoscopic, open, and converted appendectomy for perforated appendicitis. Surg Endosc 2001;15:660–2.
2. Gerring EL, Hunt JM. Pathophysiology of equine postoperative ileus: effect of adrenergic blockade, parasympathetic stimulation and metoclopramide in an experimental model. Equine Vet J 1986;18:249–55.
3. Cohen ND, Lester GD, Sanchez LC, et al. Evaluation of risk factors associated with development of postoperative ileus in horses. J Am Vet Med Assoc 2004; 225:1070–8.
4. Blikslager AT, Bowman KF, Levine JF, et al. Evaluation of factors associated with postoperative ileus in horses: 31cases (1990–1992). J Am Vet Med Assoc 1994; 205:1748–52.
5. Morton AJ, Blikslager AT. Surgical and postoperative factors influencing short-term survival of horses following small intestinal resection: 92 cases (1994–2001). Equine Vet J 2002;34:450–4.
6. Roussel AJ, Hooper RN, Cohen ND, et al. Prokinetic effects of erythromycin on the ileum, cecum, and pelvic flexure of horses during the postoperative period. Am J Vet Res 2000;61:420–4.
7. King JN, Gerring EL. Detection of endotoxin in cases of equine colic. Vet Rec 1988;123:269–71.
8. Livingston EH, Passaro EP. Postoperative ileus. Dig Dis Sci 1990;35:121–32.
9. Fukuda H, Tsuchida D, Koda K, et al. Inhibition of sympathetic pathways restores postoperative ileus in the upper and lower gastrointestinal tract. J Gastroenterol Hepatol 2007;22:1293–9.
10. Lester GD, Bolton JR, Cullen LK, et al. Effects of general anesthesia on myoelectric activity of the intestine in horses. Am J Vet Res 1992;53(9):1553–7.
11. Kurz A, Sessler DI. Opioid-induced bowel dysfunction: pathophysiology and potential new therapies. Drugs 2003;63:649–71.
12. Uemura K, Tatewaki M, Harris MB, et al. Magnitude of abdominal incision affects the duration of postoperative ileus in rats. Surg Endosc 2004;18(4):606–10.
13. Schmidt J, Stoffels B, Nazir A, et al. Alvimopan and COX-2 inhibition reverse opioid and inflammatory components of postoperative ileus. Neurogastroenterol Motil 2008;20:689–99.
14. De Winter BY, Boeckxstaens GE, De Man JG, et al. Effect of adrenergic and nitrergic blockade on experimental ileus in rats. Br J Pharmacol 1997;120:464–8.
15. Cannon WB, Murphy FT. Physiologic observations on experimentally induced ileus. J Am Med Assoc 1907;49:840–3.
16. deJonge WJ, van den Wijngaard RM, The FO, et al. Postoperative ileus is maintained by intestinal immune infiltrates that activate inhibitory neural pathways in mice. Gastroenterology 2003;125(4):1137–47.
17. Kalff JC, Schwarz NT, Walgenbach KJ, et al. Leukocytes of the intestinal muscularis externa: their phenotype and isolation. J Leukoc Biol 1998;63:683–91.
18. Kalff JC, Schraut WH, Simmons RL, et al. Surgical manipulation of the gut elicits an intestinal muscularis inflammatory response resulting in postsurgical ileus. Ann Surg 1998;228(5):652–63.
19. Bauer AJ. Mentation on the immunological modulation of gastrointestinal motility. Ann Surg 2008;228(5):652–63.
20. Kalff JC, Carlos TM, Schraut WH, et al. Surgically induced leukocytic infiltrates within the rat intestinal muscularis mediate postoperative ileus. Gastroenterology 1999;117:378–87.

21. Kreiss C, Birder LA, Kiss S, et al. COX-2 dependent inflammation increases spinal Fos expression during rodent postoperative ileus. Gut 2003;52(4):527–34.
22. Kalff JC, Türler A, Schwarz NT, et al. Intra-abdominal activation of a local inflammatory response within the human muscularis externa during laparotomy. Ann Surg 2003;237(3):301–15.
23. The FO, Bennink RJ, Ankum WM, et al. Intestinal handling-induced mast cell activation and inflammation in human postoperative ileus. Gut 2008;57(1):33–40.
24. Van Hoogmoed LM, Rakestraw PC, Snyder JR, et al. Evaluation of nitric oxide as an inhibitory neurotransmitter in the equine ventral colon. Am J Vet Res 2000; 61(1):64–8.
25. Rakestraw PC, Snyder JR, Woliner MJ, et al. Involvement of nitric oxide in inhibitory neuromuscular transmission in equine jejunum. Am J Vet Res 1996;57: 1206–13.
26. Little D, Tomlinson JE, Blikslager AT. Post operative neutrophilic inflammation in equine small intestine after manipulation and ischaemia. Equine Vet J 2005; 37(4):329–35.
27. Schwarz NT, Kalff JC, Türler A, et al. Selective jejunal manipulation causes postoperative pan-enteric inflammation and dysmotility. Gastroenterology 2004;126: 159–69.
28. Türler A, Moore BA, Pezzone MA, et al. Colonic postoperative inflammatory ileus in the rat. Ann Surg 2002;236:56–66.
29. Türler A, Schnurr C, Nakao A, et al. Endogenous endotoxin participates in causing a panenteric inflammatory ileus after colonic surgery. Ann Surg 2007; 245(5):737–44.
30. Sagrada A, Fargeas MJ, Bueno L. Involvement of 1 and 2 adrenoceptors in the postlaparotomy intestinal motor disturbances in the rat. Gut 1987;28:955–9.
31. Kreiss C, Toegel S, Bauer AJ. α_2-Adrenergic regulation of NO production alters postoperative intestinal smooth muscle dysfunction in rodents. Am J Physiol Gastrointest Liver Physiol 2004;287:G658–66.
32. Shen HM, Sha LX, Kennedy JL, et al. Adrenergic receptors regulate macrophage secretion. Int J Immunopharmacol 1994;16:905–10.
33. Hamano N, Inada T, Iwata R, et al. The a2-adrenergic receptor antagonist yohimbine improves endotoxin-induced inhibition of gastrointestinal motility in mice. Br J Anaesth 2007;98(4):484–90.
34. Traub RJ, Herdegen T, Gebhart GF. Differential expression of Fos and c-jun in two regions of the rat spinal cord following noxious colorectal distention. Neurosci Lett 1993;160:121–5.
35. Birder LA, de Groat WC. Increased Fos expression in spinal neurons after irritation of the lower urinary tract in the rat. J Neurosci 1992;12:4879–89.
36. Schwarz NT, Kalff JC, Turler A, et al. Prostanoid production via COX-2 as a causative mechanism of rodent postoperative ileus. Gastroenterology 2001;121: 1354–71.
37. Hunt JM, Gerring EL. The effect of prostaglandin E1 on motility of the equine gut. J Vet Pharmacol Ther 1985;8(2):165–73.
38. Zühlke HV, Lorenz EP, Harnoss BM, et al. Endotoxinemia and bacteremia in manual oral decompression of ileus. Chirurgia 1988;59:349–56.
39. King JN, Gerring EL. The action of low dose endotoxin on equine bowel motility. Equine Vet J 1991;23(1):3–4.
40. Eades SC, Moore JN. Blockade of endotoxin-induced cecal hypoperfusion and ileus with an α_2 antagonist in horses. Am J Vet Res 1993;54(4):586–90.

41. Meisler SD, Doherty TJ, Andrews FM, et al. Yohimbine ameliorates the effects of endotoxin on gastric emptying of the liquid marker acetaminophen in horses. Can J Vet Res 2000;64:208–11.
42. Eskandari MK, Kalff JC, Billiar TR, et al. LPS-induced muscularis macrophage nitric oxide suppresses rat jejunal circular muscle activity. Am J Physiol 1999; 277:G478–86.
43. Beutler B, Du X, Poltorak A. Identification of Toll-like receptor 4 (Tlr4) as the sole conduit for LPS signal transduction: genetic and evolutionary studies. J Endotoxin Res 2001;7:277–80.
44. Hoshino K, Takeuchi O, Kawai T, et al. Cutting edge: Toll-like receptor 4 (TLR4)-deficient mice are hyporesponsive to lipopolysaccharide. Evidence for TLR4 as the Lps gene product. J Immunol 1999;162:3749–52.
45. Eskandari MK, Kalff JC, Billiar TR, et al. Lipopolysaccharide activates the muscularis macrophage network and suppresses circular smooth muscle activity. Am J Physiol 1997;273:G727–34.
46. Mircica E, Clutton RE, Kyles KW, et al. Problems associated with perioperative morphine in horses: a retrospective case analysis. Vet Anaesth Analg 2003;30: 147–55.
47. Senior JM, Pinchbeck GL, Dugdale AH, et al. Retrospective study of the risk factors and prevalence of colic in horses after orthopaedic surgery. Vet Rec 2004;155:321–5.
48. Andersen MS, Clark L, Dyson SJ, et al. Risk factors for colic in horses after general anaesthesia for MRI or nonabdominal surgery: absence of evidence of effect from perianaesthetic morphine. Equine Vet J 2006;38(4):368–74.
49. Boscan P, Van Hoogmoed LM, Farver TB, et al. Evaluation of the effects of the opioid agonist morphine on gastrointestinal tract function in horses. Am J Vet Res 2006;67(6):992–7.
50. Delesalle C, Dewulf J, Lefebvre RA, et al. Use of plasma ionized calcium levels and Ca2+ substitution response patterns as prognostic parameters for ileus and survival in colic horses. Vet Q 2005;27(4):157–72.
51. Dart AJ, Snyder JR, Spier SJ, et al. Ionized calcium concentration in horses with surgically managed gastrointestinal disease: 147 cases (1988–1990). J Am Vet Med Ass 1992;201(8):1244–8.
52. Garcia-Lopez JM, Provost PJ, Rush JE, et al. Prevelance and prognostic importance of hypomagnesemia and hypocalcemia in horses that have colic surgery. Am J Vet Res 2001;62:7–12.
53. Mecray PM, Barden RP, Ravdin IS. Nutritional edema: its effect on the gastric emptying time before and after gastric operations. Surgery 1937;1:53–64.
54. Moore-Olufemi SD, Xue H, Allen SJ, et al. Inhibition of intestinal transit by resuscitation-induced gut edema is reversed by L-NIL. J Surg Res 2005;129(1):1–5.
55. Lobo DN, Bostock KA, Neal KR, et al. Effect of salt and water balance on recovery of gastrointestinal function after elective colonic resection: a randomised controlled trial. Lancet 2002;359:1812–8.
56. Ke QH, Zheng SS, Liang TB, et al. Pretreatment of hypertonic saline can increase endogenous interleukin 10 release to attenuate hepatic ischemia reperfusion injury. Dig Dis Sci 2006;51(12):2257–63.
57. Oreopoulos GD, Hamilton J, Rizoli SB, et al. In vivo and in vitro modulation of intercellular adhesion molecule (ICAM)-1 expression by hypertonicity. Shock 2000;14(3):409–14.

58. Attuwaybi B, Kozar RA, Gates KS, et al. Hypertonic saline prevents inflammation, injury, and impaired intestinal transit after gut ischemia/reperfusion by inducing HO-1. J Trauma 2004;56(4):749–58.

59. Ross JW. Hypertonic saline in adynamic ileus. Can Med Assoc J 1926;16(3): 241–4.

60. Lv R, Zhou ZQ, Wu HW, et al. Hydroxyethyl starch exhibits antiinflammatory effects in the intestines of endotoxemic rats. Anesth Analg 2006;103(1):149–55.

61. Nohé B, Burchard M, Zanke C, et al. Endothelial accumulation of hydroxyethyl starch and functional consequences on leukocyte-endothelial interactions. Eur Surg Res 2002;34(5):364–72.

62. Kelley MC, Hocking MP, Marchand SD, et al. Ketolorac prevents postoperative small intestinal ileus in rats. Am J Surg 1993;165:107–12.

63. Valk N, Doherty TJ, Blackford JT, et al. Phenylbutazone prevents the endotoxin-induced delay in gastric emptying in horses. Can J Vet Res 1998;62(3):214–7 Erratum in: Can J Vet Res 1998;62(4):320.

64. King JN, Gerring EL. Antagonism of endotoxin-induced disruption of equine bowel motility by flunixin and phenylbutazone. Equine Vet J Suppl 1989;7:38–42.

65. Groudine SB, Fisher HA, Kaufman RP Jr, et al. Intravenous lidocaine speeds the return of bowel function, decreases postoperative pain, and shortens hospital stay in patients undergoing radical retropubic prostatectomy. Anesth Analg 1998;86(2):235–9.

66. Koppert W, Ostermeier N, Sittl R, et al. Low-dose lidocaine reduces secondary hyperalgesia by a central mode of action. Pain 2000;85(1–2):217–24.

67. Hollmann MW, Durieux ME. Local anesthetics and the inflammatory response: a new therapeutic indication? Anesthesiology 2000;93(3):858–75.

68. Rimbäck G, Cassuto J, Tollesson PO. Treatment of postoperative paralytic ileus by intravenous lidocaine infusion. Anesth Analg 1990;70(4):414–9.

69. Brianceau P, Chevalier H, Karas A, et al. Intravenous lidocaine and small-intestinal size, abdominal fluid, and outcome after colic surgery in horses. J Vet Intern Med 2002;16(6):736–41.

70. Durando MM, MacKay RJ, Linda S, et al. Effects of polymyxin B and Salmonella typhimurium antiserum on horses given endotoxin intravenously. Am J Vet Res 1994;55(7):921–7.

71. Van Hoogmoed LM, Nieto JE, Snyder JR, et al. Survey of prokinetic use in horses with gastrointestinal injury. Vet Surg 2004;33:279–85.

72. Milligan M, Beard W, Kukanich B, et al. The effect of lidocaine on postoperative jejunal motility in normal horses. Vet Surg 2007;36:214–20.

73. Malone E, Ensink J, Turner T, et al. Intravenous continuous infusion of lidocaine for treatment of equine ileus. Vet Surg 2006;35(1):60–6.

74. Catchpole BN. Ileus: use of sympathetic blocking agents in its treatment. Surgery 1969;66(5):811–20.

75. Tanila H, Kauppila T, Taira T. Inhibition of intestinal motility and reversal of postlaparotomy ileus by selective alpha 2-adrenergic drugs in the rat. Gastroenterology 1993;104(3):819–24.

76. Tonini M. Recent advances in the pharmacology of gastrointestinal prokinetics. Pharm Res 1996;33(4–5):217–26.

77. Dart AJ, Peauroi JR, Hodgson DR, et al. Efficacy of metoclopramide for treatment of ileus in horses following small intestinal surgery: 70 cases (1989-1992). Aust Vet J 1996;74(4):280–4.

78. Doherty TJ, Andrews FM, Abraha TW, et al. Metoclopramide ameliorates the effects of endotoxin on gastric emptying of acetaminophen in horses. Can J Vet Res 1999;63(1):37–40.

79. Lippold BS, Hildebrand J, Straub R. Tegaserod (HTF 919) stimulates gut motility in normal horses. Equine Vet J 2004;36(7):622–7.

80. Lester GD, Merritt AM, Neuwirth L, et al. Effect of erythromycin lactobionate on myoelectric activity of ileum, cecum, and right ventral colon, and cecal emptying of radiolabeled markers in clinically normal ponies. Am J Vet Res 1998;59(3): 328–34.

81. Ringger NC, Lester GD, Neuwirth L, et al. Effect of bethanechol or erythromycin on gastric emptying in horses. Am J Vet Res 1996;57(12):1771–5.

82. Lester GD, Merritt AM, Neuwirth L, et al. Effect of alpha 2-adrenergic, cholinergic, and nonsteroidal anti-inflammatory drugs on myoelectric activity of ileum, cecum, and right ventral colon and on cecal emptying of radiolabeled markers in clinically normal ponies. Am J Vet Res 1998;59(3):320–7.

83. Adams SB, MacHarg MA. Neostigmine methylsulfate delays gastric emptying of particulate markers in horses. Am J Vet Res 1985;46(12):2498–9.

Acute Diarrhea in Hospitalized Horses

Ann M. Chapman, DVM, MS

KEYWORDS

• Horses • Diarrhea • Nosocomial • *Salmonella*
• *Clostridium difficile*

The development of diarrhea among hospitalized horses is a major concern for equine veterinary hospitals and referral centers. It is a potential complication of hospitalization for surgical or medical procedures and can contribute to the morbidity and mortality of horses with gastrointestinal and nongastrointestinal diseases. Unfortunately, it can be difficult to pinpoint the exact cause of acute diarrhea or colitis, and in most cases, the specific etiologic agent is presumptive or undetermined. A complete review of colitis with particular attention to advance diagnostics and therapeutics has been published.[1] This article discusses the major etiologic agents of diarrhea in hospitalized horses, considers factors that place hospitalized horse at special risk for diarrhea, and examines several infectious colitis outbreaks that have occurred at veterinary referral centers.

Acute diarrhea and colitis can be especially alarming to owners and veterinarians when it occurs in horses admitted to a veterinary hospital for routine or elective procedures, particularly procedures not related to gastrointestinal disease. Close monitoring during the hospital stay is important for early recognition of a developing colitis. Clinical parameters that should be monitored narrowly include rectal temperature, heart rate, respiratory rate, hydration, mucous membrane color and quality, capillary refill time, appetite, and fecal character and frequency. If the fecal character becomes softer or more liquid but the defecation frequency and clinical parameters remain normal, then this may represent mild diarrhea of minimal consequence. Watery feces with blood or a foul odor that persists and is accompanied by fever, tachycardia, tachypnea, injected hyperemic mucous membranes, dehydration, loss of appetite, depression, and signs of abdominal discomfort suggests the existence of a more serious condition. In most cases, abnormal clinical parameters precede the onset of diarrhea. In such a case, diagnostics should be pursued immediately to identify the hemodynamic status of the patient and determine if intervention is required.

Department of Veterinary Clinical Sciences, School of Veterinary Medicine, Louisiana State University, Baton Rouge, LA 70803, USA
E-mail address: achapman@vetmed.lsu.edu

Vet Clin Equine 25 (2009) 363–380
doi:10.1016/j.cveq.2009.05.001
0749-0739/09/$ – see front matter © 2009 Elsevier Inc. All rights reserved.

vetequine.theclinics.com

Causes for diarrhea may be classified as noninfectious and infectious. Determining whether infectious diarrhea or colitis was community acquired or hospital acquired (nosocomial) can be important when implementing infectious disease control measures in a facility. Nosocomial disease is defined as one that was neither present nor incubating at the time of hospital admission but occurred 72 hours after admittance. Defining nosocomial or hospital-acquired infection is complicated by the fact that a horse with a community-acquired infection may be incubating the disease on admission and manifest clinical signs during hospitalization.[2] If community-acquired, hospital-expressed infection is not properly identified, it may lead to incorrect estimates of noscomial infection rates.[2] An extensive review of surveillance for nosocomial diarrhea or colitis in veterinary hospitals has been published.[3]

Most university veterinary teaching hospitals and large private referral hospitals have an active surveillance program that targets the subset of patients that are at greatest risk, such as horses with colic and other gastrointestinal disease. Others may use a global surveillance program for infectious colts by examining the entire population of horses admitted.[3] For example, at the Veterinary Teaching Hospital and Clinics at Louisiana State University, all patients admitted to the hospital are screened for *Salmonella* fecal shedding by obtaining daily fecal specimens until five samples are tested (**Box 1**). These programs are costly, however, and many smaller referral hospitals do not have the budget or workforce to implement such a large-scale active surveillance protocol. Rather they collect passive surveillance data from horses that develop diarrhea.

Noninfectious causes of diarrhea include antimicrobial-associated colitis, nonsteroidal anti-inflammatory drug (NSAID)–associated colitis (eg, right dorsal colitis), feed-related causes (carbohydrate overload, dietary change), peritonitis, toxicosis (cantharidin, arsenic, mercury), sand enteropathy, neoplasia, and inflammatory bowel disease. Among these causes, this article concentrates on the most common iatrogenic causes of diarrhea (antimicrobial associated, NSAID associated, feed related). Major subpopulations of hospitalized horses receive antimicrobials either therapeutically to treat known infections or prophylactically before surgical procedures. NSAIDs are frequently given to horses for analgesia before presentation, upon admission, and throughout the hospital stay. An overdose of NSAIDs predictably induces severe colitis; however, more recent reports in the literature demonstrate that NSAID-associated colitis may occur in horses receiving the recommended dose of phenylbutazone[4] and that gastrointestinal tract ulceration and inflammation can be evident as early as 3 days from the onset of therapy.[5] Prostaglandins are important inhibitors of intestinal inflammation and help maintain mucosal blood flow; blocking the formation of these substances may increase the severity of colitis.

Finally, despite efforts to replicate the normal diet of the equine patient, many horses undergo a significant change in diet during hospitalization. Horses that present for colic are frequently anorexic before admission, and feed is typically withheld for variable periods of time before and after surgical procedures. Loss of appetite and feed alterations do not cause severe colitis, but evidence indicates that changes in the diet composition may alter enteric flora[6,7] and contribute to disease.[8]

Infectious causes of diarrhea in horses include *Salmonella*, clostridial enterocolitis (*Clostridium difficile, Clostridium perfringens*), *Neorickettsia risticii*, and cyathostomiasis. Infectious etiologies of acute diarrhea are of notable concern because they pose a threat for hospital-wide spread. This article focuses on salmonellosis and clostridial enterocolitis because these infectious agents have been isolated from the hospital environment and have the potential to cause colitis in hospitalized horses. Although *N risticii* is an important cause of acute colitis (Potomac horse fever) in adult horses, infection requires the accidental ingestion of infected digenetic nematodes in first or intermediate hosts. Although an outbreak of Potomac horse fever has occurred at racetracks,[9] hospital-acquired infection has not been documented. Community-acquired, hospital-expressed Potomac horse fever and cyathostomiasis may occur in horses at veterinary hospitals and referral centers, but these diseases have been reviewed elsewhereand are not covered in this article.[10,11]

It is important to note that the development of colitis in hospitalized horses may be multifactorial and occur in conjunction with gastrointestinal and nongastrointestinal diseases. Infectious and noninfectious factors may have a combined or synergistic effect to induce disease.

NONINFECTIOUS CAUSES OF DIARRHEA: DIETARY ALTERATIONS AND CARBOHYDRATE OVERLOAD

The colonic liquor of the horse is a complex, dynamic microbiologic ecosystem composed of several hundred species of resident and transient bacteria, protozoa, and fungi.[12] (See the article by Al Jassim and Andrews elsewhere in this issue for details on the bacterial community in the horse gastrointestinal tract.) Commensal and pathologic bacteria populate the equine colon, of which gram-negative rods predominate (50%), followed by gram-positive rods (23%), gram-positive cocci (22%), and finally gram-negative cocci (4%).[12] Anaerobic bacteria are highly abundant and play a vital role in hindgut fermentation. In healthy horses, commensal organisms must compete with pathogenic bacteria for survival in a delicate balance that can be disrupted easily by various circumstances. Studies have demonstrated that alterations in intestinal microbial composition can occur with changes in season[7] and alterations in diet.[8,13] For example, the addition of barley to the diet of ponies increased lactate-utilizing bacteria (*Streptococcus* spp and *Lactobacillus* spp), decreased cellulolytic bacteria, altered the volatile fatty acid ratio, and decreased colonic pH.[13] As discussed later, a variety of intestinal luminal conditions (bacterial populations, pH, nutrients, oxygen tension) may affect the ability of pathogenic micro-organisms to invade.

In the hospital setting, horses are inevitably subject to a change in diet, unless the owner provides a supply of the normal feedstuff for the hospitalization period. It is generally recommended to mimic the native diet as much as possible and avoid drastic changes, especially in the amount of concentrates offered during the hospital stay. Minor diet changes typically do not cause profound diarrhea, as can be seen with severe carbohydrate overload. Subtle changes in enteric bacterial flora may occur, however, and could play a role in opportunistic infections with enteric pathogens such as *Salmonella*.

Conversely, some hospitalized equine patients may have a reduction in dietary intake either voluntarily (hypophagia, anorexia) or because of imposed feed withdrawal before surgical procedures. Extended feed-withholding may be necessary in horses with dysphagia or intestinal dysfunction and gastric reflux (eg, ileus, duodenitits proximal jejunitis). Detrimental changes in the intestinal microflora (such as defaunation) or villous atrophy of the intestinal mucosa may occur with prolonged fasting (>72 hours), resulting in severe diarrhea. When voluntary intake is contraindicated or not possible, parenteral or enteral nutrition (when intestinal function is present) is recommended to prevent fasting-induced diarrhea. A complete review of enteral and parenteral nutrition is published;[14,15] however, caution is needed when initiating an enteral nutrition program, because overaggressive feeding after an extended period of feed withdrawal may lead to severe colitis.

Box 1
Examples of equine surveillance programs for Salmonella

Active surveillance for Salmonella

Patient selection

Outpatients: Fecal samples are not collected routinely, unless salmonellosis is a differential diagnosis.

Inpatients: All horses entering hospital as inpatients must have fecal samples submitted to an approved diagnostic laboratory for *Salmonella* culture. A *Salmonella* surveillance tracking form is included in the patient record on admission.

Sample collection

Fecal samples are collected:

On the day of admission

Every 24 hours until a total of five samples are collected (including weekends and holidays)

If the patient remains hospitalized beyond 5 days, fecal samples are collected every 7 days thereafter, regardless of whether the patient's location within the hospital changes during this time.

At least 10 g of fresh feces (one large fecal ball) should be collected and placed in a clean unused specimen cup. The sample should be properly labeled with date of collection, patient name, signalment, and patient case number and submitted to the diagnostic laboratory as soon as possible.

Samples that are collected on weekends or holidays should be stored in a dedicated refrigerator and submitted the next available business day.

Surveillance data

Surveillance information is collected on each patient including:

Date of sample collection

Stall location

Presenting complaint

Antibiotics administered

Surgical procedures performed

Changes in fecal consistency and frequency

Isolation of suspected horses

Horses that culture positive for *Salmonella* without clinical signs are placed in isolation immediately.

A hospitalized horse is moved to isolation ward if it develops:

Loose or watery feces

Fever

Leukopenia or neutropenia

A hospitalized horse that develops diarrhea that persists for >24 hours regardless of body temperature or white blood cell results also must be moved to the isolation ward.

A hospitalized horse without fever or leukopenia that develops projectile diarrhea (<24 h) that exits the stall must be moved to the isolation ward.

Passive surveillance for Salmonella

Patient selection

Hospitalized horses that develop:

Loose or watery feces

± fever

± leukopenia or neutropenia

Fecal samples should be submitted to an approved diagnostic laboratory for *Salmonella* culture and PCR. Culture results are needed to provide antibiotic sensitivities and identify multidrug-resistant *Salmonella*. However, PCR may provide a more rapid diagnosis.

If *Salmonella* is identified in the affected horse, daily fecal samples should be collected from the remainder of horses in the facility.

Sample collection

Fecal samples are collected:

On development of diarrhea

Every 24 hours until a total of five samples are collected (including weekends and holidays)

At least 5–10 g of fresh feces should be collected and placed in a clean unused specimen cup. The sample should be properly labeled with date of collection, patient name, signalment, and patient case number and submitted to the diagnostic laboratory as soon as possible.

Samples that are collected on weekends or holidays should be stored in a dedicated refrigerator and submitted the next available business day.

Isolation of suspected horses

Affected horses should be moved to a separate isolation facility or strictly confined to their stall.

Hospitalized horses that are clinically normal should be monitored closely for evidence of impending diarrhea by recording:

Fecal consistency

Rectal temperature (at least twice daily)

Attitude

Appetite

Adapted from Guidelines for the control of large animal infectious diseases. Louisiana State University, Veterinary Teaching Hospital & Clinics, Baton Rouge, LA, 2006.

NONINFECTIOUS CAUSES OF DIARRHEA: ANTIMICROBIAL-ASSOCIATED DIARRHEA

In a hospital environment, antimicrobial therapy may be necessary to treat known infections or may be needed prophylactically to prevent infection during surgical procedures.[16] Perioperative antibiotics play an important role in reducing surgical infections and improving patient outcomes; however, they are not without risk in equine patients. Antibiotics can have an adverse effect on the distribution and number of normal bacteria and protozoa in the cecum and colon by disrupting the balance of commensal and pathogenic organisms, which can permit the overgrowth of pathogenic species.[17] Consequently, certain antibiotics with poor intestinal absorption, such as macrolides (erythromycin[18]) and lincosamides (lincomycin[19] and clindamycin) have been associated with severe antibiotic-induced colitis when administered orally in experimental models, even at low dosages.

Administration of oral oxytetracycline to horses caused a marked change in the fecal bacteria populations within 24 hours of the first dose.[20] In this study, after oxytetracycline administration, *Veillonella* sp, a normal intestinal flora, disappeared, whereas coliforms, *Streptococcus* spp and *Bacteroides* spp, and pathogenic bacterial species (such as *Clostridium perfringens* type A) increased significantly.[20] Other studies demonstrated that mares were at risk for developing clostridial enterocolitis when their foals were treated with erythromycin and rifampin for *Rhodococcus equi* infection.[21] Experimentally, colitis has been induced in adult horses when low doses of these drugs are administered; hospitalized mares should be monitored closely when accompanying foals that are receiving macrolide therapy.

Parenteral antibiotics also are capable of causing diarrhea or colitis. Some parenteral antimicrobials undergo enterohepatic circulation or biliary excretion and are able to affect intestinal microflora. In one study, hospitalized horses that received parenteral antibiotics were 10.9 times more likely to have positive fecal *Salmonella* culture results when compared with horses that did not receive parental antibiotics.[22] This finding suggests that antibiotics change the antagonistic relationship of intestinal microflora to favor overgrowth of pathogenic strains. Essentially, all antibiotics are capable of causing diarrhea in horses, and owners should be warned of the potential complication of colitis before the initiation of antimicrobial therapy. If diarrhea develops shortly after the initiation of antimicrobial therapy, then antibiotic-associated colitis should be suspected.[23]

A retrospective study by Cohen and Woods[24] demonstrated that horses with acute diarrhea were 4.5 times less likely to survive if they had a previous exposure to antimicrobial agents compared with horses that did not. In this study, potentiated sulfonamides or penicillin G were the antimicrobials most commonly administered before the development of diarrhea. The relationship between antibiotics and colitis is not always consistent, however. Another retrospective study found no significant difference between historical and documented evidence of antimicrobial use and nonsurvival in horses with acute idiopathic enterocolitis.[25] The relationship between antimicrobial agents and diarrhea is complex. Most controversy in using antimicrobial agents exists with indiscriminate use in horses without documented evidence of bacterial infection or with the excessive use of critical antimicrobials. Extensive evidence suggests that inappropriate use of antibiotics contributes to the emergence of multidrug-resistant bacteria,[26] most concerning of which in equine gastrointestinal disease is multidrug-resistant *Salmonella*. The association between antimicrobial agents and infectious colitis is discussed later.

NONSTEROIDAL ANTI-INFLAMMATORY DRUGS

Diarrhea associated with overdose of NSAIDs has been documented experimentally and retrospectively in horses.[27,28] NSAID-associated enteropathy may occur when these drugs are administered at an appropriate dosage and for short periods of time,[4,5] which may suggest an idiosyncratic response. Recent studies have shown that colonic acetic acid concentration decreased significantly in horses administered phenylbutazone for 21 days. Colonic volatile fatty acid s are important byproducts of bacterial fermentation and are important in facilitating absorption of water in the colon. Prolonged phenylbutazone therapy, at a dose of 4.4 mg/kg orally, may predispose the colon to inflammation.[5] Because hospitalized horses may receive NSAID therapy for prolonged periods to alleviate pain and decrease clinical signs associated with endo-toxemia, they may be at risk for NSAID-induced enteropathy. Severe diarrhea may not be the hallmark of this disease initally, but recognition of the early signs, such as leth-argy, anorexia, reduced fecal outpu,t and colic, is imperative to initiate treatment and prevent further complications.[29]

Periodic laboratory monitoring of hospitalized horses that receive NSAID therapy is recommended to detect subtle indicators of intestinal inflammation (hypoalbumine-mia, hypoproteinemia, anemia, and neutropenia). Efforts should be made by clinicians to limit the use of NSAIDs to the lowest dose possible that provides the desired pain relief in the patient yet minimizes unwanted side effects, particularly to the gastrointes-tinal tract. Alternative methods of analgesic therapy might be considered in hospital-ized horses, including different routes of analgesia, such as local or topical therapy, different classes of analgesics, such as opiates or α-2 agonists, and finally, the use of newer cyclooxygenase-1 sparing NSAIDs, such as firocoxib (Equioxx, Merial Limited, Decatur, Georgia), which may prove beneficial in some horses.

INFECTIOUS CAUSES OF DIARRHEA: SALMONELLOSIS

Equine salmonellosis has long been recognized as an important infectious cause of colitis in adult horses.[30,31] *Salmonella* belongs to the family of bacteria called Entero-bacteriaceae, which is comprised of facultative anaerobic, gram-negative bacillus (or rods). The taxonomic nomenclature of *Salmonella* has suffered numerous revisions throughout the years, which has led to much confusion in scientific reports and publi-cations. In 2003, the Centers for Disease Control and Prevention (CDC) adopted the Kauffmann-White Scheme for identifying serotypes.[32] Under this system, salmonellae in subspecies *S enterica* (subspecies *enterica*) are named, whereas organisms in other subspecies are identified by an antigenic formula. The primary mode of transmission of *Salmonella* is the fecal-oral route; however, airborne transmission has been demon-strated in some species.

Oliveira and colleagues[33] found that pigs could be experimentally infected by inhaling *Salmonella* over short distances; however, aerosol transmission has never been demonstrated in horses. Both nonspecific and specific host defenses attempt to limit infection by pathogenic organisms. After ingestion, the organism must survive the acid milieu of the gastric fluid. Most of the bacteria perish in the stomach, but with a large inoculum, enough bacteria survive to reach the distal small intestine and colon. One study in mice suggested that gut luminal contents and composition may be critical to establishing infection in the intestinal epithelium.[34]

It stands to reason that changes in intestinal contents and composition of nutrients (amino acids composition, carbohydrates) may be needed for *Salmonella* to receive physiologic and environmental cues to invade intestinal epithelium. By sequentially up-regulating the genetic components of *Salmonella* pathogenicity island-1, including the subunits of the type III secretory system system and a complex hierarchy of effector proteins,[35] *Salmonella* is able to enter into nonphagocytic cells. Once internalized into cells, *Salmonella* has the capacity to efficiently replicate and then disseminate through a complex series of cellular translocations. By exploitating phagocytic cells, *Salmonella* can spread to extraintestinal sites. This fact is evidenced by experimental infection of *Salmonella typhimurium* in ponies, which revealed positive cultures of the mesenteric lymph nodes 20 hours after surgical inoculation of the dorsal colon.[36]

The classic feature of clinical salmonellosis in most vertebrate species is profuse, voluminous watery diarrhea. This diarrhea occurs as a result of intestinal fluid losses by two mechanisms: (1) active fluid loss through secretory hyperstimulation and

(2) passive fluid loss by inflammation-mediated malabsorption. Mucosal and submucosal edema, microvascular changes, and neutrophilic inflammation can be observed secondary to experimental infection with *Salmonella* in ponies.[36] *Salmonella* also produces various virulence factors, including exotoxin, cytotoxin, and enterotoxin that mediate the development of diarrhea.[37] Milder infections are usually self-limiting, and patients usually show clinical improvement in a relatively brief period of time. Another important clinical feature of salmonellosis is the potential for some infected animals to shed the organism without demonstrating clinical signs of the disease (silent shedder).[38]

In highly concentrated populations of horses, *Salmonella* infection is of particular concern. Outbreaks have occurred at veterinary referral hospitals, on breeding farms, and at racetracks. Veterinary referral centers are of particular concern because congregations of potentially susceptible animals are subject to comingling in these facilities. Horizontal disease transmission is of particular concern in these situations. There have been numerous reports of *Salmonella* outbreaks among veterinary hospitals,[39–54] and most of these infection outbreaks are caused by multidrug-resistant strains of *Salmonella* (**Table 1**). Studies of salmonellosis in horses at veterinary referral centers have identified risk factors that increase the likelihood of infection during hospitalization[55–60] or during an outbreak.[50,51,61] Despite some inconsistencies between these studies, possibly because of the differences in sample populations and sampling techniques, many similar risk factors exist. Horses that received antibiotic therapy[56,58,60] and were undergoing feed restriction or diet change[58,61] were at greater risk for developing salmonellosis. This is most likely because of alterations in enteric microflora. In another study, foals were at greater risk for *Salmonella* infection,[60] most likely because of reduced immunocompetency, lack of competing enteric microflora, and coprophagia.

Stress also may play a role in *Salmonella* infection because several studies found that prolonged transport[55,62] or heat exposure[58] increased the likelihood of salmonellosis. Other stressors that have been identified include major surgery, particularly abdominal surgery,[60,63–65] gastrointestinal disease (colic),[22,55,56,60,66] and respiratory disease.[59] Drawing universal conclusions from these studies examining risk factors is difficult, because sample size, study populations, and temporal relationships are markedly different. To add to the confusion, a recent study that examined the development of nosocomial diarrhea in hospitalized horses failed to identify *Salmonella* from either case or control horses.[65] Overall, these studies suggested that the factors that influence infection are not exclusive and may vary within and between veterinary hospitals. Facilities must maintain vigilant biosecurity measures to reduce nosocomial disease.

SALMONELLA PREVALENCE

Prevalence is defined as the total number of cases of a disease in the population at a given time. The unanswered question that worries most equine hospitals is the prevalence of *Salmonella* infection among the horse population in the local geographic area. The entry of horses with community-acquired *Salmonella* into the hospital is a particular concern, especially if the organism is multidrug resistant. Numerous studies have examined the prevalence *Salmonella* shedding in a variety of horse populations (**Table 2**).[55,57–61,64,67–79] Reported prevalences in these studies vary substantially, which may be because of differences in the inclusion criteria for the subjects and the type and number of fecal samples obtained. The United States Department of Agriculture, Animal Plant Health Inspection Service reported prevalence of *Salmonella*

Table 1
Reported outbreaks of *Salmonella* spp that have occurred among horses

References	Dates of Outbreak	Location	*Salmonella* Serotype	Comment
[39]	September–October 1967	Liverpool, England	*Salmonella typhimurium*	Infection introduced from infected cow
[40]	May 1971–April 1972	Missouri	*Salmonella typhimurium*	8 horses
[41]	1980–1984	Kentucky	*Salmonella agona*	87 cases on 56 farms 52 deaths
[22,42,43]	June 1981–March 1982	California	*Salmonella* Saint-Paul *Salmonella* Krefeld	47 horses
[44]	1985–1986 2 years	Central Kentucky	*Salmonella* Saint-Paul	108 isolates
[45]	March–April 1988 1 month	Georgia	*Salmonella give* (3), *Salmonella newport* (7), *Salmonella anatum* (3)	13 horses
[46,47]	April 1991–August 1992 1.5 years	Wisconsin	*Salmonella anatum*	Introduced from private veterinary clinic
[48]	October 1991–May 1992 8 months	California	*Salmonella* Krefeld	ICU study, 20 horses
[49]	1992–1997 6 years	Victoria, Australia	*Salmonella* Heidelberg	31 cases of multidrug-resistant *Salmonella*
[50]	June–September 1996 13 weeks	Colorado	*Salmonella infantis*	25% nosocomial rate
[51]	May 1996–January 1997 9 months	Michigan	*Salmonella typhimurium*	28 horses, 46% case fatality
[52]	1997–2000 3 years	Ontario	*Salmonella typhimurium* DT104	17 horses, 29% case fatality
[53]	August–December 1999 April–November 2000	Indiana	*Salmonella typhimurium*	33 cases, 42% mortality
[54]	July 2003–May 2004	Pennsylvania	*Salmonella newport*	—

shedding, by a single fecal culture, in 8417 horses from the US general horse population to be 0.8%.[78] Based on that study, it is believed that active shedding of *Salmonella* occurs rather infrequently in adult horses in the general population. Several studies have evaluated the prevalence of *Salmonella* fecal shedding among horses admitted to veterinary teaching hospitals (see **Table 2**). The reported prevalence

Table 2
Reported prevalence of *Salmonella* identification in various populations of horses

Reference	Study Period	Location	Sample	Detection Method	Population	Horses Sampled	Prevalence (%)
64	1975	California	Feces	Culture	General hospitalized	1451	3.2
67	1980–1981	Pennsylvania	Feces or rectal swab	Culture	Admitted for colic	100	13
61	1984–1986	Colorado	Feces	Culture	General hospitalized (>3 d)	246	7
68	1985–1986	Sydney, Australia	Feces	Culture	General hospitalized & mares on farm	250 (hospital) 75 (farm)	2.8 (hospital), 0 (farm)
69	1989	Oklahoma	Lymph node	Culture	Slaughterhouse	70	71.4
70	1990–1991	Utrecht, the Netherlands	Feces	Culture	Admitted for diarrhea	380	54 (direct culture), 46 (with selenite)
57	1992–1996	California	Feces	Culture	Hospitalized ICU or isolation	1446	6.3
58	1993–1996	California	Feces	Culture	Hospitalized in ICU	1429	5.46
71	1993	Melbourne, Australia	Ileum swab	Culture	Slaughterhouse	143	27
72	1994–1995	Texas	Feces	Culture and PCR	Outpatient	152	0 (culture), 17 (PCR)
72	1994–1995	Texas	Feces	Culture and PCR	Inpatient	110	10 (culture), 64 (PCR)
73	1994	California	Lymph node	Culture	Necropsy	102	1.96
74	1995–1996	Montreal, Canada	Feces	Culture	General hospitalized	613	1.7

	Years	Location	Sample	Method	Population	Number	Percentage
75	1996–1999	Michigan	Feces	Culture	Hospitalized with gastrointestinal disease or at risk	638	5.5
55	1997–1999	Colorado	Feces	Culture	Hospitalized for colic	246	9
59	2000–2001	Indiana	Feces or tissue	Culture	General hospitalized (in and outpatient)	230	5.6
76	2001	Indiana	Feces or tissue	Culture and PCR	Isolation patients	34	26 (culture), 68 (PCR)
77	2001–2002	Indiana	Feces	Culture and PCR	Hospitalized for nongastrointestinal disease	116	9.5 (culture), 75 (PCR)
60	2002	Florida	Feces	Culture	Hospitalized with gastrointestinal disease	1750	13
78	1998–1999	28 states	Feces	Culture	Resident horses on farms	8417	0.8
79	2002–2004	Colorado	Feces	Culture	General hospitalized	1290	4.0

ranged from 1.7% to 10% of those studies examining general equine admissions (inpatient and outpatient).[59,61,64,68,72,74,77,79] The prevalence of *Salmonella* shedding in horses admitted to intensive care units (ICUs) ranged from 5.46% to 6.3%,[57,58] and those admitted for gastrointestinal disease (including colic) ranged from 5.5% to 13%.[55,60,67,75] The prevalence of *Salmonella* shedding in patients increased during hospitalization from 0.4% positive upon admission to 4.35% positive during hospitalization.[59] With all the reports in the literature, it is difficult to draw universal conclusions about the shedding rates of *Salmonella* among all horses because prevalence studies by their very nature only examine a defined population of horses at a given point in time. There is a trend for *Salmonella* to be isolated more frequently from horses admitted for gastrointestinal disease and those admitted for ICU treatment, however.

The incidence of zoonotic infection in people who handle horses infected with *Salmonella* is unknown. In one study, however, *Salmonella* was not isolated from the feces of personnel associated with an equine veterinary teaching hospital during an outbreak of salmonellosis.[50] Another study found that *Salmonella* was identified in the households of personnel who have regular contact with infected livestock.[80] Also, multidrug-resistant *Salmonella typhimurium* was the cause of clinical illness in 18 people who were either employees or clients of four small animal facilities in the United States.[81] It has been suggested that *Salmonella* enteritis in people is underreported and that differentiating zoonotic transmission from food-borne disease may be difficult; the true risk for transmission of the organism from horses to people remains elusive.

CLOSTRIDIAL ENTEROCOLITIS

Clostridium difficile is an obligate anaerobic endospore-forming, gram-positive rod. Like *Salmonella*, transmission of the organism occurs by the oral-fecal route; however *C difficile* infection may occur by ingestion of either the vegetative organism or the resistant endospores. As an obligate anaerobe, the vegetative form of the bacteria does not survive well under aerobic conditions; however, endospores are capable of surviving under adverse conditions environmentally in soil and water. One study examining the presence of *C difficile* spores in a veterinary hospital isolated the organism from stalls, floors, medical equipment, and the footware of medical personnel.[66] The organism is more frequently identified in soil samples from studfarms (11%) than farms with only mature horses (1%).[82] The same study detected *C difficile* in the feces of healthy horses and foals, suggesting that healthy foals may serve as a potential reservoir for the organism.[82]

Toxin production is an important component of the virulence of *C difficile*. At least five toxins have been identified, of which toxin A and B are the most studied and most clearly understood. Toxin A is an effective enterotoxin which is capable of causing intestinal fluid accumulation and initiating inflammation, whereas toxin B is a potent cytotoxin.[83] The toxin A and B genes are identified from the majority of *C difficile* isolates from horses with acute enteric disease; however toxin A+/B- strains and toxin A-/B+ strains have been described.[84] Identification of the toxin genes does not always correspond to toxin detection by immunoassay. This may be caused by gene silence, defective toxin production, or minuscule gene expression (and thus below the level of immunoassay detection).[84] Detecting clostridial toxins in feces by immunoassays or cytotoxicity assay (toxin B) is necessary in establishing *C difficile*-associated diarrhea.[85]

In people, a strong relationship between *C difficile* and antimicrobial-associated diarrhea is well established,[86] and in recent years this association has been proven in horses.[87–91] Antimicrobial-induced changes in intestinal microflora may have a permissive role in the establishment or proliferation of *C difficile*; however, cases of *C difficile*-associated diarrhea that are not related to antibiotic therapy are recognized. Several antibiotics that have been implicated in the development of *C difficile*-associated diarrhea include included β-lactam antibiotics,[87,88,90] erythromycin,[18,21] gentamicin,[90] and potentiated sulfonamides.[87,90] In an experimental model, *C difficile* enterocolitis was induced in pony foals by inoculation with either endospores or vegetative bacterial cells. An important factor in the induction of *C difficile*-associated diarrhea with endospores in these foals was disruption of normal gastrointestinal flora with clindamycin administration.[91] This most likely mimics naturally acquired disease because endospores are more persistent in the environment than vegetative cells. Recent studies have shown that toxigenic *C difficile* obtained from horses with antibiotic-associated diarrhea showed a preferential attachment to equine intestinal cells versus human intestinal cells in vitro,[92] suggesting that a host-species dependency and preference may exist. Also, one strain of *C difficile* that was nontoxigenic showed no intestinal cell attachment in vitro, suggesting that the ability of the bacteria to produce toxin may have a relationship to its ability to colonize gastrointestinal epithelium.[92]

The development of *C difficile*-associated diarrhea in hospitalized horses has been examined in the literature. There was no significant difference between the development of nosocomial diarrhea and the identification of *C difficile* in a prospective study of 81 horses.[93] An outbreak of *C difficile*-associated diarrhea developed in nine hospitalized horses within 2 days in another report.[94] Although it was determined that several different strains of *C difficile* were responsible for the development of diarrhea, a cluster of cases warrants attention. Risk factors for *C difficile*-associated diarrhea are similar to those discussed for Salmonellosis (eg, antimicrobials, diet change, surgery) and are most likely related to factors that alter cecocolic microflora and allow colonization, proliferation, and production of toxin production. Most of these associations are anecdotal, and further studies are needed to expand our understanding of nosocomial clostridial infection.

SUMMARY

Although noninfectious and infectious causes of diarrhea have been identified in hospitalized horses, many times a specific etiologic agent cannot be found. A definitive link between this condition and pathogenic bacteria cannot always be made,[93] so it seems likely that diarrhea or colitis in the hospitalized horse is multifactorial. These factors include host factors (immunocompentency, stress), bacterial virulence factors, dietary changes, antimicrobial administration, and NSAID therapy. Despite years of extensive research, many mysteries still exist, and predicting when hospitalized horses will develop diarrhea appears complex. Early recognition of the clinical signs and initiation of therapy is essential for a positive outcome, because case fatality rate for hospitalized horses that develop acute diarrhea ranges from 25% to 42%.[23,24] Understanding of the relationship between the etiologies presented here and the risk factors for the development of nosocomial diarrhea is essential to prevent this potentially serious complication of hospitalization. Additional research is needed to determine how these factors cause diarrhea and which horses are likely to develop diarrhea once hospitalized.

REFERENCES

1. Fieary DJ, Hassel DJ. Enteritis and colitis in horses. Vet Clin North Am Equine Pract 2006;22:437–79.

2. Traub-Dargatz JL, Dargatz DA, Morley PS, et al. An overview of infection control strategies for equine facilities with an emphasis on veterinary hospitals. Vet Clin North Am Equine Pract 2004;20(3):507–20.

3. Morley PS. Surveillance for nosocomial infections in veterinary hospitals. Vet Clin North Am Equine Pract 2004;20(3):561–76.

4. Cohen ND, Carter GK, Mealey RH, et al. Medical management of right dorsal colitis in 5 horses: a retrospective study (1987–1993). J Vet Intern Med 2008; 19(4):272–6.

5. McConnico RS, Morgan TW, Williams CC, et al. Pathophysiologic effects of phenylbutazone on the right dorsal colon in horses. J Am Vet Med Assoc 2008;69(11): 1496–505.

6. Moore BE, Dehority BA. Effects of diet and hindgut fermentation on diet digestibility and microbial concentrations in the cecum and colon in the horse. J Anim Sci 1993;71:3350–8.

7. Kobayash Y, Koike S, Miyaji M, et al. Hindgut fermentation and their seasonal variations in Hokkaido native horses compared to light horses. Ecol Res 2006; 21(2):285–91.

8. Goodson J, Tyznik WJ, Cline JH, et al. Effects of an abrupt diet change from hay to concentrate on microbial numbers and physical environment in the cecum of the pony. Appl Environ Microbiol 1988;54:1946–50.

9. Rikihisa Y, Reed SM, Sama RA, et al. Serosurvey of horses with evidence of equine monocytic erlichiosis. J Am Vet Med Assoc 1990;197:1327–32.

10. Palmer JE. Potomac horse fever. Vet Clin North Am Equine Pract 1993;9(2): 399–410.

11. Lyons ET, Drudge JH, Tolliver SC. Larval cyathostomiasis. Vet Clin North Am Equine Pract 2000;16(3):501–13.

12. Maczulak AE, Dawson KA, Baker JP. Nitrogen utilization in bacterial isolates from the equine cecum. Appl Environ Microbiol 1985;50(6):1439–43.

13. Julliand V, de Fombelle A, Drogoul C, et al. Feeding and microbial disorders in horses: part 3. Effects of three hay:grain ratios on microbial profile and activities. J Equine Vet Sci 2001;21(11):543–6.

14. Magdesian K. Nutrition for critical gastrointestinal illness: feeding horses with diarrhea or colic. Vet Clin North Am Equine Pract 2003;19(3):617–44.

15. Sweeny RW, Hansen TO. Use of a liquid diet as a sole source of nutrition in six dysphagic horses and as a dietary supplement in seven hypophagic horses. J Am Vet Med Assoc 1990;197(8):1030–2.

16. Southwood LL. Principles of antimicrobial therapy: what should we be using? Vet Clin North Am Equine Pract 2006;22:279–96.

17. Papich MG. Anitmicrobial therapy for gastrointestinal disease. Vet Clin North Am Equine Pract 2003;19:645–63.

18. Gustafsson A, Baverud V, Gunnarsson A, et al. The association of erythromycin ethylsuccinate with acute colitis in horses in Sweden. Equine Vet J 1997;29(4): 314–8.

19. Raisbeck MF, Holt GR, Osweiler GD. Lincomycin-associated colitis in horses. J Am Vet Med Assoc 1981;179(4):362–3.

20. White MA, Prior SD. Comparative effects of oral administration of trimethoprim/ sulphadiazine or oxytetracyline on faecal flora of horses. Vet Rec 1982;111: 316–8.

21. Baverud V, Franklin A, Gunnarsson A, et al. *Clostridium difficile* associated with acute colitis in mares when their foals are treated with erythromycin and rifampin for *Rhodococcus equi* pneumonia. Equine Vet J 1998;30:482–8.

22. Hird DW, Pappaioanou M, Smith BP. Case-control study of risk factors associated with isolation of *Salmonella* Saint-Paul in hospitalized horses. Am J Epidemiol 1984;120(6):852–64.
23. Buechner V. The use of antimicrobial therapy in gastrointestinal disease in the adult horse. Equine Pract 1989;11(10):9–14.
24. Cohen ND, Woods AM. Characteristics and risk factors for horses with acute diarrhea to survive: 122 cases (1990–1996). J Am Vet Med Assoc 1999;214(3): 382–90.
25. Stampfli HR, Townsend HG, Prescott JF. Prognostic features and clinical presentation of acute idiopathic enterocolitis in horses. Can Vet J 1991;32:232–7.
26. Dargatz DA, Traub-Dargatz JL. Multidrug-resistant *Salmonella* and nosocomial infections. Vet Clin North Am Equine Pract 2004;20(3):587–600.
27. MacAllister CG, Morgan SJ, Borne AT, et al. Comparison of adverse effects of phenylbutazone, flunixin meglumine, and ketoprofen in horses. J Am Vet Med Assoc 1993;202:71–7.
28. Collins LG, Tyler DE. Phenylbutazone toxicosis in the horse: a clinical study. J Am Vet Med Assoc 1984;184:699–703.
29. Cohen ND. Right dorsal colitis. Equine Vet Educ 2002;14(4):212–9.
30. Smith BP. Equine salmonellosis: a contemporary view. Equine Vet J 1981;13(3): 147–51.
31. Bryans J, Fallon EH, Shephard BP. Equine salmonellosis. Cornell Vet 1961;51: 467–77.
32. Centers for Disease Control. *Salmonella* surveillance: annual summary, 2004. Atlanta (GA): US Department of Health and Human Services, CDC; 2006.
33. Oliveira CJ, Carvalho LF, Garcia TB. Experimental airborne transmission of *Salmonella agona* and *Salmonella typhimurium* in weaned pigs. Epidemiol Infect 2006;134(1):199–209.
34. Clark MA, Hirst BH, Jepson MA. Inoculum composition and *Salmonella* pathogenicity island 1 regulate M-cell invasion and epithelial destruction by *Salmonella typhimurium*. Infect Immun 1998;66(2):724–31.
35. Gruenheid S, Finlay BB. Microbial pathogenesis and cytoskeletal function. Nature 2003;422(6933):775–81.
36. Murray MJ, Dodran RE, Pfeiffer CJ, et al. Comparative effects of cholera toxin, *Salmonella typhimurium* culture lysate, and viable *Salmonella typhimurium* in isolated colon segments in ponies. Am J Vet Res 1989;50(1):22–8.
37. Murray MJ. *Salmonella*: virulence factors and enteric salmonellosis. J Am Vet Med Assoc 1986;189(2):145–7.
38. Smith BP, Reina-Guerra M, Hardy AJ, et al. Equine salmonellosis: experimental production of four syndromes. Am J Vet Res 1979;40(8):1072–7.
39. Baker JR. An outbreak of salmonellosis involving veterinary hospital patients. Vet Rec 1969;85:8–10.
40. Dorn CR, Coffman JR, Schmidt DA, et al. Neutropenia and salmonellosis in hospitalized horses. J Am Vet Med Assoc 1975;166:65–7.
41. Donahue JM. Emergence of antibiotic-resistant *Salmonella agona* in horses in Kentucky. J Am Vet Med Assoc 1986;188(6):592–4.
42. Ikeda JS, Hirsh DC. Common plasmid encoding resistance to ampicillin, chloramphenicol, gentamicin, and trimethoprim-sulfadiazine in two serotypes of *Salmonella* isolated during an outbreak of equine salmonellosis. Am J Vet Res 1985; 46(4):769–73.
43. Carter JD, Hird DW, Farver TB, et al. Salmonellosis in hospitalized horses: seasonality and case fatality rates. J Am Vet Med Assoc 1986;188(2):163–7.

44. Powell DG, Donahue M, Ferris K, et al. An epidemiological investigation of equine salmonellosis in central Kentucky during 1985 and 1986. In: Powell DG, editor. Equine infectious diseases V: Proceedings of the 5th International Conference. Lexington (KY): The University Press of Kentucky; 1988. p. 231–5.

45. Castor ML, Wooley RE, Schotts EB, et al. Characteristics of *Salmonella* isolated from an outbreak of equine salmonellosis in a veterinary teaching hospital. Journal of Equine Veterinary Science 1989;9(5):236–41.

46. Hartmann FA, West SE. Antimicrobial susceptibility profiles of multidrug-resistant *Salmonella anatum* isolated from horses. J Vet Diagn Invest 1995;7(1):159–61.

47. Hartmann FA, Callan RJ, McGuirk SM, et al. Control of an outbreak of salmonellosis caused by drug-resistant *Salmonella anatum* in horses at a veterinary hospital and measures to prevent future infections. J Am Vet Med Assoc 1996; 209(3):629–31.

48. Pare J, Carpenter TE, Thurmond MC. Analysis of spatial and temporal clustering of horses with *Salmonella Krefeld* in an intensive care unit of a veterinary hospital. J Am Vet Med Assoc 1996;209(3):626–8.

49. Amavisit P, Markham PF, Lightfoot D, et al. Molecular epidemiology of *Salmonella* Heidelberg in an equine hospital. Vet Microbiol 2001;80(1):85–98.

50. Tillotson K, Savage CJ, Salman MD, et al. Outbreak of *Salmonella infantis* infection in a large animal veterinary teaching hospital. J Am Vet Med Assoc 1997; 211(12):1554–7.

51. Schott HC, Ewart SL, Walker RD, et al. An outbreak of salmonellosis among horses at a veterinary teaching hospital. J Am Vet Med Assoc 2001;218(7):1152–9.

52. Weese JS, Baird JD, Poppe C, et al. Emergence of *Salmonella typhimurium* definitive type 104 (DT104) as an important cause of salmonellosis in horses in Ontario. Can Vet J 2001;42:788–92.

53. Ward MP, Brady TH, Couetil LL, et al. Investigation and control of an outbreak of salmonellosis caused by multidrug-resistant *Salmonella typhimurium* in a population of hospitalized horses. Vet Microbiol 2005;107(3–4):233–40.

54. Rankin SC, Whichard JM, Joyce K, et al. Detection of bla_{SHV} extened-spectrum β-lactamase in *Salmonella enterica* serovar Newport MDR-AmpC. J Clin Microbiol 2005;43(11):5792–3.

55. Kim LM, Morley PS, Traub-Dargatz JL, et al. Factors associated with *Salmonella* shedding among equine colic patients at a veterinary teaching hospital. J Am Vet Med Assoc 2001;218(5):740–8.

56. Hird DW, Casebolt DB, Carter JD, et al. Risk factors for salmonellosis in hospitalized horses. J Am Vet Med Assoc 1986;188(2):173–7.

57. Mainar-Jaime RC, House JK, Smith BP, et al. Influence of fecal shedding of *Salmonella* organisms on mortality in hospitalized horses. J Am Vet Med Assoc 1998;213(8):1162–6.

58. House JK, Mainar-Jaime RC, Smith BP, et al. Risk factors for among nosocomial *Salmonella* infection among hospitalized horses. J Am Vet Med Assoc 1999; 214(10):1511–6.

59. Alinovi CA, Ward MP, Couetil LL, et al. Risk factors for fecal shedding of *Salmonella* from horses in a veterinary teaching hospital. Prev Vet Med 2003;60(4):307–17.

60. Ernst NS, Hernandez JA, MacKay RJ, et al. Risk factors associated with fecal *Salmonella* shedding among hospitalized horses with signs of gastrointestinal tract disease. J Am Vet Med Assoc 2004;225(2):275–81.

61. Traub-Dargatz JL, Salman MD, Jones RL. Epidemiologic study of salmonellae shedding in the feces of horses and potential risk factors for development of the infection in hospitalized horses. J Am Vet Med Assoc 1990;196(10):1617–22.

62. Owen RA, Fullerton J, Barnum DA. Effects of transportation, surgery, and antibiotic therapy in ponies infected with *Salmonella*. Am J Vet Res 1983;44(1):46–50.
63. Baker JR. Salmonellosis in the horse. Br Vet J 1970;126:100–5.
64. Smith BP, Reina-Gurerra M, Hardy AJ. Prevalence and epizootiology of equine salmonellosis. J Am Vet Med Assoc 1978;172(3):353–6.
65. Ekiri A, Mackay R, Gaskin J, et al. Nosocomial *Salmonella* infections in hospitalized horses. In: 9th International Equine Colic Research Symposium. Liverpool, UK; 2008. p. 131–2.
66. Weese JS, Staempfli HR, Prescott JF. Isolation of environmental *Clostridium difficile* from a veterinary teaching hospital. J Vet Diagn Invest 2000;12: 449–52.
67. Palmer JE, Benson CE, Whitlock RH. *Salmonella* shed by horses with colic. J Am Vet Med Assoc 1985;187(3):256–7.
68. Begg AP, Johnston KG, Hutchins DR, et al. Some aspects of the epidemiology of equine salmonellosis. Aust Vet J 1988;65(7):221–3.
69. McCain CS, Powell KC. Asymptomatic salmonellosis in healthy adult horses. J Vet Diagn Invest 1990;2:236–7.
70. van Duijkeren E, Sloet van Oldruitenborgh-Oosterbaan MM, Houwers DJ, et al. Equine salmonellosis in a Dutch veterinary teaching hospital. Vet Rec 1994; 135:248–50.
71. Bucknell DG, Gasser RB, Irving A, et al. Antimicrobial resistance in *Salmonella* and *Escherichia coli* isolated from horses. Aust Vet J 1997;75(5):355–6.
72. Cohen ND, Martin LJ, Simpson RB, et al. Comparison of polymerase chain reaction and microbiological culture for detection of salmonellae in equine feces and environmental samples. Am J Vet Res 1996;57(6):780–6.
73. House JK, Smith BP, Wildman TR, et al. Isolation of *Salmonella* organisms from the mesenteric lymph nodes of horses at necropsy. J Am Vet Med Assoc 1999; 215(4):507–10.
74. Ravary B, Fecteau G, Higgins R, et al. [Prevalence of *Salmonella* spp. infections in cattle and horses from the veterinary teaching hospital of the faculty of veterinary medicine, University of Montreal]. Can Vet J 1998;39:566–72 [in French].
75. Ewart SL, Schott HC, Robison RL, et al. Identification of sources of *Salmonella* organisms in a veterinary teaching hospital and evaluation of the effects of disinfectants on detection of *Salmonella* organisms on surface materials. J Am Vet Med Assoc 2001;218(7):1145–51.
76. Alinovi CA, Ward MP, Couetil LL, et al. Detection of *Salmonella* organisms and assessment of a protocol for removal of contamination in horse stalls at a veterinary teaching hospital. J Am Vet Med Assoc 2003;223(11):1640–4.
77. Ward MP, Alinovi CA, Couetil LL, et al. Evaluation of a PCR to detect *Salmonella* in fecal samples of horses admitted to a veterinary teaching hospital. J Vet Diagn Invest 2005;17(2):118–23.
78. Traub-Dargatz JL, Garber LP, Fedorka-Cray PJ, et al. Fecal shedding of *Salmonella* spp by horses in the United States during 1998 and 1999 and detection of *Salmonella* spp in grain and concentrate sources on equine operations. J Am Vet Med Assoc 2000;217(2):226–30.
79. Morley P, Dunowska M. Surveillance for *Salmonella* shedding in large animal patients [abstract #267]. In: Proceedings of the 22nd Annual Forum of American College of Veterinary Internal Medicine. Minneapolis; 2004. p. 881.
80. Rice DH, Hancock DD, Roozen PM, et al. Household contamination with *Salmonella enterica*. Emerg Infect Dis 2003 [serial online]. Available from: http://www.cdc.gov/ncidod/EID/vol9no1/02-0214.htm. Accessed December 1, 2008.

81. Wright JG, Tengelsen LA, Smith KE. Multidrug-resistant *Salmonella typhimurium* in four animal facilities. Emerg Infect Dis 2005;119(8):1235–41.

82. Baverud V, Gustafsson A, Franklin A, et al. *Clostridium difficile*: prevalence in horses and environment, and antimicrobial susceptibility. Equine Vet J 2003; 35(5):465–71.

83. Lyerly DM, Lockwood DE, Richardson SH, et al. Biological activities of toxins A and B of *Clostridium difficile*. Infect Immun 1982;35:1147–50.

84. Magdesian KG, Dujowich M, Madigan JE, et al. Molecular characterization of *Clostridium difficile* isolates from horses in an intensive care unit and association of disease severity with strain type. J Am Vet Med Assoc 2006;228(5):751–5.

85. Baverud V. *Clostridium difficile* diarrhea: infection control in horses. Vet Clin North Am Equine Pract 2004;20:615–30.

86. Barbut F, Petit JC. Epidemiology of *Clostridium difficile*–associated infections. Clin Microbiol Infect 2001;7:405–10.

87. Baverud V, Gustafsson, Franklin A, et al. *Clostridium difficile* associated with acute colitis in mature horses treated with antibiotics. Equine Vet J 1997;29(4): 279–84.

88. Gustafsson A, Baverud V, Gunnarsson A, et al. Study of faecal shedding of *Clostridium difficile* in horses treated with penicillin. Equine Vet J 2004;36(2):180–2.

89. Weese JS, Staempfli HR, Prescott JF. A prospective study of the roles of *Clostridium difficile* and enterotoxigenic *Clostridium perfringens* in equine diarrhea. Equine Vet J 2001;33(4):403–9.

90. Magdesian KG, Hirsh DC, Jang SS, et al. Characterization of *Clostridium difficile* isolates from foals with diarrhea: 28 cases (1993–1997). J Am Vet Med Assoc 2002;220(1):67–73.

91. Arroyo LG, Weese S, Stampfli HR. Experimental *Clostridium difficile* enterocolitis in foals. J Vet Intern Med 2004;18:734–8.

92. Taha S, Johansson O, Jonsson SR, et al. Toxin production by and adhesive properties of Clostridium difficile isolated from humans and horses with antibiotic-associated diarrhea. Comp Immunol Microbiol Infect Dis 2007;30:163–74.

93. Scantlebury CE, Pinchbeck GL, Clegg PD, et al. Case-control study investigating risk factors for nosocomial diarrhea in horses. In: 9th International Equine Colic Research Symposium. Liverpool, UK; 2008. p. 43–4.

94. Madewell BR, Tang YL, Jang S, et al. Apparent outbreak of *Clostridium difficile*-associated diarrhea in horses in a veterinary medical teaching hospital. J Vet Diagn Invest 1995;7:343–6.

Equine Grass Sickness: Epidemiology, Diagnosis, and Global Distribution

Claire E. Wylie, BVM&S, MSc, MRCVS[a,*],
Chris J. Proudman, MA, VetMB, PhD, FRCVS[b]

KEYWORDS

• Equine grass sickness • Dysautonomia • Mal seco
• Botulism • *Clostridium botulinum* • Epidemiology

Equine grass sickness (EGS) is recognized as a debilitating and predominantly fatal neurodegenerative disease affecting grazing equids. The most severely affected body system is the gastrointestinal tract. The condition is often termed equine dysautonomia, reflecting extensive autonomic dysfunction; however, it is more accurately considered a polyneuronopathy affecting the central and peripheral nervous system.[1] EGS occurs most frequently within Great Britain, although it is also recognized in regions of mainland Europe. It affects predominantly young horses with access to pasture in the springtime. The condition "mal seco," regularly diagnosed in regions of South America, is generally regarded as the same disease. Although EGS has been recognized for nearly 100 years the cause has not been definitively determined. There is strong historical and modern evidence suggesting EGS may be the result of exotoxins produced within the gastrointestinal tract by the bacterium *Clostridium botulinum* (ie, toxicoinfectious botulism rather than ingestion of preformed botulinum toxin) suggesting that prevention by vaccination may be possible.

CLINICAL SIGNS

There are two distinct clinical presentations of EGS. The first form, acute grass sickness, presents as colic, with rapid development of clinical signs. This form is invariably fatal and all cases die or require euthanasia, usually within 7 days.[2] Some practitioners use the term subacute grass sickness to describe horses presenting with moderately

[a] Epidemiology and Disease Surveillance, Animal Health Trust, Centre for Preventive Medicine, Lanwades Park, Kentford, Newmarket, Suffolk CB8 7UU, England
[b] Department of Veterinary Clinical Science, Faculty of Veterinary Science, University of Liverpool, Leahurst, Neston, Wirral CH64 7TE, England
* Corresponding author.
E-mail address: claire.wylie@aht.org.uk (C.E. Wylie).

Vet Clin Equine 25 (2009) 381–399
doi:10.1016/j.cveq.2009.04.006
0749-0739/09/$ – see front matter © 2009 Elsevier Inc. All rights reserved.

severe colic of more than 2 days' duration. For the purposes of this article subacute grass sickness is considered the same as acute grass sickness, because these two distinct classifications are difficult to accurately distinguish. The second clinical presentation of EGS is chronic grass sickness and has a more insidious onset of clinical signs, which are mainly characterized by weight loss or dysphagia. The clinical course of most cases of chronic grass sickness exceeds 7 days, and survival of this form may be possible in appropriately selected and managed cases.[2] The spectrum of disease of EGS includes peracute cases, which present as sudden death, and it is postulated that subclinical cases may occur.[3] It is unusual for EGS to recur in recovered individuals, although there are sporadic unconfirmed reports.[4]

Most presenting clinical signs are associated with failure of normal gastrointestinal function (**Figs. 1** and **2**) (**Table 1**).[2,5,6] Other systemic clinical signs are attributable to damage beyond the gastrointestinal tract (**Fig. 3**) (**Table 2**).

PATHOLOGIC FINDINGS

Pathologic findings differ between acute and chronic cases. Acute grass sickness cases have notable gastrointestinal pathology, characterized by gastric and small intestinal distension. In longer duration cases the colon and cecum are obstructed by dehydrated intestinal contents, with a severe, firm pseudoimpaction apparent. The mucosa and gut contents often have a black coating, representing adhesion of blood products.[6] Cases of acute grass sickness may have distal esophageal ulceration due to reflux oesophagitis.[7] Pathologic findings in a chronic grass sickness case are often unremarkable, with the exception of notable emaciation. Other nonspecific pathologic changes are variably displayed and include, but are not restricted to: pneumonia,[7] hepatic pathology,[7–9] splenomegaly,[7,10] and swollen, hemorrhagic adrenal glands.[7]

Histopathologic lesions have been identified in the nerve cell bodies of peripheral[9,11,12] and central[1,9,11,13,14] neurons. Evidence that lesions are also found in the somatic efferent lower motor neurons suggest that the term dysautonomia is incomplete, and the disease is more accurately considered a polyneuronopathy.[1,2] The pathognomonic ganglionic changes for EGS are chromatolysis (loss of Nissl substance leading to cytoplasmic eosinophilia) with nuclear eccentricity, pyknosis, and karyorrhexis (**Fig. 4**).[7] Neuronophagia occurs after cell death often initiating an increase in capsule/satellite cells.[7] Cytoplasmic vacuolation and the presence of

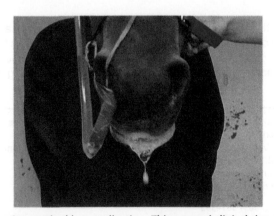

Fig. 1. A horse showing marked hypersalivation. This unusual clinical sign is commonly seen in cases of acute grass sickness.

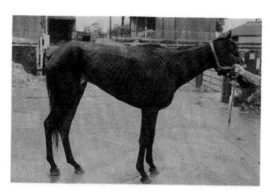

Fig. 2. The typical clinical presentation of a chronic grass sickness case displaying marked weight loss and the appearance of a "wasp-waist."

smooth round eosinophilic bodies/spheroids within or adjacent to perikarya are two additional features often recognized.[7]

DIAGNOSIS

The diagnosis of EGS in the live horse is often presumptive based on the unique combination of clinical signs and epidemiology. It has been proposed that rhinitis

Table 1		
Clinical signs associated with failure of normal gastrointestinal function in acute and chronic equine grass sickness		
Clinical Signs	**Acute Grass Sickness**	**Chronic Grass Sickness**
Colic	Continuous or intermittent, moderate pain	Variable. Possible mild colic following feeding
Dysphagia	Present but often impossible to assess because of colic	Present in varying degrees
Hypersalivation (see **Fig. 1**)	Present: often marked	Not present
Inappetence	Complete anorexia	Present: often complete
Nasogastric reflux	High volumes (up to 12 L) foul-smelling fluid. May be spontaneous or may only occur after nasogastric intubation	Not present
Abnormal abdominal shape	Abdominal distension may be present	Rapid, severe weight loss rapidly developing to emaciation and development of a "wasp-waist" (see **Fig. 2**)
Absence of gut sounds	Complete	Partial
Abnormal feces	Absence of feces or small, hard, dry pellets covered in white mucus-like coating	Absence of feces or small, hard, dry pellets covered in white mucus-like coating
Rectal examination	Palpable distension of small intestine. Corrugated secondary impaction of the cecum and large colon	Flaccid, empty gastrointestinal tract

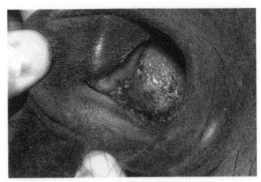

Fig. 3. Rhinitis sicca evident in the nostrils of a chronic grass sickness case. (*Courtesy of Professor Bruce McGorum, MRCVS, Edinburgh, Scotland.*)

Table 2
Systemic clinical signs not directly attributable to gastrointestinal tract dysfunction in acute and chronic equine grass sickness

Clinical Signs	Acute Grass Sickness	Chronic Grass Sickness
Depression	Profound	Present
Dehydration	Present: often severe	Mild
Sweating: predominantly flanks, neck, base of the ears and below the tail[2]	Patchy or generalized	Patchy
Bilateral ptosis	Often present	Often present
Tachycardia: often substantially higher than expected for degree of hypovolemia	Marked: 60–120 bpm[2]	Moderate: 50–60 bpm[2]
Hyperemic membranes	Present, with poor jugular filling	Absent
Rhinitis sicca (bilateral discharge of thick tenacious mucus, or accumulation of drying mucus casts within the nasal passages) (see Fig. 3)[2]	Absent	Often present. May cause snuffling respiration[2]
Piloerection	May be present	May be present
Muscle tremors (fasciculations): predominantly triceps, flanks, quadriceps	Present	Present
Abnormal stance	May have a base-narrow stance	Base-narrow stance: "elephant on a tub"
Behavioral changes	"Play" with drinking water	Play with water, chew slowly, back into walls
Paraphimosis	Absent	Commonly present in entire males

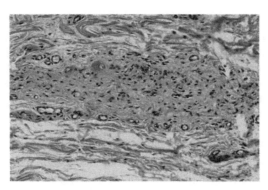

Fig. 4. Chromatolytic neurons visible from ganglionic histopathologic examination of an equine grass sickness case.

sicca is a pathognomonic clinical sign,[2] but its appearance is variable. Hypersalivation and tachycardia in the absence of hypovolemia are unusual clinical signs that are characteristic of acute grass sickness.

Further evidence may be obtained by performing ancillary tests including the following.

Rectal Examination

Acute grass sickness cases, characterized by ileus of the small intestine, often have small intestinal distension palpable on rectal examination. The clinical challenge with such cases is to differentiate them from other causes of small intestinal obstruction. Over time, dry, hard feces accumulate in the large colon and the collapse of colonic sacculations onto the fecal mass leads to a corrugated feel to the colon. Rectal examination of chronic cases reveals a flaccid, empty gastrointestinal tract.

Nasogastric Intubation

Acute grass sickness cases may give rise to gastric reflux on intubation if intestinal obstruction has been present for sufficient time. The absence of reflux does not preclude this diagnosis, particularly in acute cases. The volume of reflux obtained reflects the duration and completeness of ileus. Chronic grass sickness cases do not give rise to significant volumes of gastric reflux.

Abdominal Paracentesis

Abdominal paracentesis is valuable to rule out other conditions. Frequently paracentesis reveals no abdominal fluid in EGS cases; however, fluid that is obtained may reveal a raised protein level.

Hematology/Biochemistry

Individual assessment of hematology and biochemistry is of limited diagnostic value. In combination, a packed cell volume greater than 0.40 L/L, cortisol greater than 400 nmol/L and urea greater than 10 mmol/L indicates acute grass sickness.[15] Variable changes in blood catecholamines,[16] haptoglobin,[17] and orosomucoid[17] may also occur but are rarely measured in clinical cases.

Administration of the α₁-Adrenergic Agonist Phenylephrine to Evaluate Ptosis

Bilateral ptosis is a common clinical signs resulting from paralysis of one of the smooth muscles of the upper eyelid (Müller superior tarsal muscle).[18] Subjective assessment of ptosis can be complemented by the topical administration of 0.5% phenylephrine to one eye, which causes the eyelashes to rise within approximately 30 minutes of administration (**Fig. 5**).[18] Sedation interferes with the functioning of phenylephrine; therefore this test should be performed in the nonsedated horse.[18]

Exploratory Laparotomy

Exploratory surgery of the abdomen is frequently indicated to rule out cases of small intestinal obstruction, which present with clinical signs similar to acute grass sickness.[19] At surgery, conditions such as anterior enteritis, ileal impaction, and idiopathic focal eosinophilic enteritis are identified if present. In the absence of such lesions, findings consistent with acute grass sickness include small intestinal distension with no physical obstruction, uncoordinated spasms of small intestinal motility, and gastric distension. Characteristic surgical findings in a longer duration acute grass sickness case are: severe secondary impaction of the large colon, especially the left ventral colon, and black coating to the mucosa and contents.[6]

Less commonly used diagnostic techniques include abdominal ultrasonography, endoscopy, the assessment of esophageal function by barium swallows and subsequent contrast radiography,[20,21] urine analysis,[22] and quantitative EMG.[23] These techniques have been largely superseded by those described earlier.

DEFINITIVE DIAGNOSIS

Histopathologic examination of autonomic neurons for chromatolytic changes presents the only widely accepted method of obtaining a definitive diagnosis of EGS.[24]

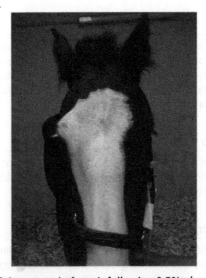

Fig. 5. Demonstration of the reversal of ptosis following 0.5% phenylephrine administration in the right eye, highlighting asymmetry of the angle of the eyelashes. (*Courtesy of* Caroline Hahn, MRCVS, Edinburgh, Scotland.)

Antemortem diagnosis is confirmed by histopathologic examination of the nerve cell bodies within the myenteric or submucosal plexus, achieved by ileal biopsy by way of midline laparotomy.[24] Ileal biopsy is recommended because pathology is seen most consistently at this site.[3,7,24,25] In the author's clinic (C.J.P.) many horses are taken to surgery to harvest an ileal biopsy for definitive diagnosis. With rapid processing a histologic diagnosis can be available within 6 hours. Although some clinicians have expressed reservations about this approach[26,27] it is becoming widely accepted as an appropriate means of making a definitive diagnosis in acute cases, usually before a decision for euthanasia.

More accessible antemortem biopsy sites have been considered, including nasal and rectal biopsies. The antemortem evaluation of nasal biopsies has not been fully investigated.[28] Although postmortem studies of rectal biopsy samples suggested they may play a role in obtaining a diagnosis,[29] a recent study suggests they are unreliable for the diagnosis of EGS in the live horse.[30]

Postmortem diagnosis is confirmed by histopathologic examination of ileal sections, the peripheral sympathetic celiacomesenteric, or the more easily located cranial cervical ganglia.[4,9]

DIFFERENTIAL DIAGNOSIS

Differential diagnoses frequently associated with EGS include botulism, peritonitis, esophageal choke, and strangulating lesions of the small intestine. The possible spectrum of clinical signs observed may require consideration of any causes of colic, dysphagia, or weight loss.

There have been previous suggestions of a relationship between EGS and equine motor neuron disease, a neurodegenerative disorder related to periods of oxidative stress. At one stage these two conditions were considered to represent different ends of a scale of disease, with some overlap within the clinical signs.[6,31] Significant pathologic and epidemiologic differences have led to the conclusion that the two conditions are indeed distinct, however.[32]

Similarities between acute EGS and atypical myopathy have recently been described in the literature.[33] There are several similarities in the clinical signs and risk factors for these two conditions, both of which cause sudden deaths of horses at pasture. It remains unclear whether the two conditions have a common cause, but because of distinct pathologic changes they are currently considered most likely to be two distinct disease entities.[33]

TREATMENT/MANAGEMENT

All cases of acute grass sickness are currently considered incurable and therefore require euthanization on humane grounds on diagnosis.[2,26] A proportion of chronic grass sickness cases respond to symptomatic, empiric treatment. Nutritional support is perhaps the most important factor because affected horses have a highly capricious appetite. Access to fresh grass, succulents (apples and carrots), and various compounded feeds and forage maximizes the chance of the horse eating. A clean, deep bed encourages the horse to lie down and light exercise in the form of in-hand walking may stimulate appetite and intestinal motility. Fecal output should be monitored and enteral fluids administered to soften ingesta if necessary. Attentive nursing and human contact, including frequent hand-feeding, are anecdotally associated with increased recovery rates.[31]

Postprandial discomfort is an occasional feature and may be controlled by phenylbutazone or flunixin meglumine analgesia at half the recommended dose.[31] Liquid paraffin is occasionally required in the early stages of recovery to aid gastrointestinal tract lubrication. Other therapeutics have been evaluated, including gut motility enhancers (cisapride),[20] appetite stimulants (valium, brotizolam, diazepam),[31,34] nandrolone steroids, antioxidants (acetylcysteine),[34] and aloe vera gel,[34] with no clear beneficial effects, and they are therefore not used routinely. Probiotics may have beneficial effects, although they have not been scientifically evaluated.[31]

PROGNOSIS

Only mildly affected chronic grass sickness cases have a chance of survival.[27] The following findings indicate a poor prognosis and may preclude successful treatment for that individual: severe dysphagia requiring stomach tubing or intravenous fluids, complete anorexia, severe colic requiring analgesia, ileus with complete absence of gut sounds and the failure to pass feces unaided, severe rhinitis sicca, marked depression, and weakness with the inability to stand unaided.[26] The amount of weight lost in the initial stages of the disease does not determine outcome, and age should not prejudice the decision to attempt treatment.[35] The survival rate for appropriately selected chronic grass sickness cases is considered to be around 70%.[31] In the clinic of one of the authors (C.J.P.), survival rate of all grass sickness cases is only 5%, but most cases present with acute signs and are not candidates for treatment. It is important that the owners/trainers of horses with a positive diagnosis of grass sickness are given a realistic prognosis for survival. If treatment/nursing is considered an option, the caregivers should be counseled regarding the effort involved, the timescale for recovery, and the probability of survival.

Recovery is extremely variable and each horse can show an irregular pattern of behavior day to day.[36] Cases that are likely to survive generally gain weight in the first 5 weeks following diagnosis, with return to normal body weight taking an average of 9 months. A proportion of surviving horses retain residual signs, including poor appetite,[35] degrees of dysphagia,[35] mild colic,[35] sweating,[35] and coat abnormalities (textural or color changes).[2] The return to high-performance activity may be possible following a prolonged convalescent period.[26,35] Recognized complications include choke, diarrhea, and inhalation pneumonia.[37] Although choke is often self-limiting, the development of diarrhea and pneumonia adversely affect prognosis.[37]

GEOGRAPHIC DISTRIBUTION

EGS occurs most frequently in Great Britain, where the first outbreak was recognized in eastern Scotland in 1909.[38,39] Epidemiologic studies have suggested there are identifiable high-risk areas throughout the United Kingdom,[40,41] with a high proportion of cases occurring in Scotland, but with cases also occurring in England and Wales.[42–45] EGS is considered to occur rarely in Ireland, with only three reported cases, which is surprising considering its close proximity to Great Britain, the abundance of grass (the proposed main risk factor for EGS), and the frequency with which horses are transported to and from the mainland.[46,47]

EGS has also been reported in many countries in Western Europe, including France,[48] Germany,[49,50] Hungary,[51] Norway,[52] Sweden,[53] Austria,[54] Switzerland,[55] The Netherlands,[56] Belgium,[57] Denmark,[9,58] Finland, Cyprus, and Luxembourg (Chris J. Proudman, MA, VetMB, PhD, FRCVS, personal communication, 2006). The prevalence is considered to be highest in countries geographically close to Great Britain, in particular Germany and Belgium (**Fig. 6**). There are reports of single cases occurring in Australia,[59] the Falkland Islands,[60] and Africa (Ethiopia), and the authors are aware of a credible but unpublished report from the United States (Missouri). There have been no reports of EGS occurring in any parts of Asia.

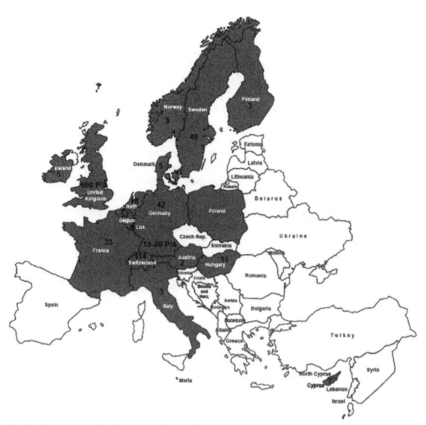

Fig. 6. The European distribution of EGS. The figures refer to the number of histopathologically confirmed cases from each country.

Mal seco is a predominantly fatal polyneuropathy affecting horses in South America. It is diagnosed regularly within the Patagonia, Mendoza, and San Juan areas of Argentina and southern Chile.[61,62] There are two common presentations: mal hinchado, or swollen sickness, which presents with the same clinical signs as acute grass sickness, and a chronic form called mal seco, which presents similarly to chronic grass sickness.[61] Rhinitis sicca is not a common presenting sign with chronic mal seco; otherwise, the clinical findings, gross postmortem, and histopathologic changes are extremely similar to EGS.[61,63–65] Further similarities to EGS extend to the etiologic factors, with the condition commonly occurring in grazing horses during periods of low temperature and cold winds.[62] The similarities between these two conditions suggest they are the same, differing only in the global terminology used to describe them.[6,43,62]

SURVEILLANCE WITHIN GREAT BRITAIN

Although EGS has been recognized in Great Britain for almost 100 years the full extent of the condition and its impact on equine mortality has been poorly understood. To address this, a multicenter collaborative project for the surveillance of EGS within Great Britain was developed in 2007, based at the Animal Health Trust, Newmarket. The ongoing project aims are to collate details of clinical cases occurring prospectively within Great Britain and retrospective information about cases occurring since 2000 to investigate changes in the distribution and frequency of the disease.

Preliminary results from the surveillance scheme need to be interpreted with care because no reference to the general equine population within Great Britain has so far been possible. The preliminary results suggest there has been an average of at least 154 cases per year in Great Britain since 2000. Analysis of the distribution of cases reported to the surveillance scheme suggests that since 2000, 57% of cases originated from England, 40% from Scotland, and 3% from Wales. Certain geographic regions produce higher numbers of cases than others and EGS seems to recur on premises more frequently within Scotland than elsewhere in Great Britain (**Fig. 7**). Acute grass sickness cases occur more commonly (66%) in comparison with chronic cases (34%). The reported fatality rate seems to be lower than most previous reports with 84% of cases resulting in death or euthanasia, and 16% of horses survive, although this may be because of reporting bias of surviving cases. Results support previous reports of a strong seasonal occurrence of EGS, with most cases reported in the springtime, May in particular (**Fig. 8**). A range of ages has been reported to the surveillance scheme with histopathologically confirmed cases reported to have occurred in horses ranging from 2 months to 27 years old, and unconfirmed cases in horses from 2 months to 47 years. Most cases reported to the surveillance scheme occur in horses aged 5 to 6 years old. Male and female horses are equally represented and a wide range of breeds are affected (58% pure breeds and 42% cross breeds).

RISK FACTORS

EGS affects many horse and pony breeds with no identified breed predisposition, although heavy draft breeds may be at increased risk.[42] There are also confirmed cases in the donkey,[40] Przewalski horse,[66] and domestic zebra.[66,67] Mares may be slightly protected in comparison with geldings and stallions.[42] EGS has a well-documented age predisposition. Although the disease has been diagnosed in all ages of horses (up to 20+ years old), risk is highest in young animals.[68] McCarthy and colleagues[69] reported highest risk in animals aged 4 years old, decreasing thereafter. Clinically the age category most commonly affected is 2 to 7[40] years old with horses older than 10 years rarely affected.[42] It has been proposed that the disease is rare in older animals because of the development of immunity or tolerance to the causative agents, and is rare in very young animals because of insufficient ingestion of grass (the main risk factor) or the presence of maternal antibodies.

As the name suggests, there is a strong association between the development of EGS and access to grazing.[40–42] There are only rare isolated reports of cases in horses without access to fresh grass.[58,70] There is a strong seasonal distribution to EGS with the spring, especially May, consistently producing the greatest number of cases in Great Britain.[41,42,44,71] Cases can arise in any month of the year, however, with a second smaller peak often reported in the autumn.[41,71] The reasons for this marked seasonality are unknown. Several manageable risk factors for EGS have been identified (**Table 3**).

Manipulation of the listed risk factors is the main preventive strategy for EGS. Identification of high-risk horses should be undertaken to prioritize changes in management to this group, and should include new arrivals, especially young horses (2–7 years) within the high-risk season (March–June). The following recommendations, based on epidemiologic evidence, can be made to owners of horses on high-risk premises (ie, premises that have recently given rise to one or more grass sickness case): (1) avoid dietary change during the high-risk spring period, (2) offer grazing horses supplementary forage, (3) avoid pasture disturbance, and (4) avoid overuse of anthelmintics and tolerate low levels of intestine parasitism.

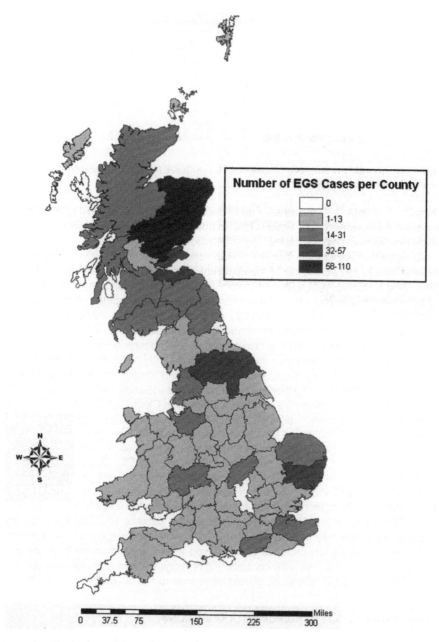

Fig. 7. The distribution of EGS cases reported to the nationwide surveillance scheme in Great Britain since the year 2000.

ETIOLOGY

Consideration of the risk factors identified for EGS suggests an etiologic agent is ingested during grazing, which produces a potent neurotoxin under certain environmental conditions. Identification of the specific cause for EGS remains elusive. The role of various agents has been postulated, including toxic plants,[10,38,58,72] bacteria,[10,38,72–74] viruses,[10]

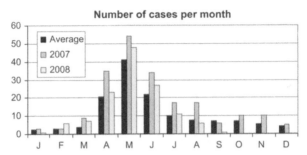

Fig. 8. The monthly occurrence of cases of EGS in Great Britain, as reported to the nation-wide surveillance scheme.

fungi,[10,72,75] molds,[10,76] parasites,[72] and insects.[39,77] Currently the most popular hypothesis is that EGS is a toxicoinfectious form of botulism caused by *C botulinum* type C and local production of its associated potent neurotoxins.[46,68,78,79]

A possible association between EGS and *C botulinum* was suggested by researchers in 1923 because of the apparent pathologic and clinical similarities with the disease botulism.[38,80] An organism with similar morphology and toxicity to *C botulinum* was isolated from the gastrointestinal tract and spleen of affected cases, although it could not be conclusively characterized.[38,39] In 1922 and 1923 two vaccination trials in Scotland assessed the protective effects of vaccination with antitoxin-neutralized *C botulinum* toxin vaccine.[38] Although reanalysis of data using modern methods indicates that vaccination significantly reduced the mortality rates, the results were unjustly dismissed at the time and studies subsequently ended.[39] Within the last decade further evidence of an association with *C botulinum* has been presented, including (1) a prominent increase in Clostridial species in EGS cases compared with controls,[81] (2) a strong correlation between histologically confirmed EGS cases and detection of the C1 neurotoxin (BoNT/C) in the ileal contents and feces,[79] (3) lower serum concentrations of IgG antibodies to surface antigens of *C botulinum* type C and C1 neurotoxin (BoNT/C) in EGS cases compared with controls,[78] and (4) evidence that horses with low systemic antibody (IgG) levels to *C botulinum* type C and *Clostridium novyi* type A surface antigens and the C1 neurotoxin (BoNT/C) are at increased risk for EGS.[45] Because the ileum has been identified as the likely site of toxin absorption it is logical to assume mucosal immunity (IgA) plays a significant role in EGS. IgA levels to the surface antigen and neurotoxin of *C botulinum* have been found to be increased in the small intestine of acute grass sickness cases compared with controls.[82] It remains unclear why high mucosal antibody levels against *C botulinum* should be related to the development of EGS.

COMPARATIVE ASPECTS OF NEUROMUSCULAR BOTULISM

The suggestion that EGS may be caused by *C botulinum* draws comparisons to the disease botulism. Botulism is a highly fatal neuromuscular disease of horses characterized by flaccid paralysis following intoxication with *C botulinum*. Botulism occurs following toxicosis by one of three routes[83]: (1) ingestion of preformed toxin in contaminated feed (classic botulism or forage poisoning), (2) contamination of wounds by spores[84,85] (wound botulism), and (3) ingestion of spores with local toxin production and absorption in the gastrointestinal tract (toxicoinfectious botulism).

The main presenting signs of botulism in the adult horse are generalized, symmetric myasthenia or dysphagia, frequently leading to recumbency and respiratory failure

Table 3
Manageable risk factors (and references) for equine grass sickness

Risk Factor	Findings
Access to grazing	Part-stabling results in EGS occurring almost as infrequently as in horses with no access to fresh grass.[40]
Grazing type	Horses grazing on sand or loam soil types are at an increased risk for EGS, whereas horses grazing on chalk soils are at decreased risk.[68] Soils high in nitrogen have also been found to be a risk for EGS.[69]
Previously affected premises/paddocks	EGS tends to recur on previously affected grazing,[40,42,68,69] with the incidence on previously affected premises estimates at two cases per 100 horse-years at risk.[68] There is evidence of space-time clustering with cases occurring more frequently within 20 days of the last case.[44] Cases are most likely to occur within 2 years of a previous case.[40,42]
Pasture disturbance	Recently disturbed pasture (construction work or mole activity) increases the risk for EGS development threefold.[69] One study found that the use of machinery on the pasture (mechanical feces removal, harrowing) increased the risk for recurrence, possibly because of pasture disturbance.[68]
Premises type	Stud farms and livery yards are at increased risk, possibly associated with increased horse numbers.[68]
Pasture feces removal	In one study the mechanical removal of feces was found to increase the risk for recurrence, whereas manual removal of feces was protective.[68] In the same study grass cutting was found to be protective, and it was postulated these features may be reflective of reduced overgrazing.[68]
Other grazing stock	In one study on EGS recurrence on previously affected premises the risk increased with the presence of domesticated and game birds and decreased when co-grazing with ruminants was used.[68]
Previously affected horses	Reports of the disease occurring in the same horse more than once are rare, and there are no reports of histopathologic diagnosis being made in the same horse more than once. Contact with a previous case reduces the risk for EGS development 10-fold in co-grazers.[42]
Recent movement	Movement from one premises or paddock to another increases the risk, with occurrence commonly within 2 to 4 weeks.[41,42]
Dietary change	Inconsistent evidence that absence of supplementary feed increases risk[40,42] with the provision of preserved forage found to be protective.[45] Change in the quality and quantity of feeding increases the risk.[39,45]
Anthelmintic strategy	Increased frequency of worming, especially the use of ivermectin-based wormers in succession, may increase the risk.[42,45]
Body condition	Inconsistent evidence that horses in good-fat body condition are at increased risk.[41,42]

culminating in death or the need for euthanasia.[83] The following clinical signs are common to both botulism and EGS: anorexia, colic, dysphagia, ileus, fasciculations, hypersalivation, tachycardia, and weight loss. Mydriasis, profound myasthenia, and respiratory distress are features unique to botulism, whereas rhinitis sicca and increased sweating are associated with EGS but are not recognized features of botulism. Unlike EGS, the gross postmortem changes of botulism are unremarkable and there are no consistent histopathologic lesions.

The toxicoinfectious form of botulism is considered to be limited to foals because the normal intestinal flora of adult horses inhibits spore growth and subsequent toxin production within the gastrointestinal tract.[86] As with adult horses, the predominant feature is the onset of generalized, symmetric myasthenia. The initial presenting sign is often the onset of muscle tremors leading to recumbency; hence, another name for the disease is shaker foal syndrome. Most cases of toxicoinfectious botulism (70%) occur in foals between 2 and 5 weeks of age.[83] There are no confirmed reports of toxicoinfectious botulism in foals in the United Kingdom, with the exception of one case report describing clinico-pathologic features of both EGS and toxicoinfectious botulism in the same foal.[87] EGS has not been authentically reported in foals less than 4 months old and the reasons for the discrepancy in age predisposition of toxicoinfectious botulism and EGS are unclear. It is postulated that EGS may occur as a form of toxicoinfectious botulism in older horses following a trigger factor that compromises the normal intestinal microbiota.

Botulism in the horse is caused by toxins from *C botulinum* types A, B, and C.[83] Types D through G cause botulism in other species but have not been previously identified in the horse.[88,89] There is evidence to suggest that EGS may be due to toxicoinfection with *C botulinum* type C. *C botulinum* type C is commonly associated with botulism caused by either decomposing carcasses[90] or the transportation of toxin by birds,[91] unlike types A and B, which are typically associated with silage and hay stored in plastic bags or tubes.[92] Type C botulism is known to present in atypical forms; there are reports of cases occurring with no evidence of dysphagia, and another form causing severe edema to the muzzle and face leading to respiratory distress. It is plausible that EGS may be an atypical presentation of type C toxicoinfectious botulism. Alternatively, the clinical discrepancies between EGS and botulism may suggest the involvement of novel toxin production.

There are geographic differences in the distribution of botulism and EGS.[83,93] Botulism is a common disease in parts of the United States, especially the east coast, where most cases are caused by types A and B. Despite type C being frequently isolated from soil samples it is not a common cause of clinical botulism cases in the United States. In Europe botulism cases are often caused by type C; however, the disease does not have a high frequency within Great Britain, in contrast to EGS. The geographic discrepancies between EGS and botulism may suggest the involvement of novel toxins, or may reflect the geographic distribution of specific trigger factors or bacterial types required for the development of EGS.

Control of botulism in endemic areas is undertaken by vaccination. A *C botulinum* type B toxoid is available in the United States and is believed to provide complete protection.[83] No multivalent or licensed type C toxoids for horses are available in North America or the United Kingdom, although in certain parts of the United States horses are often vaccinated with a type C toxoid manufactured for mink.[83]

PROSPECTS FOR PREVENTION OF EQUINE GRASS SICKNESS

The successful prevention of botulism by vaccination suggests EGS may also be controlled in the same way.[4] Studies are currently evaluating the immunogenicity and safety of a recombinant protein-based type C botulinum toxin vaccine with that of the type C vaccine licensed for use in mink in North America. It is proposed that following these trials a randomized, controlled, field trial will be performed on premises within Great Britain identified to be at high risk by means of the nationwide surveillance scheme. Successful vaccination trials within Great Britain will provide evidence to demonstrate causation between C botulinum type C and EGS, and provide a feasible and reliable mechanism of prevention.[4]

SUMMARY

This article described EGS, a predominantly fatal disease of grazing horses that occurs with the greatest frequency in Great Britain. Historical and modern evidence suggests an association between EGS and toxicoinfection by the bacterium C botulinum, with the specific involvement of the type C toxins. This article reviewed clinical aspects, epidemiology, and global distribution of EGS, and described the proposed association with C botulinum and the future prospects for disease prevention.

REFERENCES

1. Hahn CN, Mayhew IG, de Lahunta A. Central neuropathology of equine grass sickness. Acta Neuropathol 2001;102(2):153–9.
2. Pirie RS. Grass sickness. Clin Tech Equine Pract 2006;5(1):30–6.
3. Doxey DL, Milne EM, Woodman MP, et al. Small intestine and small colon neuropathy in equine dysautonomia (grass sickness). Vet Res Commun 1995;19(6): 529–43.
4. Hedderson EJ, Newton JR. Prospects for vaccination against equine grass sickness. Equine Vet J 2004;36(2):186–91.
5. Scholes SF, Vaillant C, Peacock P, et al. Enteric neuropathy in horses with grass sickness. Vet Rec 1993;132(26):647–51.
6. Cottrell DF, McGorum BC, Pearson GT. The neurology and enterology of equine grass sickness: a review of basic mechanisms. Neurogastroenterol Motil. 1999; 11(2):79–92.
7. Whitwell K. Histopathology of grass sickness—comparative aspects of dysautonomia in various species (equine, feline, canine, leporids). In: Hahn C, Gerber V, Mayhew IG, et al., editors. Proceedings of the 1st International Workshop on Grass Sickness, equine motor neuron disease and related disorders. Newmarket (UK): Equine Veterinary Journal Ltd; 1997. p. 18–20.
8. Marrs J, Small J, Milne EM, et al. Liver and biliary system pathology in equine dysautonomia (grass sickness). J Vet Med A Physiol Pathol Clin Med 2001; 48(4):243–55.
9. Obel AL. Studies on grass disease: the morphological picture with special reference to the vegetative nervous system. J Comp Pathol 1955;65(4):334–46.
10. Pool WA. "Grass disease" in horses. Vet Rec 1928;8(2):23–30.
11. Gilmour JS. Observations on neuronal changes in grass sickness of horses. Res Vet Sci 1973;15(2):197–200.
12. Perkins JD, Bowen IM, Else RW, et al. Functional and histopathological evidence of cardiac parasympathetic dysautonomia in equine grass sickness. Vet Rec 2000;146(9):246–50.
13. Barlow RM. Neuropathological observations in grass sickness of horses. J Comp Pathol 1969;79(3):407–11.
14. Wright JA, Hodson NP. Pathological changes in the brain in equine grass sickness. J Comp Pathol 1988;98(2):247–52.

15. Doxey DL, Milne EM, Gilmour JS, et al. Clinical and biochemical features of grass sickness (equine dysautonomia). Equine Vet J 1991;23(5):360–4.

16. Hodson NP, Wright JA, Hunt J. The sympatho-adrenal system and plasma levels of adrenocorticotropic hormone, cortisol and catecholamines in equine grass sickness. Vet Rec 1986;118(6):148–50.

17. Milne EM, Doxey DL, Kent JE, et al. Acute phase proteins in grass sickness (equine dysautonomia). Res Vet Sci 1991;50(3):273–8.

18. Hahn CN, Mayhew IG. Phenylephrine eyedrops as a diagnostic test in equine grass sickness. Vet Rec 2000;147(21):603–6.

19. Edwards GB. "Equine dysautonomia." Grass sickness of horses: clinical picture and management. J Small Anim Pract 1987;28(5):364–8.

20. Milne EM, Doxey DL, Woodman MP, et al. An evaluation of the use of cisapride in horses with chronic grass sickness (equine dysautonomia). Br Vet J 1996;152(5): 537–49.

21. Greet TR, Whitwell KE. Barium swallow as an aid to the diagnosis of grass sickness. Equine Vet J 1986;18(4):294–7.

22. Marrs J, John H, Milne E, et al. Urine analysis in equine grass sickness. Vet Rec 1999;144(26):734–5.

23. Wijnberg ID, Franssen H, Jansen GH, et al. The role of quantitative electromyography (EMG) in horses suspected of acute and chronic grass sickness. Equine Vet J 2006;38(3):230–7.

24. Scholes SF, Vaillant C, Peacock P, et al. Diagnosis of grass sickness by ileal biopsy. Vet Rec 1993;133(1):7–10.

25. Murray A, Cottrell DF, Woodman MP. Cholinergic activity of intestinal muscle in vitro taken from horses with and without equine grass sickness. Vet Res Commun 1994;18(3):199–207.

26. Milne EM, Woodman MP, Doxey DL. Use of clinical measurements to predict the outcome in chronic cases of grass sickness (equine dysautonomia). Vet Rec 1994;134(17):438–40.

27. Doxey DL, Johnston P, Hahn C, et al. Histology in recovered cases of grass sickness. Vet Rec 2000;146(22):645–6.

28. Prince D, Corcoran BM, Mayhew IG. Changes in nasal mucosal innervation in horses with grass sickness. Equine Vet J 2003;35(1):60–6.

29. Wales AD, Whitwell KE. Potential role of multiple rectal biopsies in the diagnosis of equine grass sickness. Vet Rec 2006;158(11):372–7.

30. Kelley AM, Mair TS, Pearson GR. The value of rectal biopsies in the diagnosis of grass sickness in the live horse. In: Proceedings of the 9th International Equine Colic Research Symposium. Liverpool, UK: Equine Veterinary Journal Ltd; 2008, p. 130.

31. Milne EM. Grass sickness: an update. In Pract. 1997;19(March):128–33.

32. Divers TJ, Cummings JF, Mohammed HO, et al. Equine motor neuron disease in the eastern United States—clinical and laboratory findings. In: Hahn C, Gerber V, Mayhew IG, et al, editors. Proceedings of the 1st International Workshop on grass sickness, EMND and related disorders. Newmarket (UK): Equine Veterinary Journal Ltd; 1997. p. 9–11.

33. Vercauteren G, van der Heyden S, Lefere L, et al. Concurrent atypical myopathy and equine dysautonomia in two horses. Equine Vet J 2007;39(5):463–5.

34. Fintl C, McGorum BC. Evaluation of three ancillary treatments in the management of equine grass sickness. Vet Rec 2002;151(13):381–3.

35. Doxey DL, Milne EM, Ellison J, et al. Long-term prospects for horses with grass sickness (dysautonomia). Vet Rec 1998;142(9):207–9.

36. Doxey DL, Milne EM, Harter A. Recovery of horses from dysautonomia (grass sickness). Vet Rec 1995;137(23):585–8.

37. Doxey DL, Tothill S, Milne EM, et al. Patterns of feeding and behaviour in horses recovering from dysautonomia (grass sickness). Vet Rec 1995;137(8):181–3.

38. Tocher JF, Brown W, Tocher JW, et al. "Grass sickness" investigation report. Vet Rec 1923;3:37–45, 75-89.

39. Begg GW. "Grass disease" in horses. Vet Rec 1936;48(21):655–63.

40. Gilmour JS, Jolly GM. Some aspects of the epidemiology of equine grass sickness. Vet Rec 1974;95(4):77–81.

41. Doxey DL, Gilmour JS, Milne EM. A comparative study of normal equine populations and those with grass sickness (dysautonomia) in eastern Scotland. Equine Vet J 1991;23(5):365–9.

42. Wood JL, Milne EM, Doxey DL. A case-control study of grass sickness (equine dysautonomia) in the United Kingdom. Vet J 1998;156(1):7–14.

43. McCarthy HE, Proudman CJ, French NP. Epidemiology of equine grass sickness: a literature review (1909-1999). Vet Rec 2001;149(10):293–300.

44. French NP, McCarthy HE, Diggle PJ, et al. Clustering of equine grass sickness cases in the United Kingdom: a study considering the effect of position-dependent reporting on the space-time K-function. Epidemiol Infect 2005;133(2): 343–8.

45. McCarthy HE, French NP, Edwards GB, et al. Equine grass sickness is associated with low antibody levels to Clostridium botulinum: a matched case-control study. Equine Vet J 2004;36(2):123–9.

46. Collier DS, Collier SO, Rossdale PD. Grass sickness—the same old suspects but still no convictions!. Equine Vet J 2001;33(6):540–2.

47. McFarlane A. Suspected cases of grass disease in Northern Ireland. Vet Rec 1941;53:762–3.

48. Lhomme C, Collobert-Laugier C, Amardeilh MF, et al. [Equine dysautonomia, an anatomoclinical study of 8 cases]. Revue de Medecine Veterinaire 1996;147(11): 805–12 [in French].

49. Mayer H, Valder WA. [Grass sickness in Germany]. Berl Munch Tierarztl Wochenschr 1968;91:147–8 [in German].

50. Schulze C, Venner M, Pholenx J. [Chronic grass sickness (equine dysautonomia) in a 2½-year-old Icelandic mare on a north Frisian island]. Pferdeheilkunde 1997; 13:345–50 [in German].

51. Voros K, Bakos Z, Albert M, et al. [Occurrence of grass sickness in Hungary]. Magyar Allatorvosok Lapja 2003;91(2):67–74 [in Hungarian].

52. Baustad B, Bakken TK, Kolbjornsen O, et al. [Grass sickness in horses (equine dysautonomia). Case reports and literature review]. Norsk Veterinaertidsskrift 1994;106(2):97–105 [in Norwegian].

53. Green B. [Equine grass sickness. A review of 40 cases]. Svensk Veterinartidning 1976;28:739–47 [in Swedish].

54. Wlaschitz S, Url A. [The first case of chronic grass sickness in Austria]. Wien Tierarztl Monatsschr 2004;91(2):42–5 [in German].

55. Arnold P, Gerber H, Schuler T, et al. [Grass sickness in the horse]. Schweiz Arch Tierheilkd 1981;123(7):383–5 [in German].

56. Leendertse IP. [A horse with grass sickness]. Tijdschr Diergeneeskd 1993; 118(11):365–6 [in Dutch].

57. Middlem A, Jonckheere J. [Grass sickness in Belgium]. Annales de Médecine Vétérinaire 1930;75:193–8 [in French].

58. Lannek N, Lindberg P, Persson F. A grass disease enzootic in stable-fed horses with an investigation of the aetiological role of the food. Vet Rec. 1961;73(24): 601–3.

59. Stewart WJ. A case of suspected acute grass sickness in a thoroughbred mare. Aust Vet J 1977;53(4):196.

60. Woods JA, Gilmour JS. A suspected case of grass sickness in the Falkland Islands. Vet Rec 1991;128(15):359–60.

61. Uzal FA, Robles CA. Mal seco, a grass sickness-like syndrome of horses in Argentina. Vet Res Commun 1993;17(6):449–57.

62. Araya O, Vits L, Paredes E, et al. Grass sickness in horses in southern Chile. Vet Rec 2002;150(22):695–7.

63. Uzal FA, Doxey DL, Robles CA, et al. Histopathology of the brain-stem nuclei of horses with "Mal seco", an equine dysautonomia. J Comp Pathol 1994;111(3):297–301.

64. Uzal FA, Robles CA, Olaechea FV. Histopathological changes in the coeliaco-mesenteric ganglia of horses with "mal seco," a grass sickness-like syndrome, in Argentina. Vet Rec 1992;130(12):244–6.

65. Uzal FA, Woodman MP, Giraudo CG, et al. An attempt to reproduce "mal seco" in horses by feeding them festuca Argentina. Vet Rec 1996;139(3):68–70.

66. Ashton DG, Jones DM, Gilmour JS. Grass sickness in two non-domestic equines. Vet Rec 1977;100(19):406–7.

67. Wales AD, Blunden AS, Hosegood OM. Grass sickness with atypical presentation in a young zebra. Vet Rec 2001;148(26):818–9.

68. Newton JR, Hedderson EJ, Adams VJ, et al. An epidemiological study of risk factors associated with the recurrence of equine grass sickness (dysautonomia) on previously affected premises. Equine Vet J 2004;36(2):105–12.

69. McCarthy HE, French NP, Edwards GB, et al. Why are certain premises at increased risk of equine grass sickness? A matched case-control study. Equine Vet J 2004;36(2):130–4.

70. Forsyth AA. Grass disease in a coalmine. Vet J 1941;97:26–8.

71. Archer DC, Pinchbeck GL, Proudman CJ, et al. Is equine colic seasonal? Novel application of a model based approach. BMC Vet Res 2006;2:27.

72. Greig JR. Acute "grass disease": an interpretation of the clinical symptoms. Vet Rec 1928;8(2):31–4.

73. Ochoa R, de Velandia S. Equine grass sickness: serologic evidence of association with Clostridium perfringens type A enterotoxin. Am J Vet Res 1978;39(6): 1049–51.

74. Gilmour JS, Brown R, Johnson P. A negative serological relationship between cases of grass sickness in Scotland and Clostridium perfringens type A entero-toxin. Equine Vet J 1981;13(1):56–8.

75. Robb J. Isolation and testing of potential fungal causal agents. Paper presented at: Grass Sickness Symposium 1996; Penicuik: Equine Grass Sickness Fund; 1996.

76. Doxey DL. "Mal seco" and grass sickness. Vet Rec 1992;131(9):204.

77. Lloyd DC. Preliminary notes on grass disease investigations in South West Wales. Welsh Agricultural J 1934;10:317–9.

78. Hunter LC, Poxton IR. Systemic antibodies to Clostridium botulinum type C: do they protect horses from grass sickness (dysautonomia)? Equine Vet J 2001; 33(6):547–53.

79. Hunter LC, Miller JK, Poxton IR. The association of Clostridium botulinum type C with equine grass sickness: a toxicoinfection? Equine Vet J 1999;31(6):492–9.

80. Walker AB. The relationship between grass disease of horses and botulism. Br J Exp Pathol 1929;10:352–60.
81. Garrett LA, Brown R, Poxton IR. A comparative study of the intestinal microbiota of healthy horses and those suffering from equine grass sickness. Vet Microbiol 2002;87(1):81–8.
82. Nunn FG, Pirie RS, McGorum B, et al. Preliminary study of mucosal IgA in the equine small intestine: specific IgA in cases of acute grass sickness and controls. Equine Vet J 2007;39(5):457–60.
83. Whitlock RH, McAdams S. Equine botulism. Clin Tech Equine Pract 2006;5(1): 37–42.
84. Bernard W, Divers TJ, Whitlock RH, et al. Botulism as a sequel to open castration in a horse. J Am Vet Med Assoc 1987;191(1):73–4.
85. Mitten LA, Hinchcliff KW, Holcombe SJ, et al. Mechanical ventilation and management of botulism secondary to an injection abscess in an adult horse. Equine Vet J 1994;26(5):420–3.
86. Swerczek TW. Experimentally induced toxicoinfectious botulism in horses and foals. Am J Vet Res 1980;41(3):348–50.
87. McGorum BC, Kyles KW, Prince D, et al. Clinicopathological features consistent with both botulism and grass sickness in a foal. Vet Rec 2003;152(11):334–6.
88. Allison MJ, Maloy SE, Matson RR. Inactivation of Clostridium botulinum toxin by ruminal microbes from cattle and sheep. Appl Environ Microbiol 1976;32(5): 685–8.
89. Galey FD. Botulism in the horse. Vet Clin North Am Equine Pract 2001;17(3): 579–88.
90. Galey FD, Terra R, Walker R, et al. Type C botulism in dairy cattle from feed contaminated with a dead cat. J Vet Diagn Invest 2000;12(3):204–9.
91. Schoenbaum MA, Hall SM, Glock RD, et al. An outbreak of type C botulism in 12 horses and a mule. J Am Vet Med Assoc 2000;217(3):365–8, 340.
92. Whitlock RH, Buckley C. Botulism. Vet Clin North Am Equine Pract. 1997;13(1): 107–28.
93. Steinman A, Kachtan I, Levi O, et al. Seroprevalence of antibotulinum neurotoxin type C antibodies in horses in Israel. Equine Vet J. 2007;39(3):232–5.

Index

Note: Page numbers of article titles are in **boldface** type.

A

Abdominal bandage, update on, 273–274

Abdominal incision, minimize size of, in decreasing severity of ileus, 355

Abdominal pain, after abdominal surgery, 346

Abdominal paracentesis, in EGS diagnosis, 385

Abdominal surgery
  postoperative complications
    abdominal pain, 346
    adhesions, 347–348
    catheter-related thrombophlebitis, 341–342
    ileus, 346–347
    incision-related, 342–345
    new perspectives in, **341–350**
    pneumonia, 345–346
  recent advances in, update on, **271–282**
    abdominal bandage, 273–274
    adhesion prevention, 272–273
    diaphragmatic hernia, 276–277
    HAL, 275–276
    incisional hernia, 277–279
    lactate, 271
    LCRA, 274–275
    small intestinal anastomosis, 274

Abdominal ultrasound, in IBD diagnosis, 307–308

Abdominocentesis
  in colic survival, 222
  in IBD diagnosis, 308–309

Absorption tests, in IBD diagnosis, 310–311

Acidosis, fermentative, 210–211

Acute dirrhea, in hospitalized horses, **363–380**. See also *Diarrhea, acute, in hospitalized horses.*

Adhesion(s)
  after abdominal surgery, 347–348
  prevention of, update on, 272–273

α_1-Adrenergic agonist phenylephrine, in ptosis evaluation, in EGS diagnosis, 386

Adrenoreceptor(s), postoperative ileus and, 353

Age, as factor in EGUS, 285

Anastomosis(es)
  large colon resection and, update on, 274–275
  small intestinal, update on, 274

doi:10.1016/S0749-0739(09)00057-1
0749-0739/09/$ – see front matter © 2009 Elsevier Inc. All rights reserved.
vetequine.theclinics.com

Printed and bound by CPI Group (UK) Ltd, Croydon, CR0 4YY

03/10/2024

01040444-0001

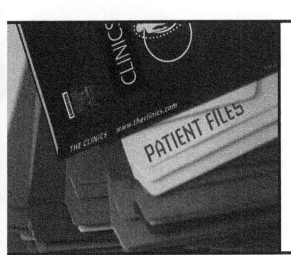
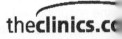

Our issues help you manage *yours.*

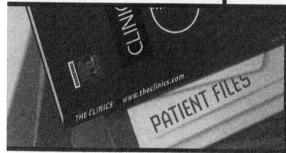

Every year brings you new clinical challenges.

Every **Clinics** issue brings you **today's best thinking** on the challenges you face.

Whether you purchase these issues individually, or order an annual subscription (which includes searchable access to past issues online), the **Clinics** offer you an efficient way to update your know how...one issue at a time.

Discover the Clinics in your specialty. Ask for them in your local medical book store • visit **www.theclinics.com** • or call 1.800.654.2452 inside the U.S. (1.314.453.7041 outside the U.S.) today!

MO23128

Moving?

Make sure your subscription moves with you!

To notify us of your new address, find your **Clinics Account Number** (located on your mailing label above your name), and contact customer service at:

E-mail: elspcs@elsevier.com

800-654-2452 (subscribers in the U.S. & Canada)
314-453-7041 (subscribers outside of the U.S. & Canada)

Fax number: 314-523-5170

Elsevier Periodicals Customer Service
11830 Westline Industrial Drive
St. Louis, MO 63146

*To ensure uninterrupted delivery of your subscription, please notify us at least 4 weeks in advance of move.